2 Minute I

concise. curated

MW00851350

2 Minute Medicine's

The Classics in Medicine™

First Edition

2 Minute Medicine™

Physician Press™

2 Minute Medicine, Inc.
PO Box 140373
Boston, MA 02114
USA

ISBN-10: 0996304290 (Paperback 1st Edition)
ISBN-13: 978-0-9963042-9-0 (Paperback 1st Edition)

About | 2 Minute Medicine is a Boston-based medical publishing company that creates and curates expert, original, and peer-reviewed medical content. As well as the present work, 2 Minute Medicine specializes in daily medical reporting of new medical studies. With thousands published medical reports updated daily on www.2minutemedicine.com, 2 Minute Medicine is your source for curated, updated and authoritative medical news.

Academics | 2 Minute Medicine conducts academic studies in medical education and has presented its data, by invitation, at numerous international peer-reviewed conferences.

For bulk orders/licenses of this, or any other 2 Minute Medicine product, please email info@2minutemedicine.com.

Cover Image: *The Anatomy Lesson of Dr. Nicolaes Tulp;* 1632, Rembrandt Harmenszoon van Rijn. Public domain work.

Introduction

Over the past 30 years, the transition from print to digital media has contributed to an exponential increase in medical literature. This information overload is revolutionizing the implementation of evidence-based medicine. Trials such as the UKPDS, ALLHAT and Child-Pugh underlie our daily decisions in clinical practice. With a plethora of landmark cases occupying isolated corners of both print and digital publications, there exists a tangible need to collect, curate, and summarize these studies in one place for the benefit of all health professionals.

In response, 2 Minute Medicine presents 160+ authoritative, physician-written summaries of the most cited landmark trials in medicine: *2 Minute Medicine's The Classics in Medicine*™. Every physician, health professional, and trainee should have a working knowledge of these trials to both understand and make daily evidence-based clinical decisions. With contributions from renowned medical faculty and practicing physicians at top institutions, *2 Minute Medicine's The Classics in Medicine* is an indispensable tool for the practicing physician or trainee.

The text is organized into 2 Minute Medicine's signature tiered writing style. This features key points, a quick "Study Rundown", and an "In-Depth" section for examining key details that one may wish to refer to when citing the study. As always, every medical summary cites the original study. In the e-book version this takes the form of a direct web link within the summary to the specific trial on the publishing journal's website in addition to a comprehensive bibliography at the end of the book. In the paperback version, references are cited at the end of each study summary as well as in a comprehensive bibliography at the end of the book.

This book is dedicated to the researchers who create the knowledge, the clinicians that practice it, the teachers who spread it, and the students that learn from it.

Sincerely,

Marc D. Succi, MD | Editor-in-Chief | Massachusetts General Hospital

Andrew Cheung, MD | Managing Editor | University Health Network, Toronto

Leah H. Carr, MD | Managing Editor | Seattle Children's Hospital

Effectively Using this Book

A note on the specialties included:

Medicine is a fluid study of the human condition. While modern medicine is segmented into various subspecialties, the reality is that illness does not respect these artificial boundaries. Thus, many of these trials could fit appropriately under the heading of several specialties in this book. In an effort to prioritize readability, the editors organized each trial under only one specialty. Furthermore, some specialties (e.g., endocrinology) do not carry their own heading. Instead, they are interspersed throughout the other specialties within this book.

A note on language:

In general, most of the trials included in this text were designed by investigators to discern causal links. These trials have generally stood the test of reproducibility over time, earning them inclusion into this collection. Thus, in many instances this text uses definitive causal terminology (e.g., "reduced", "lowered", etc.) as opposed to associative terminology (e.g., "is linked with a lower risk") to denote strong, time-tested data. While causal links by definition include an association, the inverse is not necessarily true.

A note on study abbreviations:

While one would benefit greatly from reading this book front-to-back, the summaries stand-alone. They are designed so that the reader may look up a study and read one particular summary, and thus we continually redefine abbreviations anew for each individual summary. The choice of abbreviations defined differ by study as they are tailored to individual summaries to maximize readability.

A note on references:

The e-book edition encourages efficient reading and seamless study. As such, every summarized study has a "clickable" hyperlink near the mid-page which, when "tapped" with the reader's finger, will open up the e-reader/tablet/phone internet browser and link directly to the original text by the publishing journal. This allows the reader to access the original paper instantly (journal subscription and internet access not included). The paperback edition includes full written references.

Contributors

This text is made possible by the authors and journals that published the original trials as well as the work of numerous contributors at various medical schools and hospitals.

Andrew Cheung, MD | University of Toronto

Leah H. Carr, MD | Seattle Children's Hospital

Marc D. Succi, MD | Massachusetts General Hospital

Section Contributors

Lewis R. First, MS, MD | Chair of Pediatrics at Vermont Children's Hospital | Pediatric Content

Aaron Maxwell, MD | Brown Alpert Medical School | Imaging and Intervention Content

Aimee Li, MD | University of Ottawa | Medicine Content

Milana Bogorodskaya, MD | Case Western Reserve University | Medicine Content

Evan Chen, BSc | Stanford School of Medicine | Medicine Content

Adrienne Cheung, BHSc | University of British Columbia School of Medicine | Medicine Content

Lauren Ko, BSc | Harvard Medical School | Medicine Content

Shaidah Deghan, MSc | University of Toronto School of Medicine | Medicine Content

Michael Milligan, BSc | Harvard Medical School | Medicine Content

Contents

In chronological order, by specialty:

III. Critical, Emergent and Pulmonary Care 123

VI. Imaging and Intervention 221

VII. Infectious Disease 243

I. General Chronic Disease

The HMPS I: Adverse events in patients and negligence

1. This study determined that adverse events occurred in 3.7% of hospitalizations.

2. About 28% of adverse events occurring in the hospital were attributed to negligence.

Original Date of Publication: February 1991

Study Rundown: The Harvard Medical Practical Study (HMPS) I identified a significant burden from iatrogenic injury, recognizing that a substantial proportion of adverse events in the hospital lead to permanent disability or death. Of note was the significant number of adverse events resulting from substandard care, which may be reduced by quality assurance measures. Increasing age was identified as an important risk factor for the occurrence of adverse events, likely reflecting more complicated illness and poorer health. Limitations of the study included the difficulty of evaluating negligence and degree of disability from hospital records; however, the validity and reliability of the review process were tested and found to be reasonably high with 89% sensitivity in screening for adverse events and 89% agreement on the presence of an adverse event. Other strengths of the study were the large sample size and the use of a random sample which allowed extrapolation to population estimates. In summary, the HMPS I was one of the earliest and largest efforts to quantify the incidence of adverse events and their impacts. It also determined that many adverse events were preventable, and these findings justified greater investment in quality improvement initiatives.

In-Depth [retrospective case review]: The HMPS I results are based on the review of 30 121 records from a random sample of 2 671 863 non-psychiatric patients in New York in 1984. Records were first screened by nurses and medical record analysts. Those identified as positive for the occurrence of an adverse event were independently reviewed by 2 physicians. Physicians identified 1278 adverse events, of which 306 were due to negligence. From this, the statewide incidence rate of adverse events was estimated to be 3.7%, while approximately 27.6% of these events were the result of negligence. The majority of adverse events led to disability that resolved in less than 6 months; however, 2.6% led to permanent total disability and 13.6% resulted in death. Rates of adverse events were positively correlated with increasing age ($p < 0.0001$) and negligence was more frequently implicated with increasing severity of adverse events, causing 22% of events leading to temporary disability and 51% of events resulting in death (p < 0.0001). The percentage of adverse events due to negligence did not vary between clinical specialties.

Brennan TA, Leape LL, Laird NM, Hebert L, Localio AR, Lawthers AG, et al. Incidence of Adverse Events and Negligence in Hospitalized Patients. New England Journal of Medicine. 1991 Feb 7;324(6):370–6.

The HMPS II: Characterizing adverse events in hospitalized patients

1. Drug-related complications were the most common type of adverse event in hospitalized patients.

2. Adverse events due to negligence in hospitalized patients were more likely to cause serious disability or death than adverse events not attributed to negligence.

Original Date of Publication: February 1991

Study Rundown: Many adverse events in hospitalized patients are not preventable due to current limitations in medical knowledge or capabilities. Advances in scientific knowledge and medical technology may reduce the frequency of these events over time. However, many errors in management can be prevented with the development and implementation of clinical practice guidelines and quality assurance programs. The HMPS produced reliable estimates of rates of adverse events in hospital as well as the proportion of those events attributable to management error and negligence. The study also identified high-risk groups and areas where rates of negligence were highest, both of which can be targeted with quality assurance programs. The study supports the use of systems analysis and disciplinary action in instances of negligence to minimize the significant consequences of adverse events in hospitalized patients. In summary, by further characterizing the adverse events identified in HMPS I, the findings from the HMPS II study have been fundamental in guiding the development of quality improvement initiatives by identifying priorities for the field of patient safety.

In-Depth [retrospective case review]: Published in NEJM in 1991, the results of the HMPS II further analyzed the adverse events described in HMPS I by classifying the type of adverse event, where the event occurred (inside or outside hospital), those most likely to result in serious disability, the type of management error responsible, and those most likely to be due to negligence. As described in the HMPS I summary, this investigation included a random sample of 30 195 hospital records from the state of New York in 1984. Records were reviewed independently for the occurrence of adverse events. Drug-related complications were the most common single type of adverse event. The proportion of adverse events attributed to negligence varied between categories,

22

with 17% of operative adverse events, 75% of diagnostic mishaps, and 77% of therapeutic mishaps attributed to negligent care. Adverse events due to negligence in hospitalized patients were more likely to cause serious disability or death than adverse events not attributed to negligence.

Leape LL, Brennan TA, Laird N, Lawthers AG, Localio AR, Barnes BA, et al. The Nature of Adverse Events in Hospitalized Patients. New England Journal of Medicine. 1991 Feb 7;324(6):377–84.

The DASH trial: Diet change significantly reduces blood pressure

1. A "combination" diet rich in fruits and vegetables and low in saturated and total fat significantly reduced blood pressure in comparison to the typical American diet.

2. Blood pressure reductions were observed in the setting of stable weight, unchanged sodium intake, and consumption of no more than 2 alcoholic drinks per day.

Original Date of Publication: April 1997

Study Rundown: At the time of the Dietary Approaches to Stop Hypertension (DASH) trial, national guidelines recommended reduced salt intake, weight control, and reduced alcohol consumption as nutritional means of controlling high blood pressure. Observational studies suggested that increased vegetable consumption could reduce blood pressure as well, but follow-up trials assessing the effect of individual nutrients on blood pressure were inconclusive. The DASH trial sought to assess the effect of dietary patterns, rather than individual nutrients, on blood pressure control. Results showed that, in comparison to a typical American diet low in fruits and vegetables, a diet rich in fruits and vegetables (the "fruit-and-vegetable" diet) significantly reduced systolic and diastolic blood pressure, while a "combination" diet rich in fruits and vegetables and low in saturated and total fat showed a greater reduction in blood pressure. Blood pressure reductions were greater in hypertensive participants than non-hypertensive participants. Notably, the reduction in blood pressure in hypertensive participants was similar in magnitude to reductions achieved through mono-drug therapy.

A strength of this trial was the large proportion of minorities enrolled - >60% of participants were from minority groups for all 3 experimental diets. This was done to reflect the disproportionate burden of hypertension in minority populations. Moreover, diets in the study were designed so that the salt content was kept at 3 g/day. Participants were also allowed to consume 1-2 alcoholic beverages per day, and weight-loss was not a required goal. These findings suggest that the blood pressure reduction achieved the DASH diets are meant to complement, rather than supplant, current recommendations to reduce salt and alcohol consumption. Limitations of the trial include the lack of long-term assessment of the DASH diet's efficacy, as the trial consisted only of an 11-week feeding period. Notably, patients' ease of adherence to the diet was also not evaluated. In summary, the DASH trial showed that dietary modification involving increased vegetable and fruit consumption and decreased fat consumption offers an additional approach to lowering blood pressure.

In-Depth [randomized controlled trial]: The DASH trial was a randomized, multi-centered trial that enrolled 459 participants. Eligible participants were at least 22 years of age, did not take any antihypertensive medication, and had an average systolic blood pressure (BP) greater than 160 mmHg and a diastolic BP of 80-95 mmHg. Exclusion criteria included poorly controlled diabetes, hyperlipidemia, a cardiovascular event in the previous 6 months, BMI>35, renal insufficiency, alcoholic beverage intake >14 drinks/week, and unwillingness to stop taking medications or dietary supplements. Approximately 150 participants were randomized to each of the following diets: 1) the control diet (i.e., low in vegetables and fruit with a fat content similar to the typical American diet), 2) the "vegetable-and-fruit" diet (i.e., higher in vegetables and fruit), and 3) the "combination" diet (i.e., higher in vegetables and fruit and lower in fats). For each group, participants' BPs were screened at baseline first, then all participants were given the control diet for 3 weeks. Afterward, participants in the "vegetable-and-fruit" diet and the "combination" diet were switched to their respective diet, and all diets were continued for an additional 8 weeks. Diets were designed to include commonly available foods in different forms (fresh, frozen, etc.), and all foods were prepared similarly and using the same brand-name items at each study center.

Results showed a reduction in systolic BP of 2.8 mmHg (p < 0.001) and diastolic by 1.1 mmHg (p = 0.07) in the "vegetable and fruit" diet compared to the control diet. The "combination" diet reduced systolic BP by 5.5 mmHg (p < 0.001) and diastolic BP by 3.0 mmHg (p < 0.001). For participants with hypertension, the "combination" diet reduced systolic BP by 11.4 mmHg (p < 0.001) and diastolic BP by 5.5 mmHg (p < 0.001). For participants without hypertension, the "combination" diet reduced systolic BP by 3.5 mmHg (p < 0.001) and diastolic BP by 2.1 mmHg (p = 0.003).

Appel LJ, Moore TJ, Obarzanek E, Vollmer WM, Svetkey LP, Sacks FM, et al. A Clinical Trial of the Effects of Dietary Patterns on Blood Pressure. New England Journal of Medicine. 1997 Apr 17;336(16):1117–24.

The UKPDS: Reducing diabetes-related morbidity and mortality

1. For patients with type 2 diabetes mellitus (T2DM), pharmacologic blood glucose control with sulfonylureas or insulin significantly reduced the risk of microvascular complications, but not macrovascular complications.

2. Metformin therapy significantly reduced diabetes-related and all-cause mortality.

3. Strict control of blood pressure in T2DM reduced the risk of both microvascular and macrovascular complications, along with diabetes-related mortality.

Original Date of Publication: September 1998

Study Rundown: The United Kingdom Prospective Diabetes Study (UKPDS) produced a number of publications exploring the effectiveness of different interventions in reducing diabetes-related morbidity and mortality. In this report, we highlight 3 of the most influential papers yielded from this initiative: 1) UKPDS 33, which explored the use of sulfonylureas and insulin, 2) UKPDS 34, which examined the effects of metformin, and 3) UKPDS 38, looking at the effects of tight blood pressure control in patients with T2DM.

UKPDS 33 and 34 demonstrated that intensive blood glucose control with sulfonylureas, insulin, and/or metformin significantly reduced the incidence of microvascular complications of T2DM when compared to lifestyle modifications alone (i.e., diet and weight control). In these studies, microvascular complications were defined as retinopathy, vitreous hemorrhage, neuropathy, and renal failure. Pharmacologic therapy using any of these agents was associated with significant reductions in hemoglobin A1c (HbA1c) levels. There were no significant differences between pharmacologic therapy and lifestyle modifications alone in terms of the development of macrovascular complications (i.e., coronary artery disease, peripheral arterial disease, cerebrovascular disease). Metformin, however, was shown to significantly reduce diabetes-related and all-cause mortality. With regards to blood pressure control, UKPDS 38 demonstrated that treatment with angiotensin converting enzyme (ACE) inhibitors or beta blockers to lower blood pressure below 150/85 mmHg was associated with significantly reduced microvascular complications, macrovascular complications, and diabetes-related deaths when compared to control subjects with less tight blood pressure control (i.e., <180/105 mmHg).

In summary, the use of pharmacologic agents (i.e., sulfonylureas, insulin, metformin) in patients with T2DM significantly reduced their risk for developing microvascular complications. Because metformin significantly reduced diabetes-related mortality, all-cause mortality and had low-risk of hypoglycemia, it is often considered the first-line pharmacotherapy in managing T2DM in present-day clinical practice. Moreover, tight blood pressure control was shown to reduce the incidence of microvascular and macrovascular complications, as well as diabetes-related mortality. The long duration, effective randomization, and large study population of the UKPDS are factors that have made these findings highly influential.

In-Depth [randomized controlled studies]: In UKPDS 33 and 34, patients with newly diagnosed T2DM aged 25-65 were recruited from 23 participating centers and followed over 10 years. Both papers were randomized trials that allocated patients to different treatment groups or conventional management, which involved only lifestyle modifications. UKPDS 33 demonstrated that median HbA1c levels were significantly lower in the treatment group (i.e., patients receiving sulfonylureas or insulin) at 7.0% compared to 7.9% for the control group (p < 0.0001). Moreover, the risk of microvascular complications was significantly reduced in the treatment group (RR 0.75; 95%CI 0.60-0.93). Patients in the treatment group, however, did experience significantly higher rates of hypoglycemic episodes than the control group (p < 0.0001). Similarly, treating patients with T2DM with metformin was found to be beneficial in UKPDS 34. When compared to conventional therapy (i.e., lifestyle changes alone), treatment with metformin was found to reduce diabetes-related death (RR 0.58; 95%CI 0.37-0.91) and all-cause mortality (RR 0.64; 95%CI 0.45-0.91). Moreover, metformin therapy was linked with fewer hypoglycemic episodes than treatment with sulfonylureas and insulin.

In UKPDS 38, which assessed the effects of blood pressure control, patients with newly diagnosed T2DM were again recruited from 23 participating hospitals and were followed over 10 years. Blood pressure was measured at clinic visits every 3-4 months. Patients were randomized to either tight blood pressure control (i.e., <150/85 mmHg) or less tight control (i.e., <180/105 mmHg). Patients were treated with ACE inhibitors or beta-blockers to achieve target blood pressures. It was found that patients in the tight control group experienced a 32% reduction in the risk of diabetes-related morality compared to the less tight group (p = 0.019). Diabetes-related mortality was defined as deaths resulting from myocardial infarction, sudden death, stroke, peripheral vascular disease, renal disease, hyperglycemia, or hypoglycemia. In addition, the risk of macrovascular complications was demonstrated to be 34% lower in the tight control group (p = 0.019).

UK Prospective Diabetes Study (UKPDS) Group. Intensive blood-glucose control with sulphonylureas or insulin compared with conventional treatment and risk of complications in patients with type 2 diabetes (UKPDS 33). The Lancet. 1998 Sep 12;352(9131):837–53.

UK Prospective Diabetes Study (UKPDS) Group. Effect of intensive blood-glucose control with metformin on complications in overweight patients with type 2 diabetes (UKPDS 34). Lancet. 1998 Sep 12;352(9131):854–65.

UK Prospective Diabetes Study (UKPDS) Group. Tight blood pressure control and risk of macrovascular and microvascular complications in type 2 diabetes: UKPDS 38. UK Prospective Diabetes Study Group. BMJ. 1998 Sep 12;317(7160):703–13.

Symptom-triggered benzodiazepine treatment for alcohol withdrawal

1. For patients withdrawing from alcohol, symptom-triggered pharmacologic therapy decreased detoxification time without compromising the safety or comfort of the patient.

2. Symptom-triggered individualized benzodiazepine administration significantly reduced the intensity and duration of oxazepam use during withdrawal treatment.

Original Date of Publication: May 2002

Study Rundown: Fixed doses of benzodiazepines are considered the first-line pharmacologic approach when treating patients with alcohol withdrawal. In this landmark study, withdrawing patients were randomized into 2 groups: 1) patients who underwent individualized treatment with oxazepam in response to withdrawal symptoms or 2) patients were treated with a fixed amount of oxazepam with additional doses given only as needed. It was determined that the symptom-triggered patient group not only used 6 times less oxazepam but also experienced a shorter treatment duration than did the fixed-schedule group of patients. The difference in oxazepam use was not tied to any changes in safety, withdrawal intensity, or comfort level of the patients. In summary, this study supports the use of symptom-triggered benzodiazepine administration in patients suffering alcohol withdrawal.

In-Depth [randomized controlled trial]: In this double-blinded randomized controlled trial, an uninvolved pharmacist randomized all 117 eligible patients admitted to the alcohol treatment inpatient program, a clinic associated with the Lausanne University hospital, into clusters of 10 participants to either the symptom-triggered or fixed schedule group. Fixed-schedule subjects received a 30 mg dose of oxazepam every 6 hours, and subsequently, 8 doses of 15 mg. Shortly after administration, patients would be administered additional drugs depending on their Clinical Institute Withdrawal Assessment for Alcohol Scale (CIWA-Ar) score. Symptom-triggered subjects received a placebo every 6 hours and were administered oxazepam only if their CIWA-Ar score reached certain pre-determined thresholds. In comparing the 2 groups, only 39% in the symptom-triggered group were treated with oxazepam, which stood in great contrast to the 100% treated in the fixed schedule group ($p < .001$). The mean total oxazepam dose administered to the symptom-triggered and fixed-schedule groups were 37.5 mg and 231.4 mg ($p < .001$) respectively. The mean duration of treatment in the symptom triggered group was 20.0 hours, which was significantly lower than the mean duration time of 62.7 hours in the fixed schedule group (p < .001). Despite these differences, there were no distinctions in comfort level noted between individuals in the 2 groups, as measured by comparing the CIWA-Ar scores of each patient.

Daeppen J, Gache P, Landry U, et al. Symptom-triggered vs fixed-schedule doses of benzodiazepine for alcohol withdrawal: A randomized treatment trial. Arch Intern Med. 2002 May 27;162(10):1117–21.

The CATIE trial: High rates of medication discontinuation in schizophrenic patients

1. Approximately 74% of schizophrenic patients discontinued their medications before 18 months, with the median being 6 months.

2. Olanzapine was found to have a significantly longer time to discontinuation than quetiapine or risperidone.

3. Olanzapine was associated with significantly more weight gain and increases in glycosylated hemoglobin, cholesterol, and triglycerides when compared to the other antipsychotics.

Original Date of Publication: September 2005

Study Rundown: Antipsychotic drugs form the foundation of schizophrenia management. Typical antipsychotic drugs were first developed and are highly effective in managing psychotic symptoms, though they are now linked with a high-risk of extrapyramidal side effects. Atypical antipsychotics were subsequently developed and promised lower risk of such side effects, though limited evidence existed to support these claims. This double-blind, randomized controlled study sought to compare the relative effectiveness of atypical and typical antipsychotics, in addition to evaluating claims that atypical antipsychotics have a better side effect profile. The Clinical Antipsychotic Trials of Intervention Effectiveness (CATIE) trial demonstrated that schizophrenic patients discontinued their antipsychotics at very high rates, thereby limiting the effectiveness of drug therapy. Olanzapine was found to be significantly more effective than other atypical antipsychotics (i.e., quetiapine and risperidone) in terms of time to discontinuation. However, olanzapine was associated with significantly more weight gain and increases in glycosylated hemoglobin, cholesterol, and triglyceride levels. This study was funded by the National Institute of Mental Health. Pharmaceutical companies contributed drug supplies for the study and advice regarding dosing; they were not otherwise involved in the design of the study, or the analyses and interpretation of its results.

In-Depth [randomized controlled trial]: A total of 1493 patients were recruited from 57 different centers across the United States, and were randomly assigned to receive olanzapine (7.5-30 mg daily), quetiapine (200-800 mg daily), risperidone (1.5-6 mg daily), ziprasidone (40-160 mg daily), or perphenazine (8-

32 mg daily); all medications were administered as identical-appearing capsules. Patients were included in the study if they were between 18 and 65 years of age, if they were diagnosed with schizophrenia, and if they were able to take antipsychotics. The primary outcome was the discontinuation of treatment for any reason. It was thought that this measure would represent the efficacy, safety, and tolerability of different treatment options. Secondary outcomes included reasons for discontinuation and scores on the Positive and Negative Syndrome Scale (PANSS) and the Clinical Global Impression (CGI) scale. Approximately 74% of patients discontinued their assigned treatment before the 18-month mark, with the median time to discontinuation being about 6 months. The time to discontinuation was significantly longer in the olanzapine group, when compared to the quetiapine (HR 0.63), risperidone (HR 0.75), ziprasidone (HR 0.76), and perphenazine group (HR 0.78). After adjusting for multiple comparisons, however, significant differences only remained between olanzapine and quetiapine/risperidone. The study also demonstrated that PANSS and CGI scores significantly improved over time. Notably, olanzapine was significantly associated with greater weight gain, as well as greater increases in glycosylated hemoglobin, total cholesterol, and triglycerides when compared to the other study drugs.

Lieberman JA, Stroup TS, McEvoy JP, Swartz MS, Rosenheck RA, Perkins DO, et al. Effectiveness of Antipsychotic Drugs in Patients with Chronic Schizophrenia. New England Journal of Medicine. 2005 Sep 22;353(12):1209–23.

The STAR*D trials I: Medication augmentation for depression

1. In patients who have not experienced remission of depression despite vigorous treatment with a selective serotonin-reuptake inhibitor (SSRI), augmentation of treatment by adding bupropion or buspirone achieved remission in approximately 30% of patients.

2. There were no significant differences between drug groups in terms of remission rates.

Original Date of Publication: March 2006

*The Sequenced Treatment Alternatives to Relieve Depression (STAR*D) trials explored the management of patients who had refractory depression despite treatment with a SSRI. Two papers were published based on data from the STAR*D trials in NEJM in 2006, which involved outpatients with nonpsychotic major depression who had not experienced remission with citalopram alone. In both papers, the primary outcome measure was remission with a score of <7 on the Hamilton Rating Scale for Depression (HRSD-17), while secondary outcome measurement of remission and response was done using the Quick Inventory of Depressive Symptomatology (QIDS-SR-16). Patients in this study were given the option to 1) augment their therapy by adding other agents or 2) switch to another therapy.*

Study Rundown: The use of medications to augment SSRI therapy is common practice in the treatment of depression, though no previous randomized controlled trials had explored this issue. This paper demonstrated that in patients with refractory depression despite vigorous SSRI treatment, augmenting therapy by adding bupropion or buspirone to existing SSRI therapy can help achieve remission in approximately 30% of patients. While there were no significant differences between the bupropion and buspirone groups in terms of remission rates, patients in the bupropion group were adherent to treatment for significantly longer periods of time, and experienced higher reductions in QIDS-SR-16 scores.

In-Depth [randomized controlled trial]: A total of 565 patients were recruited and randomized to either receive 1) sustained-release bupropion or 2) buspirone, in addition to citalopram, an SSRI. There were no significant differences in remission rates between the two groups based on HSRD-17 scores (29.7% for bupropion group, 30.1% for buspirone group). Similarly, remission and response rates based on QIDS-SR-16 scores were not significantly different between the groups. Patients in the bupropion group were adherent to treatment for significantly longer than those in the buspirone group (10.2 weeks vs. 9.2 weeks, p = 0.01). Moreover, patients in the bupropion group experienced significantly higher reductions in QIDS-SR-16 scores at the end of the study when compared to the buspirone group.

Trivedi MH, Fava M, Wisniewski SR, Thase ME, Quitkin F, Warden D, et al. Medication Augmentation after the Failure of SSRIs for Depression. New England Journal of Medicine. 2006 Mar 23;354(12):1243–52.

The STAR*D trials II: Switching antidepressants in depression management

1. In cases where citalopram failed or could not be tolerated, approximately 1 in 4 patients experienced remission of their depression symptoms by switching to sustained-release bupropion, sertraline, or extended-release venlafaxine.

Original Date of Publication: March 2006

Study Rundown: Apart from augmentation, switching to a different anti-depressant represents another option for managing patients who do not experience depression remission despite treatment with an SSRI. This trial examined patients suffering from refractory depression after a trial of citalopram. It demonstrated that switching to another medication resulted in approximately 1 in 4 patients experiencing remission of their symptoms with sustained-release bupropion, sertraline, or extended-release venlafaxine. A strength of the STAR*D studies is the few criteria for inclusion and exclusion, which suggests that these findings may be generalizable to an outpatient population. Limitations included the lack of a placebo control group and the fact that treatment delivery was unblinded. Interestingly, the rates of remission with switching medications were lower than the remission rates observed with augmenting therapy. Part of this may be attributed to the differences in patient pools seen in the 2 studies (i.e., the "medication switch" study having a larger proportion of patients who could not tolerate citalopram) and the inadequate doses/treatment durations. Nevertheless, this study demonstrated clinically meaningful remission rates when switching to other antidepressants.

In-Depth [randomized controlled trial]: A total of 727 outpatients with non-psychotic depression were enrolled. All patients had been previously treated with citalopram and had not experienced remission or could not tolerate citalopram. Patients were randomized to switch from citalopram to 1) sustained-release bupropion (a norepinephrine-dopamine reuptake inhibitor, NDRI), 2) sertraline (another SSRI), or 3) extended-release venlafaxine (a serotonin-norepinephrine reuptake inhibitor, SNRI). Remission rates were not significantly different between the 3 treatment groups, as measured by HSRD-17 scores (21.3% in the bupropion group, 17.6% in the sertraline group, 28.4% in the venlafaxine group). Moreover, the 3 groups were not significantly different with regards to response/remission rates, or time to response/remission, as measured by QIDS-SR-16 scores, nor were they significantly different in terms of their rates of side effects or serious adverse events.

Rush AJ, Trivedi MH, Wisniewski SR, Stewart JW, Nierenberg AA, Thase ME, et al. Bupropion-SR, Sertraline, or Venlafaxine-XR after Failure of SSRIs for Depression. New England Journal of Medicine. 2006 Mar 23;354(12):1231–42.

The ENHANCE trial: Simvastatin and ezetimibe in familial hypercholesterolemia

1. In patients with familial hypercholesterolemia, simvastatin and ezetimibe combination therapy did not result in significant differences in carotid artery thickness when compared to treatment with simvastatin alone.

2. Treatment with simvastatin and ezetimibe resulted in significantly greater reductions in low-density lipoprotein (LDL) cholesterol, triglyceride, and C-reactive protein levels as compared to treatment with simvastatin alone.

3. There were no significant differences between the 2 groups in the rates of adverse events or drug discontinuation.

Original Date of Publication: April 2008

Study Rundown: Ezetimibe is a cholesterol-absorption inhibitor that lowers plasma cholesterol by decreasing the amount of cholesterol absorption in the small intestine. This drug is often used in combination with statins, and this combination has been shown to further reduce levels of LDL when compared to statins alone. However, no prior large-scale randomized clinical trial had been conducted to assess the effect of adding ezetimibe to statins on atherosclerosis progression. In the Ezetimibe and Simvastatin in Hypercholesterolemia Enhances Atherosclerosis Regression (ENHANCE) trial, 720 patients with familial hypercholesterolemia were randomized to receive simvastatin with placebo or simvastatin with ezetimibe. After 24 months of therapy, there was no significant difference between the groups in mean change in intima-media thickness of the carotid arteries. Nevertheless, patients that took combination therapy rather than simvastatin alone experienced greater reductions in LDL cholesterol, triglyceride, and C-reactive protein levels.

In-Depth [randomized controlled trial]: This double-blinded randomized control trial was originally published in the NEJM in 2008. It was conducted at 18 centers in the United States, Canada, South Africa, Spain, Denmark, Norway, Sweden, and the Netherlands. Patients were eligible for the study if they were between 30-75 years of age and had been diagnosed with familial hypercholesterolemia by genotyping or World Health Organization diagnostic criteria. Exclusion criteria included having high-grade stenosis/occlusion of the carotid artery, a history of carotid endarterectomy/stenting, homozygous familial hypercholesterolemia, New York Heart Association class III or IV congestive heart failure, and cardiac arrhythmia. All patients underwent a screening phase, a single-blind 6-week placebo run-in period, and a double-blind study period lasting 24 months. The primary outcome was the mean change in intima-media thickness of the carotid arteries, as measured by ultrasonography of the carotid arteries.

A total of 720 patients with familial hypercholesterolemia were randomized into 2 treatment groups: 1) simvastatin 80 mg daily with placebo or 2) simvastatin 80 mg daily and ezetimibe 10 mg daily. In the simvastatin-only group, the mean change in thickness was 0.0058 ± 0.0037 mm, while it was 0.0111 ± 0.0038 mm in the simvastatin-ezetimibe group, an insignificant difference ($p = 0.29$). Patients in the simvastatin-ezetimibe group experienced a 16.5% greater reduction in LDL levels compared with the simvastatin-only group ($p < 0.01$). Patients in the combination group also experienced significantly greater reductions in triglyceride and C-reactive protein levels, when compared with simvastatin alone ($p < 0.01$). There were no significant differences between the two groups in the rates of adverse events and medication discontinuation.

Kastelein JJP, Akdim F, Stroes ESG, Zwinderman AH, Bots ML, Stalenhoef AFH, et al. Simvastatin with or without Ezetimibe in Familial Hypercholesterolemia. New England Journal of Medicine. 2008 Apr 3;358(14):1431–43.

The JUPITER: Rosuvastatin reduces the risk of major cardiovascular events in healthy patients

1. In patients with average low density lipoprotein (LDL) cholesterol levels and elevated C-reactive protein, rosuvastatin reduced the risk of a first major cardiovascular event compared to placebo.

2. Rosuvastatin therapy also significantly reduced the risk of all-cause mortality compared to placebo.

3. The study was terminated early and did not meet the prespecified number of primary endpoints needed to be sufficiently powered.

Original Date of Publication: November 2008

Study Rundown: Similarly to the present day, at the time of this study statins were commonly used medications in the treating patients with vascular disease and known hyperlipidemia. Clinical observations, however, revealed that myocardial infarctions and strokes were occurring in patients with normal levels of LDL, and in whom statin therapy would not be warranted based on consensus guidelines. Similarly, C-reactive protein, a marker of inflammation, was known to be a predictor of vascular events. The Justification for the Use of Statins in Prevention: an Intervention Trial Evaluating Rosuvastatin (JUPITER) sought to determine whether statin therapy could help prevent major cardiovascular events in patients with LDL levels below treatment thresholds, but who also had elevated CRP levels. Investigators successfully demonstrated that prescribing rosuvastatin to patients with LDL levels below treatment thresholds, but with elevated C-reactive protein levels, significantly reduced the rate of first major cardiovascular events as compared to placebo. Of note, the rates of adverse events were similar in the 2 groups. It must be noted that this trial was terminated early with a median follow-up less than 2 years. As a result, the trial did not have the prespecified 520 confirmed primary endpoints needed to be sufficiently powered.

In-Depth [randomized controlled trial]: A total of 17 802 patients were enrolled and randomized as part of the JUPITER. In order to be eligible, patients needed to meet age requirements ($\geq$50 years of age for men, $\geq$60 years of age for women), have no history of cardiovascular disease, have an LDL cholesterol <130 mg/dL, and have a high-sensitivity C-reactive protein level ≥2.0 mg/L. Exclusion criteria included previous or current use lipid-lowering therapy, current use of post-menopausal hormone-replacement therapy, evidence of hepatic dysfunction, elevated creatine kinase level, creatinine >2.0 mg/dL (176.8 μmol/L), diabetes, and uncontrolled hypertension. Moreover, patients with inflammatory conditions (e.g., severe arthritis, lupus, inflammatory bowel disease) were excluded. Eligible patients were randomized to treatment with either rosuvastatin 20 mg daily or placebo. Follow-up occurred up to 60 months after randomization. The primary outcome was the occurrence of a first major cardiovascular event (i.e., nonfatal myocardial infarction, nonfatal stroke, hospitalization for unstable angina, arterial revascularization procedure, or death from cardiovascular cause).

Patients were followed for a median of 1.9 years. The rate of the primary endpoint was significantly lower in the rosuvastatin group as compared with the placebo group (HR 0.56; 95%CI 0.46-0.69). This was driven by significant reductions in all components of the primary endpoint, except for hospitalization for unstable angina (HR 0.59; 95%CI 0.32-1.10). Notably, patients treated with rosuvastatin experienced a significant reduction in all-cause mortality when compared to those treated with placebo (HR 0.80; 95%CI 0.67-0.97). The rates of adverse events reported were similar for both groups (p = 0.60). The rates of myopathy (p = 0.82), newly diagnosed cancer (p = 0.51), gastrointestinal disorder (p = 0.43), and elevations in hepatic transaminases (p = 0.34) were similar between both groups.

Ridker PM, Danielson E, Fonseca FAH, Genest J, Gotto AM, Kastelein JJP, et al. Rosuvastatin to Prevent Vascular Events in Men and Women with Elevated C-Reactive Protein. New England Journal of Medicine. 2008 Nov 20;359(21):2195–207.

The RAVE trial: Rituximab induces remission in ANCA-associated vasculitis

1. Rituximab was non-inferior to cyclophosphamide in inducing remission of severe ANCA-associated vasculitis.

2. There were no significant differences between both groups in the rates of total, serious, or non-disease-related adverse events.

Original Date of Publication: July 2010

Study Rundown: The combination of cyclophosphamide and a glucocorticoid has long been the standard of treatment for ANCA-associated vasculitides. The Rituximab in ANCA-Associated Vasculitis (RAVE) trial demonstrated that rituximab was non-inferior to cyclophosphamide in inducing remission in severe ANCA-associated vasculitis when used alongside glucocorticoids. Moreover, there were no significant differences between the 2 groups in the rates of total, severe, or non-disease-related adverse events. The authors noted that their trial only included patients with severe ANCA-associated vasculitis, thereby limiting its generalizability. Others have also criticized this trial for its short follow-up and point to the paucity of data regarding long-term efficacy and safety. Rituximab subsequently received approval from the Food and Drug Administration for use in treating certain ANCA-associated vasculitides. One group has also recommended the use of rituximab while cautioning the lack of data about long-term effects.

In-Depth [randomized controlled trial]: The RAVE trial was a randomized, double-blind, double-dummy, non-inferiority trial examining the efficacy of rituximab in inducing remission of severe ANCA-associated vasculitis. Patients were eligible if they had Wegner's granulomatosis or microscopic polyangiitis, positive serum assays for proteinase 3-ANCA or myeloperoxidase-ANCA and a Birmingham Vasculitis Activity Score for Wegener's Granulomatosis (BVAS/WG) of 3 or more. Both patients with new diagnoses and relapsing disease were eligible for the trial. Eligible participants were randomized to receive either rituximab (375 mg/m^2 IV weekly for 4 weeks) or cyclophosphamide (2 mg/kg, with adjustments for renal insufficiency) with a subsequent switch to azathioprine if remission was achieved between 3-6 months. Both groups were also treated with glucocorticoids (i.e., 1-3 pulses of methylprednisolone, with subsequent prednisone tapered according to symptomology). The primary endpoint was a BVAS/WG score of 0 and successful completion of prednisone taper at 6 months.

A total of 197 patients with ANCA-associated vasculitis were enrolled in the trial. Approximately 64% of patients in the rituximab group and 53% of the patients in the cyclophosphamide group reached the primary endpoint, and this treatment difference met the criterion for non-inferiority (p < 0.001). The difference between the 2 groups was not statistically significant. There were no significant differences between the groups in the rates of total, severe, or non-disease-related adverse events.

Stone JH, Merkel PA, Spiera R, Seo P, Langford CA, Hoffman GS, et al. Rituximab versus Cyclophosphamide for ANCA-Associated Vasculitis. New England Journal of Medicine. 2010 Jul 15;363(3):221–32.

II. Cardiology

The V-HeFT I: Hydralazine and isosorbide dinitrate reduce mortality in heart failure

1. In patients with congestive heart failure, the combination of hydralazine and isosorbide dinitrate significantly reduced mortality compared to placebo.

2. This was one of the first large randomized trials to demonstrate a significant mortality benefit in the treatment of congestive heart failure.

Original Date of Publication: June 1986

Study Rundown: Prior to the 1980s, few options were available in heart failure treatment, with digitalis and diuretics being the only medications used to relieve symptoms. Subsequent efforts to treat heart failure focused on altering hemodynamics, and it was hypothesized that reducing preload and afterload using isosorbide dinitrate and hydralazine, respectively, could improve outcomes. The Vasodilator-Heart Failure Trial I (V-HeFT I) sought to explore the effects of using a combination of hydralazine and isosorbide dinitrate in managing heart failure. In summary, this trial demonstrated that treating patients with congestive heart failure with hydralazine-isosorbide dinitrate significantly reduced mortality compared to placebo for the initial 3-year period. This study was one of the first to demonstrate a significant reduction in mortality with heart failure treatment.

In-Depth [randomized controlled trial]: A total of 642 patients were randomized to treatment with placebo, prazosin 2.5 mg 4 times per day, or hydralazine 37.5 mg-isosorbide dinitrate 20 mg 4 times per day. Patients with chronic congestive heart failure were recruited from 11 Veterans Administration hospitals in the United States. Patients were eligible for the trial if they were male, between 18-75 years of age, and had congestive heart failure, as determined by evidence of cardiac dilatation (i.e., increased cardiothoracic size on chest x-ray, left ventricular dilatation on echocardiogram) or left ventricular impairment and reduced exercise tolerance. Patients were excluded if they had reduced exercise tolerance due to chest pain, rather than fatigue/breathlessness, myocardial infarction in the recent 3 months, or substantial disease to limit 5-year survival. Over the initial 2-year period, Cox regression demonstrated a significant 34% reduction in mortality (95%CI 4-54%) in the hydralazine-isosorbide dinitrate group compared with the placebo group. By 3 years, the hydralazine-isosorbide dinitrate group experienced a 36% reduction in mortality (95%CI 11-54%). Beyond 3 years, the data was insufficient to draw any conclusions.

Cohn JN, Archibald DG, Ziesche S, Franciosa JA, Harston WE, Tristani FE, et al. Effect of Vasodilator Therapy on Mortality in Chronic Congestive Heart Failure. New England Journal of Medicine. 1986 Jun 12;314(24):1547–52.

The CAST: Anti-arrhythmic agents increase risk of death in patients after myocardial infarction

1. The use of class IC anti-arrhythmic agents flecainide and encainide in patients following myocardial infarction with left ventricular dysfunction increased the risk of death due to arrhythmia and shock.

Original Date of Publication: March 1991

Study Rundown: Ventricular arrhythmia is a major cause of cardiac death following myocardial infarction. Thus, the Cardiac Arrhythmia Suppression Trial (CAST) sought to determine whether suppression of ventricular ectopy with class IC anti-arrhythmic drugs in patients with a recent myocardial infarction would improve outcomes, including mortality. Unfortunately, the results demonstrated an increased risk of death from arrhythmia and any cause in those patients receiving these drugs following myocardial infarction. This increased incidence of arrhythmia-associated death was not matched correspondingly with an increased incidence of non-lethal events involving arrhythmia. This study was one of the first to encourage practicing caution in the use of anti-arrhythmic drugs in patients with cardiovascular disease, including following acute myocardial infarction. In summary, this study highlighted that the use of class IC antiarrhythmic agents flecainide and encainide for suppression of ventricular ectopy should be avoided in patients post-myocardial infarction, as they carry excess risk of mortality.

In-Depth [randomized controlled trial]: This trial enrolled 1498 patients. Patients with a recent myocardial infarction, ventricular dysfunction, and asymptomatic or mildly symptomatic ventricular arrhythmia were eligible for this study. The study employed an initial open-label titration period to identify patients who responded to at least 1 drug with 80-90% suppression of ventricular arrhythmia. The patients were then randomized to receive either study drug or placebo. The primary end-point was death or cardiac arrest with resuscitation, either of which occurring secondary to arrhythmia. The trial was originally planned to last 3 years, but was discontinued a year early due to results suggesting excess death in the treatment arm. Findings demonstrated that death from arrhythmia was significantly increased in the treatment group receiving flecainide or encainide as compared to those receiving placebo (relative rate (RR) 2.64; 95%CI 1.60-4.36). Mortality from any cause was also significantly more likely in the treatment arms (RR 2.38; 95%CI 1.59-3.57).

Echt DS, Liebson PR, Mitchell LB, Peters RW, Obias-Manno D, Barker AH, et al. *Mortality and Morbidity in Patients Receiving Encainide, Flecainide, or Placebo. New England Journal of Medicine. 1991 Mar 21;324(12):781–8.*

The SOLVD trial: Enalapril reduces mortality in heart failure with reduced ejection fraction

1. Enalapril significantly reduced the risk of all-cause mortality in patients with congestive heart failure (CHF) and reduced left ventricular ejection fraction (LVEF) compared to placebo.

2. Patients being treated with enalapril had a significantly higher risk of developing elevated serum potassium levels and serum creatinine levels.

Original Date of Publication: August 1991

Study Rundown: At the time of the Studies of Left Ventricular Dysfunction (SOLVD) trial, some evidence existed to support that angiotensin converting enzyme (ACE) inhibitors improved hemodynamic stability and reduced mortality in CHF patients. One such study was the CONSENSUS trial, which was published several years before the SOLVD trial. The CONSENSUS trial, however, only included patients with New York Heart Association (NYHA) Class IV CHF. Given the results of prior studies, researchers in the SOLVD trial hypothesized that treatment with an ACE inhibitor would be beneficial to all patients with CHF with reduced ejection fraction, regardless of their NYHA classification. The SOLVD trial demonstrated that treatment with enalapril significantly reduced mortality and frequency of hospitalizations for heart failure in patients with CHF when compared with placebo. Prior to enrollment in the trial, there was a run-in period where participants received enalapril for several days followed by approximately 2 weeks of placebo. This was used as a tool to identify patients who would not tolerate the experimental drug and to assess compliance. This method, however, potentially underestimated the risks of treatment by screening out patients that may have poorly tolerated the drug. It also weakened the external validity of the trial by narrowing the study population of the trial. Nevertheless, this study demonstrated that ACE inhibitor treatment was significant beneficial for patients with all NYHA classes of CHF with reduced ejection fraction.

In-Depth [randomized controlled trial]: This study, conducted at 83 different hospitals in 3 different countries, randomized 2569 patients with LVEF ≤35% to receive either enalapril or placebo. Patients were excluded if they were already taking an ACE inhibitor as part of their CHF management, if they were >80 years of age, or if they were hemodynamically unstable or had severe co-morbidities, such as unstable angina, recent MI, severe pulmonary disease, or severe chronic kidney disease. A run-in period prior to enrollment in the trial included 2-7 days of enalapril 2.5 mg twice daily to assess for adverse reactions and noncompliance, followed by a 14-17 day placebo phase. Doses of enalapril for the treatment group varied from 2.5-10 mg twice daily and were based on the patient's tolerance of the drug by the participating physician. If a patient's heart failure worsened over the course of the study, the patient was switched over to open-label treatment.

Patients were followed for an average of 41 months. The study outcomes included all-cause mortality, specific causes of mortality, hospitalizations for heart failure, and all hospitalizations. The mortality rate in the treatment group was significantly lower than that of the placebo group (35.2% vs. 39.7%; $p < 0.0036$). The patients in the enalapril group also had a significant decrease in deaths due to progressive heart failure or arrhythmia (16.3% vs. 19.5%; $p < 0.0045$). Post-hoc sub-group analyses showed that enalapril was beneficial in all 4 NYHA classes of CHF. The enalapril group had higher incidence of elevated serum potassium levels (6.4% vs. 2.5%, $p < 0.01$) and creatinine levels (10.7% vs. 7.7%, $p < 0.01$) than the placebo group.

The SOLVD Investigators. Effect of enalapril on survival in patients with reduced left ventricular ejection fractions and congestive heart failure. New England Journal of Medicine. 1991 Aug 1;325(5):293–302.

The SAVE trial: Captopril reduces mortality after acute myocardial infarction

1. Treating patients with captopril after acute myocardial infarction (MI) with asymptomatic left ventricular (LV) dysfunction reduced mortality from cardiovascular causes (i.e., atherosclerotic heart disease, progressive heart failure).

2. The captopril group experienced lower rates of hospitalization due to heart failure and recurrent MI.

Original Date of Publication: September 1992

Study Rundown: The Survival and Ventricular Enlargement (SAVE) trial was a randomized controlled trial that sought to explore the effects of captopril on mortality and morbidity in patients suffering from acute MI and asymptomatic LV dysfunction. In previous animal studies, angiotensin converting enzyme (ACE) inhibitors like captopril were shown to delay ventricular remodeling, and help preserve function after MI. The SAVE trial was the first to demonstrate that treating patients with acute MI and asymptomatic LV dysfunction with an ACE inhibitor reduced morbidity and mortality. These benefits were thought to result from ACE inhibitors slowing the remodeling process that takes place after patients suffer MIs. The findings have since been replicated in other trials (e.g., TRACE trial), systematic reviews, and meta-analyses. In patients suffering from an acute MI and asymptomatic LV dysfunction, early initiation of and continued treatment with captopril can significantly reduce cardiovascular mortality, hospitalization due to heart failure, and recurrent MIs.

In-Depth [randomized controlled trial]: The trial was conducted at 45 centers across North America. A total of 2231 patients took part in the study and were randomized to receive either captopril or placebo. Patients were followed for a minimum of 2 years, though mean follow-up was 42 months. Inclusion criteria were age between 21-80 years, being between 3-16 days away from a recent MI, and LV ejection fraction ≤40% as determined by radionuclide ventriculography. Exclusion criteria included not being randomized within 16 days after an MI, a relative contraindication to ACE inhibitors or need for symptomatic heart failure or hypertension management, serum creatinine >221 μmol/L (or 2.5 mg/dL), and unstable post-infarction

50

course. The endpoints included all-cause mortality, death from cardiovascular causes, heart failure hospitalization, and rate of recurrent MI.

Patients randomized to receive captopril experienced a significantly reduced all-cause mortality (RRR 19%, 95%CI 3-32%, p = 0.019) and mortality from cardiovascular causes (RRR 21%, 95%CI 5-35%, p = 0.014) compared to the placebo group. Specifically, captopril was associated with significant reductions in mortality from atherosclerotic heart disease and progressive heart failure (RRR 36%, 95%CI 4-58%, p = 0.032). Moreover, the captopril group demonstrated a significant decrease in hospitalization because of heart failure (RRR 22%, 95%CI 4-37%, p = 0.019) and recurrent MIs (RRR 25%, 95%CI 5-40%, p = 0.015) compared to placebo.

Pfeffer MA, Braunwald E, Moyé LA, Basta L, Brown EJ, Cuddy TE, et al. Effect of Captopril on Mortality and Morbidity in Patients with Left Ventricular Dysfunction after Myocardial Infarction. New England Journal of Medicine. 1992 Sep 3;327(10):669–77.

The CARE trial: Pravastatin reduces risk of coronary events

1. Statin therapy reduced the risk of coronary events in patients with known coronary artery disease and low-density lipoprotein levels (LDL) >125 mg/dL.

2. The reduction in coronary events with statin therapy was found to be greater in women and patients with higher pretreatment LDL levels.

Original Date of Publication: October 1996

Study Rundown: Serum cholesterol levels have long been considered important risk factors for the development of coronary artery disease, and previous studies have demonstrated that lowering cholesterol levels in patients with high cholesterol significantly reduces the risk of coronary events. The Cholesterol and Recurrent Events (CARE) trial examined the effect of lowering LDL levels on the incidence of coronary events in patients with known coronary artery disease and average cholesterol levels. The study demonstrated that treating such patients with pravastatin to lower LDL levels significantly reduced the risk of the composite endpoint of fatal coronary artery disease or nonfatal myocardial infarction when compared to placebo. This difference was driven by a reduction in the rate of nonfatal myocardial infarctions, as there was no significant difference in mortality from coronary artery disease. Notably, women and patients with higher pretreatment LDL levels experienced significantly greater risk reductions than men and patients with lower pretreatment LDL levels, respectively. In summary, this trial supports the use of statin therapy to lower cholesterol levels patients with known coronary artery disease and LDL levels >125 mg/dL.

In-Depth [randomized controlled trial]: A total of 4159 patients from 80 centers across Canada and the United States were randomized. Patients were eligible if they had an acute myocardial infarction 3-20 months prior to randomization, were between 21-75 years of age, had total cholesterol levels of <240 mg/dL, had LDL cholesterol levels between 115-174 mg/dL, had fasting triglyceride levels <350 mg/dL, had fasting glucose levels <220 mg/dL (12.2 mmol/L), had left ventricular ejection fractions of ≥25%, and did not have symptomatic congestive heart failure. Patients were randomized to receive pravastatin 40 mg daily or placebo and followed for a median of 5.0 years. The primary endpoint was a composite of fatal coronary artery disease or nonfatal myocardial infarction.

Patients treated with pravastatin experienced significantly lower rates of the primary endpoint as compared with patients taking placebo (RR 24%; 95%CI 9-36%). This difference was driven by a significant reduction in nonfatal myocardial infarctions (RR 23%; 95%CI 4-39%), as there was no significant difference in death from coronary artery disease. The risk of revascularization (i.e., coronary artery bypass graft, percutaneous transluminal coronary angioplasty) was significantly lower in patients taking pravastatin (RR 27%; 95%CI 15-37%). Women experienced significantly larger reductions in the risk of coronary events compared to men (p=0.05 for interaction between sex and outcomes). Of note, results differed according to pretreatment LDL levels. Patients with LDL >150 mg/dL experienced a larger risk reduction compared to those with LDL between 125-150 mg/dL at baseline (35% vs. 26%, p = 0.03 for interaction between pretreatment LDL and risk reduction).

Sacks FM, Pfeffer MA, Moye LA, Rouleau JL, Rutherford JD, Cole TG, et al. The Effect of Pravastatin on Coronary Events after Myocardial Infarction in Patients with Average Cholesterol Levels. New England Journal of Medicine. 1996 Oct 3;335(14):1001–9.

The DIG trial: Digoxin reduces hospitalization in patients with systolic heart failure

1. Digoxin significantly reduced hospitalizations in patients with systolic heart failure.

2. Digoxin was most beneficial in patients with low ejection fractions (EFs) and poor functional status (NYHA III-IV).

Original Date of Publication: February 1997

Study Rundown: Digoxin, a cardiac glycoside derived from the extracts of the foxglove plant *Digitalis purpurea*, has a long history of use in the treatment of heart disease. It acts primarily as a positive inotrope by inhibiting the sarcolemmal Na-K ATPase pump and consequently increasing myocardial intracellular calcium concentrations. Prior to the Digitalis Investigation Group (DIG) trial, digoxin was commonly prescribed for patients with heart failure with the intention of improving contractility and thus cardiac output. There was no substantial evidence, however, suggesting that the use of digoxin improved long-term outcomes in patients with heart failure. This landmark randomized controlled trial enrolled 6800 patients and sought to examine the long-term effects of digoxin on mortality and hospitalization in patients suffering from systolic heart failure.

The DIG trial provided evidence that digoxin significantly reduced the number of hospitalizations in patients with heart failure. This effect was greatest for those with low ejections fractions and poor functional status. Although the study did not show any mortality benefit, digoxin was not linked to increased mortality, as had been demonstrated with other positive inotropes. This study indicated that to reduce hospitalizations, the addition of digoxin should be considered for patients with systolic heart failure (EF<0.45) who continue to have poor functional status (NYHA III-IV) and are already optimized on a beta-blocker and angiotensin converting enzyme inhibitor.

In-Depth [randomized controlled trial]: This trial was conducted at 302 clinical centers in the United States and Canada. Patients were eligible for the trial if they had heart failure with left ventricular EF ≤ 0.45 and were in normal sinus rhythm. Included patients were randomized to either receive digoxin or placebo. The primary outcome studied was death from any cardiovascular cause. Secondary outcomes included hospitalization or death from worsening of heart failure. A total of 6800 patients were randomized as part of the trial. There was no significant difference in mortality from any cause between the digoxin and placebo groups (RR 0.99; 95%CI 0.91-1.07; $p = 0.80$). Patients in the digoxin group, however, were significantly less likely to be hospitalized for worsening of heart failure (RR 0.72; 95%CI 0.66-0.79; $p < 0.001$). Subgroup analysis showed that the benefit of digoxin on a combined outcome of mortality and hospitalization for heart failure was greatest in patients with low ejection fractions (EF <0.25) and functional status (NYHA III-IV).

The Digitalis Investigation Group. The Effect of Digoxin on Mortality and Morbidity in Patients with Heart Failure. New England Journal of Medicine. 1997 Feb 20;336(8):525–33.

The MERIT-HF trial: Metoprolol reduces mortality in patients with symptomatic heart failure

1. In patients with symptomatic heart failure and reduced ejection fraction, the addition of metoprolol to standard therapy reduced all-cause mortality by 34% compared to placebo.

2. Similar findings were reported in the CIBIS-II trial.

Original Date of Publication: June 1999

Study Rundown: This trial investigated effect of adding metoprolol to standard therapy in the treatment of patients with decreased ejection fraction and symptomatic heart failure. Adding metoprolol controlled/extended release to standard optimum therapy (i.e., a diuretic and angiotensin converting enzyme (ACE) inhibitor reduced all-cause mortality by 34% in patients with symptomatic heart failure compared to placebo. Another study published around the same time, the Cardiac Insufficiency Bisoprolol Study II (CIBIS-II), reported similar findings. Of note, the study was funded by grants from a pharmaceutical company. In summary, adding metoprolol controlled release/extended release to optimum standard therapy in symptomatic heart failure (NYHA class II-IV) reduces all-cause mortality.

In-Depth [randomized controlled trial]: A total of 3991 patients were enrolled in the study and randomized to receive either metoprolol controlled release/extended release (12.5 mg for NYHA class III-IV, 25 mg for NYHA class II) once daily or placebo. The study was conducted at 313 sites in 13 European countries and the United States. Patients were included if they had symptomatic heart failure (i.e., New York Heart Association functional class II-IV) for at least 3 months, a left ventricular ejection fraction less than 0.40 in the 3 months before enrollment, a stable clinical condition in the 2 week run-in phase for the study, and were taking optimum standard therapy (i.e., combination of diuretics and ACE inhibitor).The trial was stopped early on the recommendation of the independent safety committee, as the predefined criterion for ending the study had been met. There was a significant reduction in all-cause mortality in the metoprolol group compared to the placebo group, with a relative risk of 0.66 (95%CI 0.53-0.81). Specifically, there were significantly fewer cardiovascular deaths, sudden deaths, and deaths from aggravated heart failure in the metoprolol group.

MERIT-HF Study Group. Effect of metoprolol CR/XL in chronic heart failure: Metoprolol CR/XL Randomised Intervention Trial in-Congestive Heart Failure (MERIT-HF). The Lancet. 1999 Jun 12;353(9169):2001–7.

The RALES trial: Spironolactone reduces mortality in heart failure patients

1. Adding 25 mg of spironolactone to standard therapy reduced all-cause mortality in heart failure patients with an ejection fraction <35%.

Original Date of Publication: September 1999

Study Rundown: Progression of heart failure is thought to be related to physiological neuroendocrine compensation of the body to decreased effective circulating volume - the activation of the sympathetic and renin-angiotensin-aldosterone system, which lead to myocardial remodeling and subsequent progressive reduction in cardiac output. The Randomized Aldactone Evaluation Study (RALES) trial looked at the latter system, particularly the role of aldosterone blockade in treating heart failure. At the time of this study's completion, there was controversy amongst physicians in using aldosterone-inhibitors, like spironolactone, for the treatment of heart failure as it was assumed that angiotensin converting enzyme (ACE) inhibitors, which were well established as standard of care for the condition, already offered effective aldosterone blockade by inhibiting its production. Furthermore, many clinicians exhibited caution in using spironolactone, as it was thought that adding this medication to standard therapy would increase the risk of serious hyperkalemia. Increasing evidence, however, suggested that ACE inhibitors did not effectively suppress the production of aldosterone in the long-term. Thus, the RALES trail was launched in order to investigate the role of aldosterone-receptor antagonism in the treatment of advanced heart failure. Specifically, the trial sought to determine whether spironolactone would reduce mortality in patients with advanced heart failure, who were already on standard medical therapy.

This landmark study supported the use of spironolactone, in addition to standard medical therapy, to reduce mortality and hospitalizations in patients with heart failure. Based upon the study's findings, aldosterone antagonism with spironolactone should be considered for patients with a left ventricular ejection fraction (LVEF) <35% and New York Heart Association (NYHA) Class III-IV symptoms, despite optimization of standard therapy. A subsequent study conducted in 2004 demonstrated an abrupt increase in the prescription of spironolactone after the publication of the RALES trial, and showed a rapid rise in morbidity and mortality associated with hyperkalemia. Thus, calls were made for closer monitoring of patients being prescribed spironolactone.

In-Depth [randomized controlled trial]: The study involved 1663 patients from 195 centers in 15 countries. Inclusion criteria were functional NYHA class III-IV, LVEF <35%, and current treatment with standard therapy (i.e., ACE inhibitor and loop diuretic). Most patients were also on digoxin. Patients were randomly assigned to either the treatment arm (i.e., standard therapy and spironolactone 25-50 mg daily) or the placebo arm (i.e., standard therapy and placebo). The trial was scheduled to run for 3 years, but was discontinued early at 24 months due to the clear benefit of spironolactone. Patients treated with spironolactone experienced significantly lower mortality than those treated with placebo (RR 0.70; 95%CI 0.60-0.82; p < 0.001), which was driven by significantly lower rates of death due to progressive heart failure and sudden cardiac death. The spironolactone group also had significantly lower rates of hospitalization for worsening heart failure (RR 0.65; 95%CI 0.54-0.77; p < 0.001). The rates of gynecomastia and breast pain were significantly higher in the spironolactone group (p < 0.001), while there was no difference between the groups in the risk of serious hyperkalemia.

Pitt B, Zannad F, Remme WJ, Cody R, Castaigne A, Perez A, et al. The Effect of Spironolactone on Morbidity and Mortality in Patients with Severe Heart Failure. New England Journal of Medicine. 1999 Sep 2;341(10):709–17.

The ATLAS trial: Angiotensin converting enzyme inhibitor dosing in chronic heart failure

1. When compared to a lower dose, high-dose angiotensin converting enzyme (ACE) inhibitors were associated with a significantly reduced risk of hospitalization or death in patients with chronic heart failure.

Original Date of Publication: December 1999

Study Rundown: At the time, physicians often prescribed ACE inhibitors to patients with chronic heart failure in lower doses than proven effective by large-scale studies. Nonetheless, convincing research on the comparative benefits of high dose and low dose ACE inhibitors was severely lacking. The Assessment of Treatment with Lisinopril and Survival (ATLAS) trial randomized 3164 patients to receive low- or high-dose of the ACE inhibitor lisinopril for 29-58 months. This study demonstrated that compared with those in the low-dose group, patients in the high-dose treatment group experienced a significantly lower risk of death or hospitalization for any reason. The high-dose group also had significantly fewer hospitalizations for heart failure. These findings suggested that patients with heart failure due to left ventricular systolic dysfunction should not be maintained on low doses of ACE inhibitor unless they are intolerant of higher doses. Rather, tolerant patients should be placed on a higher doses of ACE inhibitors due to increased effectiveness.

In-Depth [randomized controlled trial]: The ATLAS study randomly assigned 3164 patients with New York Heart Association (NYHA) class II to IV heart failure and an ejection fraction of ≤30% to treatment with either a high-dose (32.5-35 mg daily) or low-dose (2.5-5.0 mg daily) of lisinopril, an ACE inhibitor. The trial was conducted in 287 hospitals across 19 countries. The duration of follow-up ranged from 39 to 58 months.

The trial found that patients randomized to receive high-dose lisinopril experienced a 12% lower risk of hospitalization or death for any reason (p = 0.002) and 24% fewer hospitalizations for heart failure (p = 0.002) as compared to patients in the low-dose group. Patients in the high-dose group did experience dizziness and renal insufficiency more frequently. However, these side effects did not lead to lower compliance with medication in the high-dose group.

Packer M, Poole-Wilson PA, Armstrong PW, Cleland JGF, Horowitz JD, Massie BM, et al. Comparative Effects of Low and High Doses of the Angiotensin-Converting Enzyme Inhibitor, Lisinopril, on Morbidity and Mortality in Chronic Heart Failure. Circulation. 1999 Dec 7;100(23):2312–8.

The HOPE trial: Ramipril reduces cardiovascular events in high-risk patients with normal ejection fractions

1. Ramipril significantly reduced the risk of cardiovascular events including myocardial infarction, stroke and death in high risk-patients without left ventricular dysfunction.

Original Date of Publication: January 2000

Study Rundown: Prior to the publication of the Heart Outcomes Prevention Evaluation (HOPE) trial, the benefit of angiotensin converting enzyme (ACE) inhibitors had been well established in improving long-term outcomes for patients with heart failure associated with reduced left ventricular ejection fraction. There was also evidence of the value of these medications in controlling blood pressure, particularly in diabetic patients with microalbuminuria. At the time, however, there was limited evidence as to whether ACE inhibitors provided any cardiovascular protection in the absence of left ventricular dysfunction. That is, there was uncertainty as to whether the blockade of the renin-angiotensin system offered any inherent benefit in improving cardiac outcomes in high-risk populations, independent of its effect on blood pressure or preventing the progression of systolic heart failure. This landmark study evaluated the effect of ramipril on major cardiovascular events in high-risk patients over 55 years old with normal ejection fractions.

This trial was the first to provide evidence for the potential benefit of ACE inhibitors for vascular protection in preventing adverse cardiac outcomes among a broad range of high-risk patients with normal ejection fractions. Patients assigned to receive ramipril had significantly less cardiovascular-related complications. After its publication, there was some criticism that the blood pressure lowering effect of ramipril may have accounted for the improved cardiac outcomes, as opposed to the medication itself. However, most patients did not have baseline hypertension in this study and the difference in blood pressure between the 2 groups was minor. Even in the absence of reduced ejection fraction or high blood pressure, the addition of ramipril for high-risk patients at least 55 years of age may be considered for protection against adverse cardiovascular outcomes and death.

In-Depth [randomized controlled study]: This large, double-blind, randomized control study included 9541 patients from 281 centers internationally. Inclusion criteria were age ≥55 years, a history of coronary artery disease, stroke, peripheral vascular disease, or diabetes, and one additional cardiovascular risk factor (e.g., hypertension, dyslipidemia, cigarette smoking, documented microalbuminuria). Patients with known low ejection fraction (EF <40%), history of heart failure, or who were already on an ACE inhibitor were excluded from this study. Patients were randomized to either receive 1) placebo or 2) ramipril titrated up to 10 mg daily. Primary outcome was a composite of myocardial infarction, stroke, or death from cardiovascular causes.

The trial lasted a total of 5 years. The rate of the primary outcome was significantly lower in patients being treated with ramipril as compared with placebo (RR 0.78; 95%CI 0.70-0.86). This finding held true among a broad range of patients in this study. Subgroup analysis showed that the benefit of ramipril was consistent despite sex, age, cardiac risk factors, presence of diabetes, evidence of cardiovascular disease, baseline blood pressure, or evidence of microalbuminuria. The most common adverse effect of ramipril was cough.

Yusuf S, Sleight P, Pogue J, Bosch J, Davies R, Dagenais G. Effects of an angiotensin-converting-enzyme inhibitor, ramipril, on cardiovascular events in high-risk patients. The Heart Outcomes Prevention Evaluation Study Investigators. New England Journal of Medicine. 2000 Jan 20;342(3):145–53.

The MIRACL trial: Atorvastatin reduces recurrent ischemia after acute coronary syndrome

1. In patients with a recent acute coronary syndrome (ACS), atorvastatin 80 mg daily reduced the risk of recurrent ischemia.

2. This study did not demonstrate a significant reduction in death, cardiac arrest, or nonfatal acute myocardial infarction with statin therapy, as compared to placebo.

Original Date of Publication: April 2001

Study Rundown: Previous studies had demonstrated that reducing cholesterol levels with statins was linked to a reduction in the risk of mortality and cardiac events. The Myocardial Ischemia Reduction with Aggressive Cholesterol Lowering (MIRACL) trial demonstrated that providing atorvastatin 80 mg daily 24-96 hours after the onset of an ACS reduced the risk of recurrent ischemia as compared to placebo. In summary, treating patients with ACS with atorvastatin was associated with a significant reduction in the risk of recurrent symptomatic myocardial ischemia requiring rehospitalization in the 16 weeks following an ACS. Given that this was a large, international, multicenter trial, the findings are generalizable to patients with ACS in different settings, with different ethnicities and risk profiles. Based on these findings, statins are commonly prescribed for patients who have suffered acute coronary syndromes, in hopes of reducing the risk of recurrent ischemia.

In-Depth [randomized controlled trial]: The MIRACL trial enrolled 3086 patients from 122 centers in Europe, North America, South Africa, and Australasia. Patients were eligible if they were ≥18 years of age and had chest pain >15 minutes duration in the 24 hours prior to presentation. Exclusion criteria included serum cholesterol levels >270 mg/dL (7 mmol/L), plans for coronary revascularization at the time of screening, evidence of Q-wave myocardial infarction (MI) in the past 4 weeks, and coronary artery bypass surgery in the past 3 months. Patients were randomized to receive atorvastatin 80 mg daily or placebo for 16 weeks after an ACS. The primary endpoint was a composite of death, cardiac arrest, nonfatal acute MI, or recurrent symptomatic myocardial ischemia requiring emergency rehospitalization.

At 16 weeks, patients receiving atorvastatin had significantly lower rates of the composite endpoint compared to those taking placebo (RR 0.84; 95%CI 0.70-1.00, p = 0.048), with an absolute risk reduction of 2.6% (NNT = 38). Notably, there was no significant difference between the groups in the risk of death, nonfatal acute MI, or cardiac arrest. The difference in the primary endpoint was due to a reduction in the risk of recurrent symptomatic myocardial ischemia (RR 0.74; 95%CI 0.57-0.95). The risk of abnormal liver transaminase levels was significantly higher in the atorvastatin group (2.5% vs. 0.6%, p < 0.001).

Schwartz GG, Olsson AG, Ezekowitz MD, et al. Effects of atorvastatin on early recurrent ischemic events in acute coronary syndromes: The miracl study: a randomized controlled trial. JAMA. 2001 Apr 4;285(13):1711–8.

The CHADS2 score: Stroke risk in atrial fibrillation

1. The CHADS2 index was an accurate predictor of stroke in patients with non-rheumatic atrial fibrillation.

2. Presently, CHADS2 scores are used to aid decisions regarding the need for anti-thrombotic therapy.

Original Date of Publication: June 2001

Study Rundown: The CHADS2 index combined risk factors identified in the Atrial Fibrillation Investigators (AFI) and the Stroke Prevention and Atrial Fibrillation (SPAF) investigations to create a new clinical prediction model for stroke in patients with atrial fibrillation. This study validated the 3 tools and found that CHADS2 predicts stroke with greater accuracy than both the AFI and SPAF schemes. CHADS2 scores may be used to guide decisions regarding the need for anti-thrombotic therapy (i.e., aspirin for low-risk patients, warfarin for high-risk patients), particularly in identifying low-risk patients who may benefit from aspirin therapy. Strengths of the study include wide representation of regions within the United States and generalizability of results to frail, elderly patients. The CHADS2 index includes a limited set of risk factors for stroke and may neglect other important risk factors.

In-Depth [randomized controlled trial]: This study evaluated the predictive accuracy of the AFI and SPAF stroke classification schemes, as well as the CHADS2 index, a new stroke-risk prediction model created by combining the AFI and SPAF schemes. CHADS2 is an acronym for the risk factors considered and their score value. One point is assigned for any of the following risk factors: recent congestive heart failure, hypertension, age ≥75 years, and diabetes mellitus. Two points were added if there is a history of stroke or transient ischemic attack.

Risk factor	Points
Congestive heart failure	1
Hypertension	1
Age ≥75 years	1
Diabetes mellitus	1
Stroke or transient ischemic attack	2

The study included 1733 patients between ages 65 to 95 years with non-rheumatic atrial fibrillation. Stroke rate increased by a factor of 1.5 for each 1-point increment in CHADS2 score ($p < 0.001$) and the CHADS2 index was found to predict stroke with greater accuracy than both the AFI and SPAF schemes with a c statistic of 0.82.

CHADS2 score	Stroke rate per 100 patient-years
0	1.9
1	2.8
2	4.0
3	5.9
4	8.5
5	12.5
6	18.2

Gage BF, Waterman AD, Shannon W, Boechler M, Rich MW, Radford MJ. Validation of clinical classification schemes for predicting stroke: Results from the national registry of atrial fibrillation. JAMA. 2001 Jun 13;285(22):2864–70.

The Val-HeFT trial: Valsartan reduces morbidity in chronic heart failure

1. Valsartan, an angiotensin-receptor blocker (ARB), reduced morbidity, but not mortality, in heart failure patients when added to background therapy.

2. As an exception, valsartan was associated with increased morbidity and mortality in patients already receiving both an angiotensin converting enzyme (ACE) inhibitor and beta-blocker.

Original Date of Publication: December 2001

Study Rundown: Angiotensin II contributes to cardiac remodeling that leads to decreased left ventricular function and progressive heart failure. At the time of the study in 2001, ACE inhibitors and beta-blockers were the standard therapies for heart failure. This study demonstrated that treatment with the ARB valsartan in addition to previously prescribed therapy could further decrease patient morbidity. Patient mortality, however, was not significantly different when compared to placebo, and valsartan was linked to increased morbidity and mortality in the subgroup of patients already receiving both an ACE inhibitor and beta-blocker. The study's results do not generalize to patients already receiving ARBs, who were excluded from this study. Additionally, approximately 90% of the study's participants were white. In the study's black population, consisting of African American and South African patients, the effect of valsartan was not statistically significant. Finally, valsartan was associated with only a moderate increase in ejection fraction when compared with other prior trials involving ACE inhibitors and beta-blockers. In summary, the Val-HeFT trial demonstrated an important role for ARBs in the management of heart failure.

In-Depth [randomized controlled trial]: This randomized, double-blinded, placebo-controlled, trial involved 302 centers in 16 countries. A total of 5010 patients with documented left ventricular dilatation and at least 2 weeks of treatment with ACE inhibitors, diuretics, digoxin, or beta-blockers were stratified according to previously prescribed beta-blocker treatment and randomized to receive valsartan or placebo. Two primary endpoints were measured: 1) mortality alone and 2) the combined endpoint of mortality and morbidity (defined as cardiac arrest with resuscitation, hospitalization for heart failure, etc.). The combined endpoint of mortality and morbidity was significantly lower with valsartan (RR 0.87; 97.5%CI 0.77-0.97) than placebo, which was attributed to a decreased number of hospitalizations for heart failure (p < 0.001). There was no significant difference in mortality alone (RR 1.02; 98%CI 0.88-1.18).

Cohn JN, Tognoni G. A Randomized Trial of the Angiotensin-Receptor Blocker Valsartan in Chronic Heart Failure. New England Journal of Medicine. 2001 Dec 6;345(23):1667–75.

The MADIT-II: Prophylactic defibrillators reduce mortality in left ventricular dysfunction

1. There was a 31% reduction in the risk of death associated with implantation of a defibrillator in patients with a previous myocardial infarction and left ventricular dysfunction, when compared to conventional therapy.

2. Rates of hospitalization for heart failure were not significantly elevated in the defibrillator group.

Original Date of Publication: March 2002

Study Rundown: The Multicenter Automatic Defibrillator Implantation Trial II Investigators (MADIT-II) examined the potential survival benefit of an implantable defibrillator in patients with a previous myocardial infarction and left ventricular dysfunction (without requiring patients to undergo electrophysiological testing for inducible arrhythmias). The results indicated that an implantable defibrillator may significantly improve outcomes along with appropriate drug therapy. Of note, a slightly higher rate of hospitalization with heart failure was observed in the defibrillator group, though this did not reach statistical significance. Further investigations, including electrophysiologic testing, as inclusion criteria may help to determine the specific groups for whom implantation of a defibrillator would be most beneficial with minimal risk. In summary, the findings of this trial determined that implantation of a defibrillator should be considered in patients with myocardial infarction and reduced ejection fraction as a prophylactic measure for sudden cardiac death.

In-Depth [randomized controlled trial]: The trial assessed the survival benefit of prophylactic defibrillator implantation in patients with a previous myocardial infarction and an ejection fraction of ≤ 0.30. A total of 1232 patients were assigned to receive an implantable defibrillator or to conventional medical therapy in a 3:2 ratio. After an average follow-up of 20 months, the trial found a significant 31% reduction in risk of death in the defibrillator group compared to the conventional therapy group (HR 0.69; 95%CI 0.51-0.93, p = 0.016). Subgroup analyses did not reveal any differences in this effect based on a number of factors, including age, gender, ejection fraction, and QRS interval. Serious complications associated with defibrillator therapy were uncommon. A slightly higher, though nonsignificant, rate of hospitalization with heart failure in the defibrillator group compared to conventional therapy.

Moss AJ, Zareba W, Hall WJ, Klein H, Wilber DJ, Cannom DS, et al. Prophylactic Implantation of a Defibrillator in Patients with Myocardial Infarction and Reduced Ejection Fraction. New England Journal of Medicine. 2002 Mar 21;346(12):877–83.

The COPERNICUS trial: Carvedilol reduces mortality in severe chronic heart failure

1. Adding carvedilol to the management of patients with severe heart failure was associated with a significant, 35% relative risk reduction in mortality.

2. In this patient population, carvedilol was also associated with significantly reduced risks of hospitalization and serious adverse effects, as well as improvement in symptoms.

Original Date of Publication: October 2002

Study Rundown: The landmark Carvedilol Prospective Randomized Cumulative Survival (COPERNICUS) trial provided further support to the already established and growing body of evidence supporting the use of beta-blockers in the treatment of heart failure. Prior to COPERNICUS, the randomized controlled trials MOCHA and PRECISE had demonstrated that carvedilol was associated with reductions in mortality and hospitalizations for patients with mild-moderate heart failure. The COPERNICUS trial investigated the benefit of carvedilol in patients with severe heart failure, defined as New York Heart Association (NYHA) class III-IV and a left ventricular ejection fraction (LVEF) <25%. Results from this randomized, placebo-controlled trial showed that carvedilol therapy was associated with a 35% relative risk reduction in mortality. For this reason, the study was terminated 1 year early. Carvedilol was also associated with a similar reduction in the combined risk of death or hospitalization for cardiovascular reasons/heart failure. Patients receiving carvedilol were also significantly more likely to report improvement in symptoms. Furthermore, carvedilol was associated with significantly reduced risk of serious adverse events, including heart failure, sudden death, cardiogenic shock and ventricular tachycardia.

In-Depth [randomized controlled trial]: The COPERNICUS enrolled 2289 patients. Patients were eligible for the study if they reported symptoms of dyspnea or fatigue at minimal exertion and had a LVEF<25%. These patients were optimized medically on a diuretic and an angiotensin converting enzyme (ACE) inhibitor or angiotensin receptor II blocker (ARB) upon entry to the study. Digitalis, spironolactone, amiodarone and vasodilators were permitted but not required for eligibility. Study patients were randomized to receive either

1) carvedilol titrated to a target dose of 25mg twice per day or 2) placebo. The primary endpoint studied was all-cause mortality. Secondary endpoints were combined risk of death or hospitalization, either due to cardiovascular reason or heart failure, as well as improvement or worsening of symptoms by global patient assessment. Serious adverse events were also studied.

While the study was terminated a year early, patients were followed for a mean of 10.4 months. Results showed that risk of mortality was significantly reduced for those patients receiving carvedilol (12.8% vs. 19.7%, p = 0.00013). Carvedilol therapy was also associated with significantly reduced rates of hospitalization for heart failure (17.1% vs. 23.7%, p = 0.0001) or for any reason (32.2% vs. 38.1%, p = 0.003). These effects were consistent in the subgroup analysis, which included sex, age, location, left ventricular function, as well etiology of heart failure (i.e., ischemic vs. non-ischemic). In the global patient assessment, significantly more patients reported moderate to marked improvement in symptoms and were less likely to show moderate to marked worsening. Significantly fewer patients in the carvedilol group experienced serious adverse events, such as worsening of heart failure (p < 0.0001), sudden death (p = 0.016), cardiogenic shock (p = 0.003) and ventricular tachycardia (p = 0.019), as compared to the placebo group.

Packer M, Fowler MB, Roecker EB, Coats AJS, Katus HA, Krum H, et al. Effect of Carvedilol on the Morbidity of Patients With Severe Chronic Heart Failure Results of the Carvedilol Prospective Randomized Cumulative Survival (COPERNICUS) Study. Circulation. 2002 Oct 22;106(17):2194–9.

The ALLHAT: Thiazide diuretics as first-line antihypertensive therapy

1. There were no significant differences in the rates of fatal coronary artery disease or nonfatal myocardial infarction when comparing thiazide diuretics with angiotensin converting enzyme (ACE) inhibitors or calcium channel blockers (CCBs) for hypertension management.

Original Date of Publication: December 2002

Study Rundown: Hypertension is considered a major risk factor for cardiovascular disease and blood pressure control is an international priority. Some studies have estimated that 26.4% of the global population suffered from hypertension in 2000, and this number is expected to increase to 29.2% in 2025, affecting an estimated 1.56 billion people. While antihypertensive medication therapy has been shown to reduce the risk of adverse outcomes in hypertensive patients, there are many antihypertensive agents available and questions remained regarding the best choice for initial therapy. The earliest studies demonstrated benefits associated with using thiazides and beta-blockers (BB), though many new agents were subsequently introduced into practice, including ACE inhibitors and CCBs. The Antihypertensive and Lipid-Lowering Treatment to Prevent Heart Attack Trial (ALLHAT) focused specifically on high-risk patients - it sought to determine whether there were significant differences in rates of cardiovascular events when using different first-line antihypertensive agents, such as ACE inhibitors (i.e., lisinopril), CCBs (i.e., amlodipine), alpha-blockers (i.e., doxazosin), and thiazides (i.e., chlorthalidone). The alpha-blocker arm was terminated early, as chlorthalidone was found to be superior to doxazosin. In summary, there were no significant differences in the rates of fatal coronary artery disease (CHD) or nonfatal myocardial infarction when comparing chlorthalidone with amlodipine or lisinopril for hypertension management. Because thiazide diuretics are often cheaper than other options, it was recommended that they be considered first-line therapy for hypertension based on the findings of this study.

In-Depth [randomized controlled trial]: The study involved 33 357 participants and had a mean follow-up of 4.9 years. Patients were eligible for the study if they were ≥55 years of age and had stage 1 or 2 hypertension with ≥1 additional risk factor (i.e., previous myocardial infarction, stroke, left ventricular hypertrophy, type 2 diabetes, current cigarette smoking, low high-density lipoprotein). Exclusion criteria were a history of heart failure and/or left ventricular ejection fraction <35%. The primary outcome was fatal CHD or nonfatal myocardial infarction, while the secondary outcomes were all-cause mortality, fatal/nonfatal stroke, combined CHD, and combined cardiovascular disease.

Chlorthalidone was found to be superior to doxazosin, and the alpha-blocker arm was terminated early. In the comparison between amlodipine and chlorthalidone, there were no significant differences in the primary (RR 0.98; 95%CI 0.90-1.07) or secondary outcomes. Amlodipine, however, was associated with a significantly higher risk of heart failure, particularly hospitalized/fatal heart failure (p < 0.001). The comparison between lisinopril and chlorthalidone again demonstrated no significant differences in the primary (RR 0.99; 95%CI 0.91-1.08) or secondary outcomes; but, lisinopril use was associated with significantly elevated risk of stroke, combined cardiovascular disease, heart failure, hospitalized/treated angina, and coronary revascularization. Moreover, participants in the lisinopril group had significantly higher follow-up systolic blood pressure.

The ALLHAT Officers and Coordinators for the ALLHAT Collaborative Research Group. Major outcomes in high-risk hypertensive patients randomized to angiotensin-converting enzyme inhibitor or calcium channel blocker vs diuretic: The antihypertensive and lipid-lowering treatment to prevent heart attack trial (allhat). JAMA. 2002 Dec 18;288(23):2981–97.

The AFFIRM trial: Rate-control vs. rhythm-control in atrial fibrillation

1. Compared to rhythm-control, rate-control resulted in a lower incidence of adverse events and no significant difference in mortality in patients with atrial fibrillation.

Original Date of Publication: December 2002

Study Rundown: The Atrial Fibrillation Follow-up Investigation of Rhythm Management (AFFIRM) trial compared two common strategies for managing atrial fibrillation: rhythm-control and rate-control. Patients were anticoagulated in both approaches to address the increased risk of thromboembolic disease in atrial fibrillation. Prior to this study, both rhythm-control and rate-control were considered acceptable strategies, though rhythm-control was often the initial therapy. Rhythm-control involves the use of cardioversion and antiarrhythmic medications to maintain normal sinus rhythm, and this was thought to have benefits of lowering the stroke risk and allowing anticoagulation therapy to be discontinued. At the time of this study's publication, proponents of the rate-control method argued that rate-control medications were far less toxic than antiarrhythmics, and that there were likely no differences between the methods in terms of patient-important outcomes.

To address this conflict, the AFFIRM trial was designed to assess the differences in long-term outcomes associated with these 2 treatment approaches. Patients in the rhythm-control group could be treated with specific antiarrhythmic agents or cardioversion, as decided by their treating physician. Rate-controlled patients were managed using beta blockers (BBs), calcium channel blockers (CCBs), digoxin, or a combination of these medications. In summary, there was no significant difference between the groups in mortality or the rate of the composite secondary endpoint of death, disabling stroke, disabling anoxic encephalopathy, major bleeding, and cardiac arrest. The risk of torsade de pointes, cardiac arrest, and hospitalization, however, were significantly higher in the rhythm-control group.

In-Depth [randomized controlled trial]: A total of 4060 patients were enrolled in the trial and followed for a mean of 3.5 years. They were randomized to the rhythm-control strategy (i.e., treatment with antiarrhythmic medications) or the rate-control strategy (i.e., controlling heart rate with BBs, CCBs and digoxin). Patients were included if they were ≥65 years of age, they had atrial fibrillation that was likely to be recurrent, long-term treatment of their atrial fibrillation was warranted, and they were eligible for anticoagulation therapy. The primary endpoint was mortality. The secondary endpoint was a composite of death, disabling stroke, disabling anoxic encephalopathy, major bleeding, and cardiac arrest. There was no significant difference in mortality between the groups (HR 1.15; 95%CI 0.99-1.34). The rate of the secondary endpoint was also not significantly different between the two groups. There was a significantly higher incidence of torsade de pointes, cardiac arrest (i.e., pulseless electrical activity, bradycardia, or other rhythm), and hospitalization after baseline in the rhythm-control group compared to the rate-control group. It was also demonstrated that individuals in the rhythm-control group experienced significantly higher incidence of adverse drug events, including pulmonary events, gastrointestinal events, bradycardia, and prolongation of the QT interval (p < 0.001). There was no significant difference between the groups in the incidence of stroke.

Wyse DG, Waldo AL, DiMarco JP, Domanski MJ, Rosenberg Y, Schron EB, et al. A comparison of rate control and rhythm control in patients with atrial fibrillation. New England Journal of Medicine. 2002 Dec 5;347(23):1825–33.

The EPHESUS: Eplerenone reduces mortality in heart failure after myocardial infarction

1. Eplerenone reduced all-cause mortality in patients with heart failure and left ventricular dysfunction (LVEF ≤40%) after myocardial infarction (MI) compared with placebo.

2. Eplerenone treatment in this setting significantly reduced mortality from cardiovascular causes and hospitalizations for cardiovascular issues.

Original Date of Publication: April 2003

Study Rundown: At the time of the Eplerenone Post-Acute Myocardial Infarction Heart Failure Efficacy and Survival Study (EPHESUS), aldosterone blockade was linked to a reduced mortality in severe systolic heart failure (as demonstrated in the RALES trial) and prevented ventricular remodeling in patients after an acute MI. It was hypothesized that starting a mineralocorticoid antagonist after an acute MI would be beneficial, and the EPHESUS was designed to test this proposition. In summary, the trial demonstrated that treatment with eplerenone 3-14 days after an acute MI significantly reduced mortality and the rate of hospitalization for heart failure. It has been noted that EPHESUS started randomization several months after data from the RALES trial was published, and one criticism that has been leveled at the EPHESUS was regarding their choice of mineralocorticoid antagonist. While the rates of gynecomastia have been lower with eplerenone as compared with spironolactone, the costs of treatment with eplerenone are considerably higher. Moreover, the RALES trial had demonstrated a much larger relative risk reduction in all-cause mortality with spironolactone, thus, some have suggested that EPHESUS should have been conducted with spironolactone instead.

In-Depth [randomized controlled trial]: This multicenter, randomized controlled study was conducted at 674 centers in 37 countries. 6642 patients were recruited and randomized to treatment with either eplerenone or placebo in addition to optimal management 3-14 days after suffering an acute MI. Other inclusion criteria were LVEF ≤40% and clinical findings of heart failure (i.e., pulmonary rales, pulmonary congestion on x-ray, third heart sound). Patients with diabetes did not need clinical evidence of heart failure in order to be included because of their increased risk of cardiovascular events. Patients were excluded if they were using potassium-sparing diuretics, had a serum creatinine

>220 µmol/L, or had a serum potassium >5.0 mmol/L. There were two primary endpoints: 1) time to death from any cause and 2) time to death from cardiovascular causes or first hospitalization for a cardiovascular event.

The incidence of both primary endpoints - death from any cause (RR 0.85; 95%CI 0.75-0.96) and death from/hospitalization for cardiovascular causes (RR 0.87; 95%CI 0.79-0.95) - were significantly lower in the eplerenone group as compared to the placebo group. Patients in the eplerenone group also had a significantly lower rate of sudden cardiac death (RR 0.79; 95%CI 0.64-0.97) and significantly fewer hospitalizations for heart failure (RR 0.85; 95%CI 0.74-0.99). There were significantly more episodes of serious hyperkalemia noted in the eplerenone group compared to the placebo group (5.5% vs. 3.9%, p = 0.002). Patients receiving eplerenone also had significantly more gastrointestinal issues (19.9% vs. 17.7%, p = 0.02).

Pitt B, Remme W, Zannad F, Neaton J, Martinez F, Roniker B, et al. Eplerenone, a Selective Aldosterone Blocker, in Patients with Left Ventricular Dysfunction after Myocardial Infarction. New England Journal of Medicine. 2003 Apr 3;348(14):1309–21.

The CHARM-Preserved trial: Candesartan reduces hospitalization in heart failure with preserved ejection fraction

1. In patients with heart failure and preserved ejection fraction, candesartan was not associated with a significant reduction in the rate of cardiovascular death, but was linked to a significant reduction in the rate of hospitalization for heart failure as compared with placebo.

Original Date of Publication: September 2003

Study Rundown: A large body of evidence exists supporting various interventions to improve outcomes in heart failure with reduced left-ventricular ejection fraction (LVEF). The SOLVD and ATLAS trials demonstrated that treatment with angiotensin converting enzyme (ACE) inhibitors was linked to a significant reduction in mortality among heart failure patients with reduced LVEF. The Val-HEFT and CHARM-Alternative trials demonstrated the benefits of angiotensin-receptor blocker (ARB) therapy, while the MERIT-HF and COPERNICUS trials supported the use of beta-blockers. The RALES, EMPHASIS-HF, and EPHESUS trials provide evidence for aldosterone blockade in these patients and the MADIT-II trial found that prophylactic implantable defibrillators also reduced mortality.

At the time of the Candesartan in Heart failure: Assessment of Reduction in Mortality and morbidity (CHARM)-Preserved trial, many guidelines for heart failure management did not specifically address treating patients with preserved ejections fractions. Given that there was some evidence to support the use of ACE inhibitors in treating heart failure with preserved ejection fraction, the aim of the CHARM-Preserved trial was to explore whether angiotensin blockade using an ARB would have similar benefits. In summary, there were no significant differences between the candesartan and placebo groups in terms of the rate of cardiovascular death and hospitalization for heart failure. There was a small but significant reduction in hospitalizations for heart failure, while there was a significantly higher rate of adverse events in the candesartan group.

In-Depth [randomized controlled trial]: This trial included 3025 patients from 618 centers in 26 countries. Patients were eligible for the study if they were 18 years of age or older, had New York Heart Association (NYHA) functional class II-IV symptoms for at least 4 weeks, had a history of hospital admission for a cardiac reason, and had LVEF >40%. Eligible patients were randomized to receive either candesartan or placebo. The primary outcome was cardiovascular death or unplanned admission to hospital for the management of worsening heart failure. Secondary outcomes included several combinations of cardiovascular death, admission to hospital for heart failure, non-fatal myocardial infarction, non-fatal stroke, coronary revascularization, all-cause mortality, and new development of diabetes.

There was no significant difference between the candesartan and placebo groups in terms of the rate of the primary outcome (adjusted HR 0.86; 95%CI 0.74-1.00, p = 0.051). Specifically, there was no significant difference between the groups in terms of the rate of cardiovascular death (adjusted HR 0.95; 95%CI 0.76-1.18, p = 0.635). The rate of hospital admission for heart failure was significantly reduced in the candesartan group as compared with the placebo group (adjusted HR 0.84; 95%CI 0.70-1.00, p = 0.047). The rates of study-drug discontinuation due to adverse events or laboratory abnormalities were significantly higher in the candesartan group (17.8% vs. 13.5%, p = 0.001), with the most common causes being rising creatinine (4.8% vs. 2.4%, p = 0.0005), hypotension (2.4% vs. 1.1%, p = 0.009), and hyperkalemia (1.5% vs. 0.6%, p = 0.029), all of which were elevated in the candesartan group.

Yusuf S, Pfeffer MA, Swedberg K, Granger CB, Held P, McMurray JJV, et al. Effects of candesartan in patients with chronic heart failure and preserved left-ventricular ejection fraction: the CHARM-Preserved Trial. Lancet. 2003 Sep 6;362(9386):777–81.

The CHARM-Alternative trial: Candesartan reduces mortality in heart failure

1. Candesartan therapy significantly reduced cardiovascular death and hospital admission for chronic heart failure in patients with heart failure, reduced ventricular function, and angiotensin receptor blocker (ACE) inhibitor intolerance.

2. Candesartan was well-tolerated in patients with previous intolerance to ACE inhibitors.

Original Date of Publication: September 2003

Study Rundown: ACE inhibitors have been shown to effectively reduce morbidity and mortality in patients with symptomatic heart failure, but intolerance to ACE inhibitors occurs frequently. Angiotensin-receptor blockers (ARB) are an alternative agent that may be used to inhibit the renin-angiotensin-aldosterone system but evidence of its effectiveness in reducing long-term clinical events was limited at the time this study was conducted. The Candesartan in Heart failure: Assessment of Reduction in Mortality and morbidity (CHARM)-Alternative trial was one arm of the CHARM-Overall program assessing the effectiveness of candesartan compared to placebo in patients with symptomatic heart failure and reduced left-ventricular systolic function, who could not tolerate ACE inhibitors. Results of the study showed a significant reduction in cardiovascular death and hospital admission due to heart failure in the candesartan group. In summary, an ARB should be considered in patients with symptomatic chronic heart failure, reduced ventricular function, and an intolerance to ACE inhibitors.

In-Depth [randomized controlled trial]: This study randomized 2028 patients to receive an ARB (i.e., candesartan) or placebo and investigated the long-term clinical outcomes. The CHARM-Alternative trial included patients with symptomatic chronic heart failure and left-ventricular ejection fraction of 40% or less who had a previously documented intolerance to ACE inhibitors. The primary outcome of cardiovascular death or hospital admission for CHF occurred in 33% of patients in the candesartan group and 40% of patients in the placebo group (HR 0.77; 95%CI 0.67-0.89; p = 0.0004). This reduction in the primary outcome in the candesartan group was significant and was maintained when non-fatal myocardial infarction, non-fatal stroke and coronary revascularization were included in the composite outcome. Study drug discontinuation was similar between the treatment and placebo groups suggesting that candesartan was well-tolerated in this population of patients in spite of previously documented intolerance to ACE inhibitors.

Granger CB, McMurray JJV, Yusuf S, Held P, Michelson EL, Olofsson B, et al. Effects of candesartan in patients with chronic heart failure and reduced left-ventricular systolic function intolerant to angiotensin-converting-enzyme inhibitors: the CHARM-Alternative trial. Lancet. 2003 Sep 6;362(9386):772–6.

The PROVE IT trial: High-dose atorvastatin reduces mortality after acute coronary syndrome

1. High-dose atorvastatin was associated with a 16% reduction in death or major cardiovascular events compared to standard pravastatin therapy following an acute coronary syndrome (ACS).

2. The protective effect of intensive lipid-lowering was evident in the first 30 days of therapy and was consistent across pre-specified subgroups.

Original Date of Publication: April 2004

Study Rundown: The REVERSAL trial first suggested that intensive lipid-lowering therapy may be superior to standard therapy; however, this trial was not designed to assess clinical outcomes. The Pravastatin or Atorvastatin Evaluation and Infection Therapy (PROVE IT) trial pursued this implication by comparing the standard pravastatin dose to high-dose atorvastatin and measured a composite end point of death from all-causes and major cardiovascular events. The magnitude of the improvement with intensive lipid-lowering over standard therapy was comparable to the benefit seen when comparing statins to placebo. The effect was apparent early on after therapy initiation and was consistent over the mean 2-year follow up period. It is uncertain to what extent the difference in statins may have contributed to the difference in outcomes. Future studies may explore the effect of varying doses of a single statin. The results of the PROVE IT trial challenged guidelines at the time by suggesting that target low-density lipoprotein (LDL) levels should be lower in patients following an ACS. In summary, intensive lipid-lowering with high-dose atorvastatin may further reduce the risk of mortality or major cardiovascular events compared to a standard dose of pravastatin in patients with recent ACS.

In-Depth [randomized controlled trial]: The PROVE IT trial randomly assigned 4162 patients who had been hospitalized within the previous 10 days for an ACS to receive a standard regimen of 40 mg pravastatin daily or an intensive regimen of 80 mg atorvastatin daily. The primary outcome measured was the time to death from any cause, myocardial infarction, unstable angina requiring hospitalization, revascularization or stroke. During follow-up, the LDL cholesterol levels reached were significantly lower in the atorvastatin group, with values of 2.46 mmol/L in the pravastatin group and 1.60 mmol/L in the atorvastatin group (p < 0.001). There was a 16% reduction in the hazard ratio for the primary outcome in the atorvastatin group compared to the pravastatin group (95%CI 5-26%; p = 0.005). No significant difference was detected in the rate of discontinuation because of adverse events or patient preference; however, a significantly greater proportion of patients in the atorvastatin group had elevated alanine aminotransferase levels.

Cannon CP, Braunwald E, McCabe CH, Rader DJ, Rouleau JL, Belder R, et al. Intensive versus Moderate Lipid Lowering with Statins after Acute Coronary Syndromes. New England Journal of Medicine. 2004 Apr 8;350(15):1495–504.

The CLARITY trial: Clopidogrel reduces arterial reocclusion after myocardial infarction

1. The early addition of clopidogrel to standard therapy reduced the incidence of infarct-related arterial reocclusion within 30 days following myocardial infarction (MI).

2. The addition of early clopidogrel was associated with improved outcomes of coronary angiography and a decreased need for early/emergent angiography during the event.

3. There were no differences in major bleeding, minor bleeding, or intracranial hemorrhage incidence between the clopidogrel group and the control group.

Original Date of Publication: March 2005

Study Rundown: It is well known that platelet activation and aggregation have a significant role in the initiation and propagation of coronary artery thrombosis. As a result, antiplatelet agents are part of the standard management of acute coronary syndromes. Aspirin, which inactivates the cyclooxygenase enzyme, inhibits platelet aggregation and has been shown to help reduce the rate of reocclusion after MI. Clopidogrel is another antiplatelet agent that acts by blocking ADP receptors on platelets.

The Clopidogrel as Adjunctive Reperfusion Therapy (CLARITY-TIMI 28) trial sought to determine whether early treatment with clopidogrel in addition to standard aspirin and fibrinolytic therapy would produce better outcomes than standard therapy alone in the treatment of ST-elevation MI (STEMI). The study showed that early treatment with clopidogrel resulted in a significant improvement in outcomes. The early clopidogrel group had a significantly lower incidence of persistent arterial occlusion or reocclusion, as well as improved outcomes on all angiography measures. There was also a significant decrease in the need for early or emergent angiography in the clopidogrel group and a significant decrease in the incidence of recurrent MI within 30 days of the first event. No significant difference in 30-day mortality from cardiovascular events was shown, however this study was not powered to assess the impact of intervention on mortality. In summary, this study showed that early treatment with clopidogrel in addition to standard management of STEMI significantly improved patient outcomes in regards to coronary arterial patency. This study has had meaningful impact on STEMI management and has impacted ACCF and AHA guidelines.

In-Depth [randomized controlled trial]: This large, multicenter, double-blinded, randomized, placebo-controlled trial involved enrollment of 3491 patients with an acute STEMI at 319 sites to receive early clopidogrel or placebo along with standard therapy, including aspirin and fibrinolytic agents. Patients between the age of 18-75 years who presented with ST elevation and an episode of chest pain that lasted >20 minutes within 12 hours of randomization were eligible. Patients who had received clopidogrel in the past 7 days, had a history of coronary artery bypass grafting, presented with cardiogenic shock, or who were scheduled to receive coronary angiography within 48 hours regardless of clinical indication were excluded. Eligible patients received a 300 mg loading dose of clopidogrel followed by 75 mg daily maintenance dose, which was continued to the day of angiography. If a patient did not undergo angiography, it was continued until day 8 or discharge from hospital, whichever was sooner. Patients were followed up to 30 days after randomization. The primary outcome was evidence of infarct-related arterial occlusion on angiography or death/recurrent MI before angiography, day 8 of hospitalization, or hospital discharge. The study demonstrated that early treatment with clopidogrel resulted in a 6.7% absolute reduction of the primary end point (21.7% vs. 15%; 95%CI 24-47%, $p < 0.001$). There was no significant difference in the rate of death from any cardiovascular cause between the groups. The study also demonstrated no significant difference in incidence of major or minor bleeding or intracranial hemorrhage between the 2 groups ($p = 0.64$, $p = 0.17$, and $p = 0.38$, respectively).

Sabatine MS, Cannon CP, Gibson CM, López-Sendón JL, Montalescot G, Theroux P, et al. Addition of Clopidogrel to Aspirin and Fibrinolytic Therapy for Myocardial Infarction with ST-Segment Elevation. New England Journal of Medicine. 2005 Mar 24;352(12):1179–89.

The COMMIT: Metoprolol and clopidogrel in patients with acute myocardial infarction

1. Adding early metoprolol did not further decrease the risk of death after myocardial infarction (MI) compared to conventional fibrinolytic therapy alone.

2. Use of early metoprolol decreased the risk of reinfarction and ventricular fibrillation, but increased the risk of cardiogenic shock.

3. Adding clopidogrel to aspirin decreased the combined risk of death, reinfarction, or stroke post-MI, without significantly increasing the risk of major bleeding.

Original Date of Publication: November 2005

Study Rundown: The Clopidogrel and Metoprolol in Myocardial Infarction Trial (COMMIT) featured a 2x2 factorial design, in which patients with acute myocardial infarction were treated with 1) metoprolol or placebo and 2) aspirin plus clopidogrel or aspirin plus placebo. The study assessed the effect of adding early metoprolol (intravenous then oral) to conventional fibrinolytic therapy in patients with a recent MI. This aim was motivated by the fact that previous studies had only evaluated early beta-blockade before fibrinolytic therapy had become routine. Moreover, it was thought that beta-blockers would decrease the risk of cardiac rupture associated with fibrinolytic therapy alone. COMMIT showed that the addition of metoprolol did not result in significantly fewer deaths compared to fibrinolytic therapy alone. Use of metoprolol did decrease the rate of reinfarction and ventricular fibrillation, but this was counterbalanced by an increase in cardiogenic shock, particular in patients with moderate heart failure (i.e., Killip class II or III).

The study assessed also the effect of adding clopidogrel to aspirin in the treatment of patients with a recent MI. Aspirin, which acts by blocking the thromboxane pathway of platelet aggregation, had been previously shown to reduce mortality post-MI, and it was thought that clopidogrel, which inhibits platelet aggregation via an adenosine 5'-diphosphate-mediated pathway, might reduce mortality even further. Findings from COMMIT showed that the addition of clopidogrel resulted in a significant post-MI reduction in death, reinfarction, and stroke in patients, without a significant risk of bleeding regardless of the patient's age. A limitation of the study was the possibility that instances of rapid reduction in blood pressure might have correctly indicated to physicians that metoprolol was administered rather than placebo. In summary, the COMMIT trial suggested that beta-blocker therapy may be more appropriately started only after a patient has been stabilized hemodynamically post-MI, with the aim of preventing reinfarction and fibrillation. In contrast, adding clopidogrel to aspirin should be considered for all patients with a suspected acute MI, especially given clopidogrel's modest cost and minimal required monitoring.

In-Depth [randomized controlled trial]: The COMMIT was a large, randomized, placebo-controlled trial with a 2x2 factorial design (metoprolol vs. placebo and clopidogrel plus aspirin vs. aspirin alone) involving 45 852 patients. On-site audits were performed at hospitals, and study drug packs were systematically checked to ensure that correct contents were packaged. Patients who presented with ST elevation, ST depression, or left-bundle branch block within 24 hours of a suspected acute MI were eligible. Patients at risk of adverse effects from beta blockade (e.g., low heart rate, hypotension, cardiogenic shock) or from antiplatelet therapy (e.g., bleeding, allergic reaction) were excluded. Eligible patients received metoprolol or placebo doses for intravenous infusion, followed by a 4-week supply of 1) oral metoprolol or placebo and 2) clopidogrel plus aspirin or placebo plus aspirin. The co-primary outcomes for the assessment of both clopidogrel and metoprolol were 1) the composite of death, reinfarction, cardiac arrest (metoprolol only), and stroke (clopidogrel only), and 2) death from any cause. There was no difference in death from any cause with the use of metoprolol (OR 0.99; 95%CI 0.92-1.05). Metoprolol use was associated with a significantly decreased risk of reinfarction (OR 0.82; 95%CI 0.72-0.92) and ventricular fibrillation (OR 0.83; 95%CI 0.75-0.93), but increased risk of cardiogenic shock (OR 1.30; 95%CI 1.19-1.41). Clopidogrel use resulted in a reduction in death, reinfarction, or stroke (OR 0.91; 95%CI 0.86-0.97), without a significantly increased risk of major bleeding regardless of age.

Chen ZM, Pan HC, Chen YP, Peto R, Collins R, Jiang LX, et al. Early intravenous then oral metoprolol in 45,852 patients with acute myocardial infarction: randomised placebo-controlled trial. Lancet. 2005 Nov 5;366(9497):1622–32.

Chen ZM, Jiang LX, Chen YP, Xie JX, Pan HC, Peto R, et al. Addition of clopidogrel to aspirin in 45,852 patients with acute myocardial infarction: randomised placebo-controlled trial. Lancet. 2005 Nov 5;366(9497):1607–21.

The COURAGE trial: Percutaneous coronary intervention does not improve mortality in stable coronary artery disease

1. The addition of percutaneous cutaneous intervention (PCI) to optimal medical therapy for patients with stable coronary artery disease did not improve mortality or cardiovascular outcomes.

Original Date of Publication: April 2007

Study Rundown: The Clinical Outcomes Utilizing Revascularization and Aggressive Drug Evaluation (COURAGE) trial was the first to provide evidence that in patients with stable coronary artery disease, the addition of PCI to optimal medical therapy does not provide any mortality benefit or improve cardiovascular outcomes. A subsequent report from the COURAGE investigators demonstrated that patients who received PCI were free of angina and had improvements in various quality of life parameters at 3 months after the intervention, though this difference was not sustained at 36 months. Optimization of medical therapy alone without PCI is sufficient for initial treatment of patients with stable coronary artery disease. The addition of PCI to optimal medical therapy likely does not improve mortality or cardiovascular outcomes as evidenced by the COURAGE trial.

In-Depth [randomized controlled trial]: A total of 2287 patients with stable coronary artery disease, objective evidence of myocardial ischemia, and significant disease in at least 1 major coronary artery were enrolled in this study. Patients were randomized to 2 groups: 1) optimal medical therapy alone or 2) optimal medical therapy with PCI. All patients were optimized medically on an angiotensin converting enzyme (ACE) inhibitor or angiotensin receptor blocker (ARB), antiplatelet therapy (acetylsalicylic acid or clopidogrel), as well as a combination of beta-blockers, calcium channel blockers and nitrates. All patients also received aggressive lipid optimizing therapy. The primary outcome studied was a composite of death from any cause and non-fatal myocardial infarction. The median follow-up period was 4.6 years. In patients undergoing PCI, 89% achieved clinical success. There was no significant difference in the primary outcome between the groups (HR 1.05; 95%CI 0.87-1.27; p = 0.62). Furthermore, rates of hospitalization for acute coronary syndrome were not significantly different between the groups (HR 1.07; 95%CI 0.84-1.37; p =

0.56). The need for subsequent revascularization procedures (PCI or coronary artery bypass graft) was, however, significantly higher in the medical therapy group as compared to the PCI group (32.6% vs. 21.1%, p < 0.001).

Boden WE, O'Rourke RA, Teo KK, Hartigan PM, Maron DJ, Kostuk WJ, et al. Optimal Medical Therapy with or without PCI for Stable Coronary Disease. New England Journal of Medicine. 2007 Apr 12;356(15):1503–16.

The TRITON-TIMI 38 trial: Prasugrel reduces recurrent infarction after acute coronary syndrome

1. Prasugrel was significantly more effective than clopidogrel in reducing the incidence of recurrent myocardial infarction (MI) in patients presenting with acute coronary syndrome (ACS), though there was no difference in mortality between the groups tested.

2. Patients treated with prasugrel had a significantly higher incidence of fatal major bleeding compared to clopidogrel.

Original Date of Publication: November 2007

Study Rundown: Current ACS management guidelines call for treatment with dual antiplatelet therapy, usually consisting of aspirin and clopidogrel, a thienopyridine. However, it is known that there is much interpatient variability in the metabolism of clopidogrel, which may lead to variable efficacy of the drug in different patients. Prasugrel, a newer thienopyridine, was known to be more rapid and less variable in its platelet-binding activity. This trial sought to determine whether treatment with prasugrel and aspirin produced better outcomes than the standard treatment with clopidogrel and aspirin in the management of patients with ACS. The study demonstrated that prasugrel was significantly more effective than clopidogrel at reducing the incidence of recurrent myocardial infarctions.

Notably, the study did not show a significant mortality benefit with using prasugrel. Moreover, researchers found that prasugrel use was linked to significantly higher incidence of major bleeding, both related to instrumentation and also spontaneous bleeding. While analysis of net clinical benefit still showed preference for prasugrel, stratification of groups revealed that prasugrel showed no clinical net benefit for patients who had a prior history of a cerebral vascular accident or transient ischemic attack, are above 75 years of age, or are below 60 kg for weight. In summary, this study showed that prasugrel was more effective than clopidogrel in preventing recurrent myocardial infarctions and subsequent deaths, but also increased the risk of major bleeding. Overall, the net clinical benefit of prasugrel provides evidence for its use in ACS management, but it must be used with caution. Patients should be counseled of the increased risk of bleeding with this drug over clopidogrel.

In-Depth [randomized controlled trial]: This trial was a large, multicenter, double-blinded, randomized controlled trial that enrolled 13 608 patients with acute coronary syndrome at 707 sites to receive either prasugrel or clopidogrel along with aspirin as part of the dual antiplatelet regimen for ACS management. Patients who presented with symptoms lasting greater than 10 minutes within 72 hours of enrollment, had a TIMI score greater than 3, had >1 mm ST segment change, or had an increased blood level of biomarker of cardiac necrosis were eligible. Patients who had received any thienopyridine in the past 5 days, had an increased risk of bleeding, or another contraindication to antiplatelet therapy were excluded. Eligible patients received a loading dose of a single antiplatelet agent and were continued on daily maintenance dosing along with a low-dose aspirin (75 to 162 mg daily). Patients were followed for 6-15 months, with study visits performed at hospital discharge, 30 days, 90 days, and every 3 months after that. The primary outcome was a composite of the rate of death related to cardiovascular events, non-fatal myocardial infarction, or non-fatal stroke in the follow-up period.

The study demonstrated that treatment with prasugrel was associated with significantly reduced incidence of the primary outcome when compared to clopidogrel (HR 0.81; 95%CI 0.73-0.90). A significant reduction in the primary endpoint was seen in the prasugrel group at 3 days and the trend persisted throughout the follow-up period. The difference between the groups was attributed to a significant decrease in the rate of recurrent myocardial infarctions (HR 0.76; 95%CI 0.67-0.85) in the prasugrel group compared to the clopidogrel group. There was no significant difference between the groups in terms of mortality, though prasugrel use was linked with significantly lower rates of urgent target-vessel revascularization (HR 0.66; 95%CI 0.54-0.81) and stent thrombosis (HR 0.48; 95%CI 0.36-0.64). The prasugrel group had a significantly higher incidence of fatal major bleeding compared to clopidogrel group (0.4% vs. 0.1%, p = 0.002).

Wiviott SD, Braunwald E, McCabe CH, Montalescot G, Ruzyllo W, Gottlieb S, et al. Prasugrel versus Clopidogrel in Patients with Acute Coronary Syndromes. New England Journal of Medicine. 2007 Nov 15;357(20):2001–15.

The ONTARGET: Telmisartan non-inferior to ramipril in improving cardiovascular outcomes in high-risk populations

1. The angiotensin receptor blocker (ARB) telmisartan was non-inferior to the angiotensin converting enzyme (ACE) inhibitor ramipril in improving cardiovascular outcomes in high-risk populations.

2. Telmisartan was associated with significantly less angioedema and cough compared to ramipril.

3. The combination of telmisartan and ramipril in high-risk populations did not offer additional benefit compared to ramipril alone, and was associated with increased risk of complications.

Original Date of Publication: April 2008

Study Rundown: ARBs reduce the activation of the renin-angiotensin-aldosterone system by blocking the angiotensin-II (ANG-II) receptor. At the time of their introduction, there was uncertainty as to whether ARBs were a viable alternative to ACE inhibitors. It was thought that ARBs would be associated with fewer adverse effects, as ARBs, unlike ACE inhibitors, do not reduce bradykinin degradation (which is associated with cough and angioedema). One of the indications for ACE inhibitors is to prevent cardiac events in high-risk patients without systolic heart failure, as shown in the Heart Outcomes Prevention Evaluation (HOPE) trial. The purpose of the Ongoing Telmisartan Alone and in Combination with Ramipril Global Endpoint Trial (ONTARGET) was to determine whether the ARB, telmisartan, was a non-inferior alternative to ramipril in improving cardiac outcomes (a composite of death from cardiovascular causes, myocardial infarction, stroke, or hospitalization for heart failure) in a similar patient population. The study also investigated whether combination therapy with both telmisartan and ramipril offered additional benefit to ramipril alone.

This study demonstrated that telmisartan was a non-inferior alternative to ramipril in reducing cardiac outcomes in high-risk patients, and was associated with a significantly lower risk of cough and angioedema. Combination therapy with both drugs, however, did not appear to provide additional benefit as compared to ramipril alone and was associated with increased adverse effects including renal failure. For improving cardiac outcomes, an ARB can be considered as an alternative for high-risk patients who are not able to tolerate ACE inhibitor therapy. Combination therapy with an ARB and an ACE inhibitor should be avoided.

In-Depth [randomized controlled trial]: This trial enrolled 25 620 patients from 40 countries. Patients were eligible for inclusion if they were considered high-risk for adverse cardiac outcomes, that is if they had coronary, peripheral, or cerebrovascular disease, or diabetes mellitus with end-organ damage. Patients underwent double-blind randomization to 1 of 3 groups receiving 1) 80 mg telmisartan daily, 2) 5 mg ramipril, or 3) a combination of both drugs. The primary outcome was a composite of death from cardiovascular causes, myocardial infarction, stroke, or hospitalization for heart failure. The main secondary outcome was a composite of death from cardiovascular causes, myocardial infarction, or stroke, which was the primary outcome in the HOPE trial.

With regards to the primary outcome, telmisartan was found to be non-inferior to ramipril (p = 0.004) and also non-superior (RR 1.01; 95%CI 0.94-1.09). The rate of the main secondary outcome was also similar between the groups (RR 0.99; 95%CI 0.91-1.07; p = 0.001 for non-inferiority). Patients receiving telmisartan were significantly less likely to develop cough and angioedema than those receiving ramipril (RR 0.26; p < 0.001). The combination of the drugs, however, was non-superior to ramipril alone (RR 0.99; 95%CI 0.92-1.07). Patients receiving both drugs were more likely to develop hypotensive symptoms (RR 2.75; p < 0.001), syncope (RR 1.95; p = 0.03), diarrhea (RR 3.28; p < 0.001) and renal impairment (RR 1.58; p < 0.001) than those receiving ramipril alone.

The ONTARGET Investigators. Telmisartan, Ramipril, or Both in Patients at High Risk for Vascular Events. New England Journal of Medicine. 2008 Apr 10;358(15):1547–59.

The ACCOMPLISH trial: Benazepril plus amlodipine reduces cardiovascular events

1. Benazepril plus amlodipine offered the same effect at reducing blood pressure in hypertensive patients as benazepril plus hydrochlorothiazide (HCTZ).

2. Benazepril plus amlodipine was more effective than benazepril plus HCTZ at reducing cardiovascular events in hypertensive patients at risk for such events.

Original Date of Publication: December 2008

Study Rundown: The Avoiding Cardiovascular events through Combination therapy in Patients Living with Systolic Hypertension (ACCOMPLISH) trial sought to compare a thiazide with a calcium channel blocker (CCB) as a combination therapy with an angiotensin converting enzyme (ACE) inhibitor in reducing cardiovascular events in patients with hypertension. Patients with hypertension and cardiovascular risk factors were randomized to treatment with benazepril plus amlodipine or benazepril plus HCTZ. In summary, patients in the benazepril-amlodipine group experienced significantly lower rates of the primary outcome compared to those in the benazepril-HCTZ group. This was due to a significant reduction in the rates of fatal/nonfatal myocardial infarction, while there was no significant difference in the rate of death from cardiovascular causes. This study demonstrated that adding a CCB to an ACE inhibitor reduces the risk of myocardial infarction when compared to adding a thiazide diuretic for blood pressure control in hypertensive patients. It is important to note that a pharmaceutical company was significantly involved in the execution of the study, from coordination to data analysis. Moreover, the study was stopped early by the executive committee, as preliminary results met premature termination conditions.

In-Depth [randomized controlled trial]: A total of 11 506 patients from 548 centers in the United States, Sweden, Norway, Denmark, and Finland were randomized to receive either 1) benazepril plus amlodipine or 2) benazepril plus HCTZ. Patients were started on therapy with either benazepril 20 mg and amlodipine 5 mg daily or benazepril 20 mg and HCTZ 12.5 mg daily. Patients were eligible if they had hypertension, a history of coronary events/myocardial infarction/revascularization/stroke, impaired renal function, peripheral artery disease, left ventricular hypertrophy, or diabetes mellitus. Medication doses were adjusted in the first 3 months to maintain a blood pressure ≤140/90, or ≤130/80 in patients with diabetes and kidney disease. Patients were followed every 6 months, and dose adjustments were performed during these visits. The primary endpoint was a composite of cardiovascular events or death from cardiovascular causes. Of note, the study was funded by a pharmaceutical company, which was also involved in oversecing coordination, data gathering, and data analysis.

Mean blood pressures were 131.6/73.3 mmHg in the benazepril-amlodipine group and 132.5/74.4 mmHg in the benazepril-hydrochlorothiazide group. The mean difference in blood pressure was 0.9 mm Hg systolic and 1.1 mm Hg diastolic (p < 0.001). The trial was terminated early by the executive committee. Patients in the benazepril-amlodipine group experienced a significantly lower rate of the primary endpoint as compared with patients in the benazepril-HCTZ group (HR 0.80; 95%CI 0.72-0.90), with an absolute risk reduction of 2.2%. This difference was attributed to significantly lower rates of fatal and nonfatal myocardial infarction in the benazepril-amlodipine group (HR 0.78; 95%CI 0.62-0.99), while there was no significant difference between the 2 groups in death from cardiovascular causes.

Jamerson K, Weber MA, Bakris GL, Dahlöf B, Pitt B, Shi V, et al. Benazepril plus Amlodipine or Hydrochlorothiazide for Hypertension in High-Risk Patients. New England Journal of Medicine. 2008 Dec 4;359(23):2417–28.

The SYNTAX trial: Coronary bypass superior to percutaneous coronary intervention for triple-vessel or left main artery disease

1. In severe coronary artery disease, coronary artery bypass graft (CABG) was superior to percutaneous coronary intervention (PCI) in reducing the need for repeat vascularization.

2. This study suggested CABG should remain the standard of care for severe coronary artery disease, despite being associated with a higher risk of stroke.

Original Date of Publication: March 2009

Study Rundown: The Synergy between Percutaneous Coronary Intervention with Taxus and Cardiac Surgery (SYNTAX) trial was the first large, multicenter, randomized controlled trial comparing CABG to PCI in severe coronary artery disease. This non-inferiority trial demonstrated that CABG was superior to PCI in preventing a composite measure of death, and this was driven by a decrease in the need for repeat revascularization. CABG, however, was associated with a significantly higher rate of stroke compared to PCI. Strengths of this study included the fact that it was conducted at 85 centers across North America and Europe and that it assessed all-comers with severe coronary artery disease. Criticisms of the study included the limited follow-up of 12 months and that most study participants were male. Thus, in patients with severe coronary artery disease, the SYNTAX trial suggests that CABG remain the standard of care, given reduced rate of the primary endpoint at the 12-month mark.

In-Depth [randomized controlled trial]: The SYNTAX trial, published in 2009 in NEJM, sought to determine the optimal mode of revascularization, CABG or PCI for patients with severe coronary artery disease; that is, previously untreated triple-vessel or left main artery disease. In this non-inferiority trial, the primary endpoint was a composite of death from any cause, stroke, myocardial infarction, or repeat revascularization in the 12-month period after randomization. A total of 3075 patients were included in the trial. Of these patients, 1800 were randomized to either CABG or PCI. For the other 1275, there was only 1 suitable treatment option, and they were enrolled in registries for either CABG or PCI. The majority of patients studied were male (78%).

There were no significant differences between the groups in terms of preprocedural rates of major adverse cardiac or cerebrovascular events. At 12 months, there was a significantly lower rate of the primary endpoint in the CABG group compared to PCI (12.4% vs. 17.8%, p = 0.002), which was driven by a significant reduction in the need for repeat revascularization (5.9% vs. 13.5%, p < 0.001). Notably, when compared to PCI, there was a significantly higher rate of stroke in the CABG group.

Serruys PW, Morice M-C, Kappetein AP, Colombo A, Holmes DR, Mack MJ, et al. Percutaneous Coronary Intervention versus Coronary-Artery Bypass Grafting for Severe Coronary Artery Disease. New England Journal of Medicine. 2009 Mar 5;360(10):961–72.

The ACTIVE trial: Dual antiplatelet therapy in atrial fibrillation

1. In patients with atrial fibrillation who require anticoagulation but cannot tolerate warfarin, dual anti-platelet therapy may be a potential alternative for stroke prophylaxis.

2. Clopidogrel, in addition to daily aspirin, was associated with a significantly reduced incidence of stroke, but increased incidence of major bleeding in patients with atrial fibrillation when compared to treatment with aspirin alone.

Original Date of Publication: May 2009

Study Rundown: Atrial fibrillation is a common arrhythmia characterized by uncoordinated contractions of the atria, thereby resulting in blood stasis and increased risk of thromboembolic disease. The CHADS2 score is a commonly used score to estimate a patient's annualized risk of stroke by assessing age and comorbidities. Stroke prophylaxis with antiplatelets or anticoagulants is generally recommended with a CHADS2 score of 1 or more. While vitamin K antagonists, like warfarin, remain the most commonly used anticoagulants for stroke prophylaxis in atrial fibrillation, they are not suitable for many patients due to drug interactions, elevated risk of intracranial bleeds, and monitoring requirements, amongst other reasons. Originally published in 2009, the purpose of the Atrial Fibrillation Clopidogrel Trial with Irbesartan for Prevention of Vascular Events (ACTIVE) trial was to explore whether adding clopidogrel to aspirin for stroke prophylaxis would be more effective than aspirin alone, in patients who were considered unsuitable for warfarin. In summary, the trial found that the addition of clopidogrel significantly reduced the risk of stroke, but also significantly increased the risk of major bleeding.

In-Depth [randomized controlled trial]: The study involved 7554 participants from 580 centers in 33 countries. Patients were eligible for the trial if they had atrial fibrillation at enrolment or ≥2 episodes of intermittent atrial fibrillation in the past 6 months, and at least 1 risk factor for stroke (e.g., ≥75 years, hypertension, previous stroke, left ventricular ejection fraction <45%). Patients were excluded if they required a vitamin K antagonist or clopidogrel, or if they had risk factors for hemorrhage (e.g., peptic ulcer disease in past 6 months, previous intracerebral hemorrhage, significant thrombocytopenia, alcohol abuse). Participants were randomly assigned to receive either clopidogrel 75 mg daily or a matching placebo. All participants were also prescribed 75-100 mg of aspirin daily. Follow-up occurred over a median of 3.6 years. The primary outcome was a composite measure comprised of strokes, myocardial infarctions, non-central nervous system systemic embolism, or death from vascular causes. Patients in the clopidogrel group experienced significantly lower risk of the primary outcome compared to patients taking aspirin alone (RR 0.89; 95%CI 0.81-0.98). This difference was driven by a significant reduction in the risk of stroke (RR 0.72; 95%CI 0.62-0.83). Compared to those receiving aspirin alone, the rates of major bleeding were significantly higher in the group receiving clopidogrel (RR 1.57; 95%CI 1.29-1.92), occurring most commonly in the gastrointestinal tract.

ACTIVE Investigators, Connolly SJ, Pogue J, Hart RG, Hohnloser SH, Pfeffer M, et al. Effect of clopidogrel added to aspirin in patients with atrial fibrillation. New England Journal of Medicine. 2009 May 14;360(20):2066–78.

The RE-LY trial: Dabigatran non-inferior to warfarin for stroke prevention in atrial fibrillation

1. High-dose dabigatran was superior to warfarin in the prevention of strokes in patients with atrial fibrillation, while low-dose dabigatran was non-inferior to warfarin in preventing strokes in this population.

2. There was lower risk of major hemorrhage with low-dose dabigatran compared to warfarin, while there was similar rate of major hemorrhage with high-dose dabigatran as compared to warfarin.

Original Date of Publication: September 2009

Study Rundown: Anticoagulation with warfarin, a vitamin K antagonist, has long been the standard of care for preventing thromboembolic strokes in high-risk patients with atrial fibrillation. Warfarin, however, is limited by the need for frequent monitoring due to its narrow therapeutic window, as well as its variable pharmacokinetics and drug interactions. Furthermore, its use is associated with a significant risk of major bleeding. Dabigatran, a direct thrombin inhibitor, is a newer oral anticoagulant introduced within the last decade as a possible alternative to warfarin. There is evidence for its use in venous thromboembolism (VTE) prophylaxis after total knee or hip arthroplasty, as well as in the treatment of acute VTE. At the time of this study, no evidence, existed for the use of dabigatran in the context of atrial fibrillation in the prevention of stroke. The Randomized Evaluation of Long-Term Anticoagulation Therapy (RE-LY) trial compared low- (110 mg PO BID) and high-dose (150 mg PO BID) dabigatran with dose-adjusted warfarin in preventing stroke in at risk patients with atrial fibrillation.

Dabigatran was found to be non-inferior to warfarin in the prevention of stroke in at-risk patients with atrial fibrillation, and was associated with an overall lower risk of major bleeding and intracranial hemorrhage. For those at-risk patients requiring anticoagulation for the prevention of stroke in the context of atrial fibrillation, dabigatran could be considered as an alternative to warfarin in those patients with a creatinine clearance >30 mL/min, as dabigatran is renally cleared. A major criticism of the RE-LY trial was the high risk of bias created by the unblinded administration of warfarin. Moreover, it has been noted that the incidence of intracranial hemorrhage with warfarin observed in this study was much higher than previously reported rates and reasons for this are unclear.

In-Depth [randomized controlled trial]: This large, randomized, double-blinded, controlled trial included 18 113 patients from 951 clinical centers in 44 countries. Patients were randomized to 3 groups: 1) dose-adjusted warfarin titrated to INR of 2.0-3.0, 2) low-dose dabigatran (110 mg PO twice per day), or 3) high-dose dabigatran (150 mg PO twice per day). Patients were eligible for the trial if they had atrial fibrillation documented on electrocardiogram and at least 1 high-risk feature (e.g., previous stroke or transient ischemic attack, a left ventricular ejection fraction <40%, New York Heart Association (NYHA) class II or higher symptoms, age >75 years or between 65-74 years with diabetes mellitus/hypertension/coronary artery disease). Notably, dabigatran administration was blinded, while warfarin administration was unblinded. The primary outcome studied was stroke or systemic embolism. The primary safety outcome was major hemorrhage.

The trial lasted a total of 2 years. The rate of stroke or systemic embolism was significantly lower in patients that received high-dose dabigatran as compared to warfarin (RR 0.66; 95%CI 0.53-0.82), and there was no significant difference in major bleeding between these 2 groups (p = 0.31). Furthermore, low-dose dabigatran was non-inferior to warfarin in preventing strokes (RR 0.91; 95%CI 0.74-1.11), but it was associated with a significant reduction in risk of major bleeding (RR 0.80; 95%CI 0.69-0.93). Intracranial hemorrhage was significantly less common in both dabigatran groups compared to warfarin (p < 0.001). Rate of major gastrointestinal bleeding was significantly higher for patients receiving high-dose dabigatran as compared to the warfarin group (p < 0.001). There was no significant difference in mortality between all groups.

Connolly SJ, Ezekowitz MD, Yusuf S, Eikelboom J, Oldgren J, Parekh A, et al. Dabigatran versus Warfarin in Patients with Atrial Fibrillation. New England Journal of Medicine. 2009 Sep 17;361(12):1139–51.

The PLATO trial: Ticagrelor vs. clopidogrel for acute coronary syndrome

1. Treatment with ticagrelor significantly reduced mortality among patients with acute coronary syndrome (ACS) when compared to clopidogrel.

2. Ticagrelor treatment did not significantly increase the incidence of major bleeding.

Original Date of Publication: September 2009

Study Rundown: Clopidogrel is a commonly used medication in the management of ACS. A previous study comparing prasugrel, another oral antiplatelet agent, with clopidogrel demonstrated a significant reduction in the risk of coronary thrombotic events, but no improvement in mortality. The Platelet Inhibition and Patient Outcomes (PLATO) trial compared the use of ticagrelor, a newer and more potent oral platelet inhibitor, with clopidogrel in treating patients with ACS. In summary, patients treated with ticagrelor experienced significantly lower rates of death from vascular causes, myocardial infarction, or stroke at 12 months when compared to patients on clopidogrel. This was driven by both significant reductions in the rate of death from vascular causes and myocardial infarction. Moreover, there was no significant difference between the 2 groups in the rate of major bleeding.

In-Depth [randomized controlled trial]: This study was a multicenter trial, which randomized patients to treatment with clopidogrel or ticagrelor in addition to aspirin after ACS. Patients were eligible for the study if they were hospitalized for ACS with or without ST-segment elevation, with symptom onset in the previous 24 hours. Patients were excluded if they had contraindications to clopidogrel, they received fibrinolytic therapy in the 24 hours prior to randomization, they needed oral anticoagulation, they had an increased risk of bradycardia, or they were being treated with a strong cytochrome P-450 3A inhibitor or inducer. The primary endpoint was a composite of death from vascular causes, myocardial infarction, or stroke. Major life-threatening bleeding was defined as fatal bleeding, intracranial bleeding, intrapericardial bleeding with cardiac tamponade, shock/hypotension as a result of bleeding, hemoglobin decrease ≥ 5.0 g/dL, or need for transfusion of ≥ 4 units of packed red blood cells.

A total of 18 624 patients were recruited from 862 centers in 43 countries. At 12 months, the primary endpoint occurred significantly less in the ticagrelor group as compared with the clopidogrel group (HR 0.84; 95%CI 0.77-0.92). This difference was driven by significant reductions in rates of myocardial infarction (HR 0.84; 95%CI 0.75-0.95) and death from vascular causes (HR 0.79; 95%CI 0.69-0.91) in the ticagrelor group. The rates of major bleeding were not significantly different between the 2 groups (HR 1.04; 95%CI 0.95-1.13). Notably, the rate of fatal intracranial bleeding was significantly higher in the ticagrelor group compared to the clopidogrel group (p = 0.02).

Wallentin L, Becker RC, Budaj A, Cannon CP, Emanuelsson H, Held C, et al. Ticagrelor versus Clopidogrel in Patients with Acute Coronary Syndromes. New England Journal of Medicine. 2009 Sep 10;361(11):1045–57.

The RACE-II trial: Lenient vs. strict rate-control in atrial fibrillation

1. Lenient rate-control was found to be non-inferior to strict rate-control in managing patients with atrial fibrillation.

2. Compared to strict rate-control, lenient rate-control was achieved with lower doses of medication and fewer medications.

Original Date of Publication: April 2010

Study Rundown: Atrial fibrillation is the most prevalent sustained cardiac arrhythmia. It is a condition characterized by tachycardia and irregular heart rate, which often results due to disorganized electrical signaling in the atria. The condition is associated with an increased risk of stroke, and anticoagulation is an important management consideration. Previously, rate-control and rhythm-control were both considered acceptable options for management. The AFFIRM and RACE trials demonstrated, however, that rate-control was not inferior and was also associated with fewer adverse events compared to rhythm-control. As a result, rate-control is now often the first-line approach for treating atrial fibrillation, along with appropriate anticoagulation. While certain guidelines suggested stricter rate-control would reduce symptoms, reduce the incidence of heart failure, and improve survival, these recommendations were not evidence-based. The risk of certain adverse events was higher in patients undergoing stricter rate-control, including bradycardia and syncope. The RACE-II trial was a randomized, controlled trial designed to explore whether lenient rate-control (i.e., target resting heart rate <110 bpm) was inferior to strict rate-control (i.e., target resting heart rate <80 bpm, <110 bpm during exercise) in reducing the incidence of cardiovascular events in patients with atrial fibrillation. In summary, there was no significant difference between the strategies in the risk of death from cardiovascular causes, hospitalization for heart failure, stroke, systemic embolism, major bleeding, and arrhythmic events.

In-Depth [randomized controlled trial]: The study was conducted at 33 centers in the Netherlands and involved 614 patients. Patients were eligible if they had atrial fibrillation for up to 12 months, were ≤80 years of age, had a mean resting heart rate >80 bpm, and were using oral anticoagulation therapy. Included patients were randomized to the lenient control strategy (i.e., target resting heart rate <110 bpm) or the strict control strategy (i.e., target resting heart rate <80 bpm, <110 bpm during exercise). The primary outcome was a composite of death from cardiovascular causes, hospitalization for heart failure, stroke, systemic embolism, major bleeding, and arrhythmic events (e.g., syncope, sustained ventricular tachycardia, and cardiac arrest). Secondary outcomes included components of the primary outcome, along with all-cause mortality, symptoms, and functional status. At the end of the follow-up period, the resting heart rates were 85 ± 14 and 76 ± 14 in the lenient- and strict-control groups, respectively ($p < 0.001$). It was found that lenient control was noninferior to strict control in preventing the primary outcome (HR 0.84; 90%CI 0.58-1.21). Moreover, there was no significant difference in all-cause mortality (HR 0.91; 90%CI 0.52-1.59). There were no significant differences between the groups in symptoms associated with atrial fibrillation such as dyspnea, fatigue, and palpitations. Additionally, there was no significant difference between the groups in terms of heart failure functional status.

Van Gelder IC, Groenveld HF, Crijns HJGM, Tuininga YS, Tijssen JGP, Alings AM, et al. Lenient versus Strict Rate Control in Patients with Atrial Fibrillation. New England Journal of Medicine. 2010 Apr 15;362(15):1363–73.

The HAS-BLED score: Bleeding risk in atrial fibrillation

1. The HAS-BLED score is an easy-to-remember and easy-to-apply tool that has good predictive accuracy for the risk of major bleeding in patients with atrial fibrillation.

2. Since its publication, the HAS-BLED score has been validated in a large cohort study of 7329 patients.

Original Date of Publication: November 2010

Study Rundown: In atrial fibrillation impaired atrial contraction leads to blood stasis within the atria, thereby increasing the risk of thrombus formation and cardioembolic stroke. The CHADS2 score was developed to identify patients with atrial fibrillation who are at higher risk of stroke and who should therefore be treated with oral anticoagulation. Treatment with oral anticoagulants, however, increases one's risk of bleeding. The HAS-BLED score was developed in response to the need for tools to estimate the risk of major bleeding in patients with atrial fibrillation. Originally published in 2010, the score consists of 7 factors: hypertension, abnormal renal/liver function, stroke, bleeding history or predisposition, labile international normalized ratio (INR), elderly (>65 years), and drugs/alcohol use concomitantly. This study demonstrated that the HAS-BLED score had good predictive accuracy for major bleeding in the overall cohort of patients, but performed much better in patients on antiplatelet agents or no antithrombotic therapy. When compared to the HEMOR2RHAGES scheme, the HAS-BLED score consists of fewer factors and only requires clinical assessment or routine bloodwork. The HAS-BLED score has since been validated in a larger cohort study published in the Journal of the American College of Cardiology.

In-Depth [retrospective cohort]: This study utilized a cohort of patients that were identified from the prospectively developed Euro Heart Survey on Atrial Fibrillation database. Patients in the database were followed for 1 year to determine survival and incidence of major adverse events, including major bleeding (i.e., hemoglobin drop >2 g/L or requiring transfusion). The HAS-BLED score was constructed by identifying bleeding risk factors from a derivation cohort, and adding consistent risk factors for major bleeding found in recent systematic reviews. The final score included hypertension (systolic >160 mmHg), abnormal renal (dialysis, renal transplantation, or creatinine ≥200 umol/L) or liver function (chronic liver disease, or biochemical evidence), stroke, bleeding history or predisposition, labile INR (therapeutic time in range <60%), elderly (>65 years), drugs/alcohol use concomitantly.

Of the 5272 patients in the Euro Heart Survey on Atrial Fibrillation, 3456 did not have mitral valve stenosis or valvular surgery and were included in this study. The HAS-BLED score was compared with the HEMOR2RHAGES scheme, a previously developed tool for estimating the risk of bleeding. C statistics were calculated to determine the predictive accuracy of each model using various sets of patients. The HAS-BLED score had C statistics of 0.72 (95%CI 0.65-0.79) for the overall cohort, 0.69 (95%CI 0.59-0.80) for patients on oral anticoagulants, 0.91 for patients on antiplatelet agents (95%CI 0.83-1.00), and 0.85 for patients on no antithrombotic therapy (95%CI 0.00-1.00). The HEMOR2RHAGES scheme had C statistics of 0.66 (95%CI 0.57-0.74) for the overall cohort, 0.64 (95%CI 0.53-0.75) for patients on oral anticoagulants, 0.83 for patients on antiplatelet agents (95%CI 0.68-0.98), and 0.81 for patients on no antithrombotic therapy (95%CI 0.00-1.00). *The HAS-BLED score is detailed below:*

Clinical characteristic	Points awarded
Hypertension	1
Abnormal renal and liver function (1 each)	1 or 2
Stroke	1
Bleeding history or predisposition	1
Labile INR	1
Elderly (>65 years)	1
Drugs or alcohol (1 each)	1 or 2

HAS-BLED score	Number of patients	Bleeds per 100 patient-years
0	798	1.13
1	1,286	1.02
2	744	1.88
3	187	3.74
4	46	8.70
5	8	12.50
6	2	0.0
7	0	-
8	0	-
9	0	-

Pisters R, Lane DA, Nieuwlaat R, de Vos CB, Crijns HJGM, Lip GYH. A novel user-friendly score (has-bled) to assess 1-year risk of major bleeding in patients with atrial fibrillation: The euro heart survey. Chest. 2010 Nov 1;138(5):1093–100.

The EMPHASIS-HF trial:
Eplerenone reduces mortality in
mild systolic heart failure

1. Eplerenone significantly reduced mortality in patients suffering from heart failure with reduced systolic function (left ventricular ejection fraction [LVEF] ≤30%, or 30-35% if QRS>130 ms) and mild symptoms (New York Heart Association [NYHA] class II) when compared with placebo.

2. The incidence of hyperkalemia was significantly higher in the eplerenone group.

Original Date of Publication: January 2011

Study Rundown: Mineralocorticoid antagonists significantly improved survival in patients with severe systolic heart failure (i.e., LVEF<35% and NYHA class III/IV symptoms) in the RALES trial and in patients with heart failure after myocardial infarction in the EPHESUS trial. The purpose of the EMPHASIS-HF trial was to explore the effects of adding eplerenone, a type of mineralocorticoid antagonist, to evidence-based therapy in patients with systolic heart failure and only mild symptoms (i.e., LVEF<35% and NYHA class II symptoms). Results showed that eplerenone significantly reduced the risk of death from cardiovascular causes and hospitalization for heart failure. While there was a significantly higher risk of hyperkalemia in the eplerenone group, there were no significant differences between the groups in the rate of drug withdrawal for hyperkalemia. This study, along with the RALES and EPHESUS trials, demonstrated that mineralocorticoid antagonism in patients with symptomatic systolic heart failure was linked with improved mortality and reduced hospitalization. One criticism of the trial was that the study population only differed from the RALES population based on their subjective NYHA classification. Thus, critics argued that it was difficult to determine whether there was really a true enough difference between the study populations. While the NYHA classification is subjective, it is a strong prognostic tools for heart failure patients, and the rates of mortality observed in the EMPHASIS-HF trials were much lower than those seen in the RALES trial, suggesting there was a difference in the severity of disease.

In-Depth [randomized controlled trial]: This trial involved 2737 patients recruited at 278 centers in 29 countries. Patients were considered eligible for the trial if they were ≥55 years of age, had NYHA class II symptoms, LVEF≤30% (or 30-35% if QRS>130 ms), and were being treated with angiotensin-converting enzyme inhibitor/angiotensin receptor blocker and a beta-blocker at recommended or maximal tolerated doses, unless contraindicated. Patients were excluded if they were having acute myocardial infarction, NYHA class III/IV symptoms, serum potassium >5.0 mmol/L, glomerular filtration rate <30 mL/min/1.73m², a need for potassium-sparing diuretic, or any other clinically significant coexisting condition. The primary outcome was a composite of death from cardiovascular causes or a first hospitalization for heart failure. Secondary outcomes included hospitalization for heart failure or death from any cause, death from any cause, and death from cardiovascular causes, among others.

A total of 1364 patients were randomized to the eplerenone group, while 1373 were randomized to the placebo group. At 3 years after randomization, the eplerenone group experienced a significantly lower rate of the primary outcome (HR 0.63; 95%CI 0.54-0.74) when compared to placebo. Notably, the eplerenone group experienced significantly lower rates of both death from cardiovascular causes (HR 0.76; 95%CI 0.61-0.94) as well as hospitalization for heart failure (HR 0.58; 95%CI 0.47-0.70). Moreover, patients treated with eplerenone also experienced significantly lower rates of death from any cause (HR 0.76; 95%CI 0.62-0.93) and hospitalization for any reason (HR 0.77; 95%CI 0.67-0.88). While rates of hyperkalemia were significantly higher in the eplerenone group (8.0% vs 3.7%, p < 0.001), there were no significant differences in the rates of study drug withdrawal for hyperkalemia between the 2 groups.

Zannad F, McMurray JJV, Krum H, van Veldhuisen DJ, Swedberg K, Shi H, et al.
Eplerenone in Patients with Systolic Heart Failure and Mild Symptoms. New England
Journal of Medicine. 2011 Jan 6;364(1):11–21.

The RIVAL trial: Radial vs. femoral artery access for percutaneous coronary intervention

1. The composite outcome of death, myocardial infarction (MI), stroke, and non-coronary artery bypass graft-related major bleeding did not differ between radial and femoral access for percutaneous coronary intervention (PCI).

2. Radial artery access was associated with a significantly lower rate of vascular complications when compared to femoral access.

Original Date of Publication: April 2011

Study Rundown: For patients with acute coronary syndromes (ACS), vascular access for PCI via the femoral artery is associated with a substantial risk of bleeding, particularly at the access site. Vascular access via the radial artery may reduce bleeding risks since the site is more superficial and compressible. Observational studies suggested that radial access may also be associated with a lower risk of death and MI. The Radial Vs Femoral (RIVAL) trial was the first large, randomized, controlled trial that compared radial access for PCI to femoral access. Results revealed that radial and femoral access did not differ in the rate of the composite primary outcome, which consisted of death, MI, stroke, and non-coronary artery bypass graft (CABG)-related major bleeding. Vascular access site complications, however, were significantly reduced with radial access compared to femoral. In particular, radial access was associated with a decreased risk of developing large hematomas and pseudoaneurysms requiring closure. Finally, there was a significant interaction between the primary outcome and the volume of radial PCIs performed by the medical center. One potential limitation of the study was the overall low rate of major bleeding, which may have prevented the detection of a significant difference in non-CABG-related bleeding due to radial versus femoral access. This may have been due to the study's use of experienced, high-volume interventional cardiologists whose technical skills may be superior to those of other cardiologists. In summary, the RIVAL trial demonstrated that radial and femoral artery access for PCI are equally effective in managing ACS. Radial access, while potentially more difficult to establish, may be preferable due to the significantly lower risk of vascular complications, as compared with femoral access.

In-Depth [randomized controlled trial]: The RIVAL trial was a randomized, parallel group, multicenter trial. A total of 7021 patients were enrolled in the trial and underwent randomization. Patients were eligible if they had a diagnosis of ACS and were planning to undergo PCI. Patients were excluded if they presented in cardiogenic shock, had peripheral vascular disease, or a history of previous CABG surgery. Recruited cardiologists were required to have expertise in both radial and femoral artery access, including at least 50 radial procedures. In the end, 3507 participants were randomized to radial access and 3514 participants were randomized to femoral access. The primary outcome was a composite of death, MI, stroke, and non-CABG-related major bleeding at 30 days. There was no difference in the occurrence of the primary outcome between the radial and femoral groups (HR 0.92; 95%CI 0.72-1.17). There was an observed interaction between the primary outcome and a medical center's volume of radial access (HR 0.49, 95%CI 0.28-0.87). Radial access was associated with significantly fewer vascular complications, including development of large hematoma (HR 0.40; 95%CI 0.28-0.57) and pseudoaneurysm needing closure (HR 0.30; 95%CI 0.13-0.71).

Jolly SS, Yusuf S, Cairns J, Niemelä K, Xavier D, Widimsky P, et al. Radial versus femoral access for coronary angiography and intervention in patients with acute coronary syndromes (RIVAL): a randomised, parallel group, multicentre trial. Lancet. 2011 Apr 23;377(9775):1409–20.

The PRECOMBAT trial:
Percutaneous coronary intervention vs. coronary bypass in left main coronary artery stenosis

1. In patients with left main coronary artery stenosis, angioplasty with sirolimus-eluting stents was noninferior to coronary artery bypass grafting (CABG) in preventing subsequent cardiac and cerebrovascular events.

2. Percutaneous coronary intervention (PCI) patients experienced a significantly higher incidence of ischemia-driven target vessel revascularization compared to coronary artery bypass graft patients

3. Because of low event rates, the study was underpowered.

Original Date of Publication: May 2011

Study Rundown: The Premier of Randomized Comparison of Bypass Surgery versus Angioplasty Using Sirolimus-Eluting Stent in Patients with Left Main Coronary Artery Disease (PRECOMBAT) trial compared PCI to CABG in patients with left main coronary artery stenosis. Prior to this study, some evidence suggested that PCI may be an acceptable alternative to CABG in certain patients with left main disease, though outcomes had never been assessed in a large, randomized trial. In the PRECOMBAT trial, patients with left main coronary artery stenosis were treated with PCI with a sirolimus-eluting stent or CABG and were followed for 2 years after randomization. PCI with sirolimus-eluting stents was found to be non-inferior to CABG for left main coronary artery stenosis at 12 months with respect to the primary outcome. At 2 years, the rates of major coronary events, cerebrovascular events, and all-cause mortality were similar in patients being treated with PCI or CABG. Of note, patients treated with PCI experienced significantly higher rates of ischemia-driven target vessel revascularization when compared with CABG patients at the 2-year mark. In summary, this study shows that PCI was noninferior to CABG in treating left main coronary artery stenosis with regards to the primary composite endpoint (i.e., major adverse cardiac or cerebrovascular events). As a result of low event rates, however, the study was underpowered and the study authors have noted that these findings should not be clinically directive.

In-Depth [randomized controlled trial]: This trial was conducted at 13 centers across South Korea. Patients were eligible for the study if they were ≥18 years of age and had received a diagnosis of stable angina, unstable angina, silent ischemia, or non-ST-elevation myocardial infarction (NSTEMI), with more than 50% stenosis of the left main coronary artery. Eligible patients also needed to be candidates for CABG or PCI as determined heir treating physicians and surgeons. The primary endpoint was a composite of death from any cause, myocardial infarction, stroke, and ischemia-driven target vessel revascularization in the 12 months following randomization.

A total of 600 patients were enrolled and randomized as part of the trial. At 12 months, 8.7% of patients in the PCI group and 6.7% of patients in the CABG group experienced primary endpoints (absolute risk difference 2.0%; 95%CI -1.6 to 5.6%; p = 0.01 for non-inferiority). At 24 months, there were no significant differences between the 2 groups with regards to the primary endpoint (HR 1.50; 95%CI 0.90-2.52). Ischemia-driven target vessel revascularization (i.e., repeat revascularization with stenosis of 50% and ischemic signs/symptoms or 70% without ischemic signs/symptoms) was significantly higher in the PCI group at 24 months (HR 2.18; 95%CI 1.10-4.32).

Park S-J, Kim Y-H, Park D-W, Yun S-C, Ahn J-M, Song HG, et al. Randomized Trial of Stents versus Bypass Surgery for Left Main Coronary Artery Disease. New England Journal of Medicine. 2011 May 5;364(18):1718–27.

The ARISTOTLE trial: Apixaban superior to warfarin for stroke prophylaxis in atrial fibrillation

1. Apixaban was superior to warfarin in preventing stroke in patients with atrial fibrillation.

2. Apixaban therapy had a decreased risk of intracranial hemorrhage compared to warfarin.

3. There was no difference in gastrointestinal (GI) bleeding risk between apixaban and warfarin.

Original Date of Publication: September 2011

Study Rundown: Warfarin is a vitamin K antagonist that has long been the mainstay of anticoagulation therapy for prevention of thromboembolic stroke in patients with atrial fibrillation. Recently, apixaban, a direct Xa inhibitor, was introduced to the market. It has a much wider therapeutic range, does not require monitoring, and 25% of it is cleared by the kidneys. The Apixaban for Reduction in Stroke and Other Thromboembolic Events in Atrial Fibrillation (ARISTOTLE) was a landmark trial that sought to address whether apixaban was superior to warfarin in reducing the risk of thromboembolic stroke in patients with atrial fibrillation. The trial demonstrated that apixaban was superior in preventing thromboembolic strokes in patients with atrial fibrillation when compared to warfarin. In addition, there was a significant reduction in the risk of bleeding in patients treated with apixaban compared to warfarin. While the high cost of apixaban limits its widespread use, for patients in whom warfarin is contraindicated, apixaban offers an effective, safe anticoagulation alternative to warfarin.

In-Depth [randomized controlled trial]: This study was a multicenter, blind, randomized controlled trial that assigned 18 206 patients with atrial fibrillation to either standard warfarin therapy or apixaban therapy for thromboembolism prophylaxis. All patients had a documented history of atrial fibrillation or atrial flutter at least twice in the past 12 months and all had at least 1 additional risk factor for stroke. The primary outcome in the study was rate of thromboembolic stroke or a systemic embolism. The secondary outcome was death from all causes. Patients were followed for 1.8 years and all adverse effects of therapy were documented.

The apixaban group experienced a significant reduction in thromboembolic stroke compared to the warfarin group (HR 0.79, 95%CI 0.66-0.95) but no difference in the rate of systemic embolism (HR 0.89, 95%CI 0.44-1.75). There was also a significant reduction in all-cause mortality in the apixaban group compared to the warfarin group (HR 0.89; 95%CI 0.80-0.998). Apixaban treatment also significantly reduced the risk of major bleeding as compared to warfarin (HR 0.69, 95%CI 0.6-0.8). On further examination, the apixaban group had a significantly lower rate of intracranial bleeds but no difference in the rate of GI bleeding in comparison to warfarin. When the primary outcome results were examined in subgroups, apixaban proved to be better than warfarin in all subgroups except for the younger population (i.e., patients less than 65 years of age), who fared better with warfarin therapy.

Granger CB, Alexander JH, McMurray JJV, Lopes RD, Hylek EM, Hanna M, et al. Apixaban versus Warfarin in Patients with Atrial Fibrillation. New England Journal of Medicine. 2011 Sep 15;365(11):981–92.

The ROCKET AF: Rivaroxaban non-inferior to warfarin for stroke prophylaxis in atrial fibrillation

1. Rivaroxaban was non-inferior to warfarin in preventing strokes and systemic embolism.

2. Compared to warfarin, rivaroxaban reduced the rates of critical, fatal, and intracranial bleeding.

Original Date of Publication: September 2011

Study Rundown: Warfarin is the standard for anticoagulation in patients with atrial fibrillation to prevent thromboembolic events. However, accompanying warfarin therapy are challenging pharmacokinetics, extensive food and drug interactions, and need for international normalized ratio (INR) monitoring. In recent years, investigators have studied new oral anticoagulants for use in atrial fibrillation. A main advantage of these agents is that they do not require frequent INR monitoring. Dabigatran, a direct thrombin inhibitor, was shown to be a possible alternative to warfarin in the RELY trial. Rivaroxaban is another new oral anticoagulant. It acts to prevent thrombus formation by being a direct factor Xa inhibitor. The Rivaroxaban Once Daily Oral Direct Factor Xa Inhibition Compared with Vitamin K Antagonism for Prevention of Stroke and Embolism Trial in Atrial Fibrillation (ROCKET AF) was published in 2011. The trial demonstrated that rivaroxaban was non-inferior to warfarin in preventing stroke and systemic embolism. The use of rivaroxaban was also associated with significantly lower rates of critical bleeding, fatal bleeding, and intracranial hemorrhage when compared to warfarin. Thus, in patients with non-valvular atrial fibrillation who are at elevated risk of stroke or systemic embolism, rivaroxaban may be considered as an alternative to warfarin in those patients with a creatinine clearance >30mL/min.

In-Depth [randomized controlled trial]: This large, randomized, controlled trial included 14 264 patients from 1178 clinical centers in 45 countries. Patients were included if they had nonvalvular atrial fibrillation, demonstrated on electrocardiography, and were at moderate-to-high risk for stroke (i.e., CHADS2 score $\geq$2). Patients were randomized to 2 groups: 1) rivaroxaban 20 mg daily, or 15 mg daily if creatinine clearance was 30-49 mL/min, or 2) warfarin with dose titrated to INR of 2.0-3.0. The primary outcome studied was a composite of stroke (i.e., both ischemic and hemorrhagic) and systemic embolism. The primary safety outcome was a composite of major and non-major bleeding events that were clinically relevant. In the intention-to-treat population, there was no significant difference in the incidence of the primary endpoint between the rivaroxaban and warfarin groups, thereby demonstrating non-inferiority (HR 0.88; 95%CI 0.74-1.03). With regard to the primary safety endpoint, there was no significant difference between the 2 groups in terms of the incidence of major and non-major bleeding events that were clinically relevant (HR 1.03; 95%CI 0.96-1.11). A further analysis of major bleeding events, however, demonstrated that the rivaroxaban group experienced significantly lower rates of critical bleeding (HR 0.69; 95%CI 0.53-0.91), fatal bleeding (HR 0.50; 95%CI 0.31-0.79), and intracranial hemorrhage (HR 0.67; 95%CI 0.47-0.93) compared to the warfarin group.

Patel MR, Mahaffey KW, Garg J, Pan G, Singer DE, Hacke W, et al. Rivaroxaban versus Warfarin in Nonvalvular Atrial Fibrillation. New England Journal of Medicine. 2011 Sep 8;365(10):883–91.

III. Critical, Emergent and Pulmonary Care

Initial trial of conservative management for splenic injury

1. The conservative, symptomatic management of 16 patients following assumed splenic injury from blunt abdominal trauma resulted in normalization of hemodynamic stability within 2 days of hospital admission. Furthermore, this strategy resulted in complete normalization of clinical examination by 2 weeks post-discharge, and no hospital readmissions.

2. This approach to splenic injury management was supported by subsequent investigations, eventually leading to the acceptance of conservative management as standard of care.

Original Date of Publication: October 1971

Study Rundown: The spleen is particularly susceptible to blunt abdominal trauma and, prior to this study, splenectomy was routine following abdominal injury. However, previous anecdotal evidence of the authors linked nonoperative management to positive outcomes. With the potential for spleen salvage and a reduction in surgical and post-operative risks, this study investigated the outcomes of children who were not treated surgically for their splenic injuries. The small sample size, lack of a control group, and use of descriptive statistics as the only method for analysis limited the study. In addition, conclusions drawn from the study may be inaccurate as patients were assumed to have splenic injury from clinical examination as no method, apart from surgical exploration, could confirm injury.

At the time of its publication, the proposed conservative treatment investigated in the study differed radically from expected surgical intervention. In the present day, conservative management is the preferred method of management for children with splenic injury secondary to blunt trauma. Improved imaging techniques and technology for monitoring patient hemodynamic status now allow for better assessment of the need for surgical intervention. A recent retrospective study of the evolution of splenic injury management found hospital length of stay, transfusion requirements, and mortality decreased as conservative management of splenic injury became widely accepted.

In-Depth [case-series study]: A total of 32 children admitted to the hospital during 1948-1955 following blunt abdominal trauma with potential splenic involvement were included. Six patients underwent splenectomy, 1 patient died from a crush injury, and the remaining 25 underwent nonoperative management. Of these patients, 16 were included in the study (mean age = 10 years, 69% male) as their presentation indicated likely splenic involvement, although this was not confirmed by surgical intervention. Patients underwent standard examinations with researchers reporting close monitoring of patient vitals.

All patients were conscious upon presentation with a complaint of abdominal pain and all had significant abdominal tenderness. Three children had ecchymoses overlying the site of trauma and 3 had potential intraperitoneal fluid detected on physical exam. Patient pulses ranged from 100-140/min and 4 patients had blood pressures <90/50 mmHg. Complete blood counts included hemoglobin values ranging from 7.9-11.4 g/100 mL (mean = 9.5 g/100 mL) and white blood cell counts ranging from 8000-27 000 mm^3 (mean = 17 000 mm^3). Patient temperatures ranged from 100°F-104°F (mean = 102°F). 9 children received whole blood transfusions for hemodynamic instability and 2 received plasma. All patients received intravenous fluids. Patients were hemodynamically stable within 2 days of admission. Resolution of abdominal tenderness correlated with normalization of heart rate and body temperature. Total length of stay ranged from 4 to 42 days (mean = 16 days). Two weeks after discharge, all patients' physical examinations normalized and no patient underwent readmission.

Douglas GJ, Simpson JS. The conservative management of splenic trauma. Journal of Pediatric Surgery. 1971 Oct 1;6(5):565–70.

Davies DA, Pearl RH, Ein SH, Langer JC, Wales PW. Management of blunt splenic injury in children: evolution of the nonoperative approach. Journal of Pediatric Surgery. 2009 May 1;44(5):1005–8.

Magnesium sulfate in torsade de pointes

1. Intravenous magnesium sulfate was effective at acutely terminating torsade de pointes (TdP).

2. Intravenous magnesium sulfate was not effective in terminating other ventricular tachycardias (VTs) not associated with QT prolongation.

Original Date of Publication: February 1988

Study Rundown: TdP is distinguished from other forms of VT due to its occurrence in patients with marked QT prolongation. Because of this underlying difference, TdP responds to intravenous (IV) magnesium sulfate (MgSO4), while other forms of ventricular tachycardias do not. This article was the first case-series demonstrating the effect of MgSO4 on terminating torsade de pointes. After the publication of this article, MgSO4 became the standard therapy for treatment of TdP. While the study may be considered rudimentary, the researcher's findings were influential as all 12 subjects with TdP responded to MgSO4 and none of the 5 non-TdP VT subjects did. Weaknesses of the study included a low sample size (n = 17) and significant variability in patient demographics, cardiac history and function, baseline electrolyte levels, as well as concurrent therapy. Furthermore, no individual data was shown for the 5 non-TdP subjects. In summary, despite the many weaknesses of the paper by today's standards, this study helped establish MgSO4 as standard practice in treating TdP.

In-Depth [case-series]: A total of 12 patients with TdP and 5 patients with polymorphic VT with normal QT interval were included. These patients were treated with 25% or 50% solutions of MgSO4 and were observed for termination of arrhythmia and recurrence. The mean QT interval was 0.61s in the TdP group (mean QTc of 0.64s) and 0.46s (mean QTc not provided) in the non-TdP VT group. Magnesium levels prior to onset of arrhythmia were available for 8/12 TdP patients and 2/5 non-TdP VT patients and were all within normal limits (1.6-2.5 meq/L). Two out of 12 patients had potassium levels below 3.1 meq/L (both were 2.9 meq/L). No non-TdP VT patient had potassium levels below 3.1 meq/L. Two grams of IV MgSO4 were administered to all 12 TdP and 5 non-TdP subjects as soon as arrhythmia was recognized. Four of the TdP patients received other therapies, which were not effective, prior to MgSO4 therapy. Nine patients responded immediately to the MgSO4. The other 3 patients received a second bolus within 5-15 minutes and were started on a continuous infusion. In 2 patients, the TdP recurred 1-6 hours after infusion was begun and was abolished in both after a third bolus of IV MgSO4. MgSO4 infusion was continued until QT<0.50s. Two of the 12 patients had elevated magnesium levels (3.5 and 5 meq/L) after treatment with MgSO4. Zero out of the 5 non-TdP VT patients showed improvement with MgSO4 therapy even after 2-3 boluses. Three of the 5 patients responded to other IV antiarrhythmics (2 to lidocaine, 1 to procainamide).

Tzivoni D, Banai S, Schuger C, Benhorin J, Keren A, Gottlieb S, et al. Treatment of torsade de pointes with magnesium sulfate. Circulation. 1988 Feb 1;77(2):392–7.

The DIGAMI trial: Insulin-glucose infusion in diabetics with acute myocardial infarction

1. In diabetic patients with an acute myocardial infarction (MI), insulin-glucose infusion with subsequent long-term insulin treatment significantly reduced mortality at 1 year.

Original Date of Publication: July 1995

Study Rundown: At the time of the Diabetes Mellitus Insulin-Glucose Infusion in Acute Myocardial Infarction (DIGAMI) study (1995), studies revealed that diabetic patients had higher mortality rates post-MI than non-diabetic patients. This difference remained despite the introduction of new therapeutic measures, such as beta-blockers. Increased fatty acid metabolism in diabetes is theorized to decrease the anaerobic process of glycolysis that is important for the survival of ischemic tissue. The DIGAMI study demonstrated that, in diabetic patients already receiving beta-blockers and thrombolytic treatment, metabolic control via an insulin-glucose infusion and long-term insulin therapy further decreased post-MI mortality after 1 year. It is unclear from the study results whether the immediate insulin-glucose infusion or the subsequent multidose insulin therapy was most responsible for the decrease in post-MI mortality. The lack of free fatty acid measurements also limited the study from clarifying the mechanism of benefit from insulin treatment post-MI. The study only randomized half of the 1240 eligible patients, resulting in a relatively small sample size, wide confidence intervals, and potential bias due to the exclusion of patients unwilling to undergo aggressive insulin therapy. Lastly, >80% of patients in the study were previously non-insulin dependent, suggesting that the benefits of insulin treatment may be limited to patients with the minimal disease. In summary, the DIGAMI study demonstrated a role for insulin therapy in diabetic patients who experience acute MI.

In-Depth [randomized controlled trial]: This trial involved coronary care units in 19 Swedish hospitals. Inclusion criteria included suspected acute MI within the preceding 24 hours in a patient with previously diagnosed diabetes mellitus (DM), or in a patient with a blood glucose level >11 mmol/liter without a previous DM diagnosis. All 620 patients received thrombolytic treatment (i.e., streptokinase) and beta-blockade (i.e., metoprolol), and were randomized to additionally receive an insulin-glucose infusion with follow-up multidose insulin therapy, or conventional therapy. At 1 year, the mortality rate in the insulin group was significantly lower than that of the control group (RRR 29%, p = 0.027).

Malmberg K, Rydén L, Efendic S, Herlitz J, Nicol P, Waldenstrom A, et al. Randomized trial of insulin-glucose infusion followed by subcutaneous insulin treatment in diabetic patients with acute myocardial infarction (DIGAMI study): Effects on mortality at 1 year. J Am Coll Cardiol. 1995 Jul 1;26(1):57–65.

The NINDS trial: Tissue plasminogen activator in acute ischemic stroke improves functional outcomes

1. Treatment of acute ischemic stroke with tissue plasminogen activator (t-PA) within 3 hours of symptom onset significantly improved functional outcomes 3 months after stroke, when compared with placebo.

2. Tissue plasminogen activator significantly increased the rate of symptomatic intracerebral hemorrhage.

Original Date of Publication: December 1995

Study Rundown: Prior to the National Institute of Neurologic Disorders and Stroke (NINDS) trial, evidence that thrombolytic therapy benefitted patients with ischemic stroke existed, though intracerebral hemorrhage was a frequent complication. Several previous studies found that early treatment (i.e., thrombolytics within 3 hours of symptom onset) was associated with the greatest likelihood of recovery and lower risks of hemorrhage. The NINDS trial was a larger randomized controlled trial that sought to assess the efficacy of using t-PA in treating ischemic stroke within 3 hours of symptom onset. Results showed that the administration of t-PA within 3 hours of symptom onset in patients suffering ischemic stroke significantly improved functional outcomes, as observed at the 3-month mark. Patients treated with t-PA, however, suffered significantly higher rates of symptomatic bleeding. The NINDS trial was the first randomized controlled trial demonstrating that t-PA was beneficial in patients suffering from acute ischemic stroke. While the study used carefully selected sample of stroke cases, the findings of the NINDS trial formed as the basis for approving the use of thrombolytics in the management of acute strokes. It also informed the development of practice guidelines in centers across North America.

In-Depth [randomized controlled trial]: The trial consisted of 2 phases: 1) assessing for improvements in neurologic functioning within 24 hours of symptom onset to measure t-PA activity and 2) assessing for sustained clinical improvement at 3 months. In phase 1, there was no significant difference between the groups in terms of neurologic improvement within the first 24 hours. In phase 2, patients treated with t-PA demonstrated significant improvements on several functional assessment scales (i.e., NIHSS, Barthel, Modified Rankin, Glasgow Outcome) 3 months after the onset of stroke, when compared with patients in the placebo group. There were significantly more symptomatic intracerebral hemorrhages in the t-PA group, though the rate of asymptomatic intracerebral hemorrhages was not different.

The National Institute of Neurological Disorders and Stroke rt-PA Stroke Study Group. Tissue Plasminogen Activator for Acute Ischemic Stroke. New England Journal of Medicine. 1995 Dec 14;333(24):1581–8.

The Rockall score: Risk assessment after acute upper gastrointestinal hemorrhage

1. Age, shock, comorbidity, diagnosis, major stigmata of recent hemorrhage, and rebleeding were independent predictors of mortality following acute upper gastrointestinal hemorrhage.

Original Date of Publication: March 1996

Study Rundown: Acute upper gastrointestinal hemorrhage is a common medical emergency. Risk factors for rebleeding and death were well known at the time of this study's publication but there was previously no clinically useful tool for risk stratifying patients. The Rockall risk scoring system was found to be a good indicator of prognosis following acute upper gastrointestinal hemorrhage. Rebleeding was a particularly important risk factor associated with a 5-fold increase in mortality among middle risk groups. Current treatment protocols specifically target the prevention of rebleeding due to the increased risk of mortality. The Rockall score can be applied in disease management, determining case mix in evaluating outcomes, developing treatment protocols, and selecting patients in clinical trials.

In-Depth [randomized controlled trial]: This study produced a risk scoring system following acute upper gastrointestinal bleeding based on data from 4185 cases identified in 1993 and 1625 cases identified in 1994. In the first phase of data collection, medical staff completed a questionnaire for each identified case, which included risk factors, treatment, endoscopic findings, diagnosis, complications, and mortality. Multiple regression analysis found that the following variables were independent predictors of mortality: age, shock, comorbidity, diagnosis, major stigmata of recent hemorrhage, and rebleeding. The risk scoring system was validated using the second phase of data collection. An integer score was assigned to each category of each significant variable according to its contribution to the logistic regression model. The maximum possible score is 11 with scores of 8 or more considered very high-risk categories. Rebleeding occurred in less than 5% of cases and mortality was close to 0 in patients scoring 0, 1, or 2.

Rockall TA, Logan RF, Devlin HB, Northfield TC. Risk assessment after acute upper gastrointestinal haemorrhage. Gut. 1996 Mar 1;38(3):316–21.

The TRICC trial: Restrictive transfusion in intensive care does not increase mortality

1. Using a restrictive transfusion strategy in critically ill patients did not significantly increase 30-day mortality when compared with a liberal transfusion strategy.

2. Subgroup analyses demonstrated that a restrictive transfusion strategy was associated with a significantly lower mortality in patients with Acute Physiology and Chronic Health Evaluation (APACHE) II score ≤20 and age <55 years.

Original Date of Publication: February 1999

Study Rundown: The Transfusion Requirements in Critical Care (TRICC) trial sought to explore whether restrictive and liberal red-cell transfusion strategies in critically ill patients resulted in different outcomes. Prior to this study, there were conflicting views about liberal transfusion protocols. Several observational studies suggested that anemia was a risk factor for mortality in critically ill patients, particularly those with cardiovascular disease. It was suggested that anemia may cause excessive stress in severely ill patients, resulting in poorer outcomes. Other studies suggested that the risks of blood transfusion were elevated in the critically ill.

This randomized, controlled trial examined the risks and benefits associated with different transfusion strategies among patients in the intensive care unit (ICU). One strategy was restrictive and sought to maintain lower hemoglobin levels (target between 7.0-9.0 g/dL), while the other was liberal and maintained higher hemoglobin levels (target between 10.0-12.0 g/dL). In summary, there was no difference in 30-day mortality when comparing the groups. Moreover, the study demonstrated that survival was significantly improved when using the restrictive transfusion strategy in subgroups of patients with an APACHE II score ≤20 and age <55 years (p=0.02). This trial supported the use of a restrictive transfusion strategy in critically ill patients.

In-Depth [randomized controlled trial]: Published in 1999, this study involved 838 critically ill patients recruited from 22 tertiary-level and 3 community ICUs across Canada. Patients were included if they were expected to stay in intensive care for >24 hours, had a hemoglobin concentration ≤9.0

g/dL within 72 hours of admission, and were considered to be euvolemic by treating physicians. Exclusion criteria included age <16 years old, inability to receive blood products, active blood loss at the time of enrollment, chronic anemia, pregnancy, brain death, or imminent death. Eligible patients were then randomized to either restrictive (target hemoglobin from 7.0-9.0 g/dL) or liberal transfusion strategies (target hemoglobin 10.0-12.0 g/dL). The primary outcome measure was 30-day mortality. Secondary outcomes included 60-day mortality and mortality in intensive care/during hospitalization. There was no significant difference in 30-day mortality between the groups (ARR 4.7%; 95%CI -0.84-10.2; p = 0.11). The in-hospital mortality rate, however, was significantly lower for patients in the restrictive arm (ARR 5.8%; 95%CI -0.3-11.7; p = 0.05). In the subgroups of patients with a score on the severity-of-disease APACHE II scale of ≤20 and age <55 years, survival was significantly higher for patients in the restrictive-transfusion group (p = 0.02).

Hébert PC, Wells G, Blajchman MA, Marshall J, Martin C, Pagliarello G, et al. A Multicenter, Randomized, Controlled Clinical Trial of Transfusion Requirements in Critical Care. New England Journal of Medicine. 1999 Feb 11;340(6):409–17.

The ARMA trial: Lower tidal volume ventilation in acute respiratory distress syndrome

1. This trial was terminated early when the data demonstrated that lower tidal volume ventilator settings in acute lung injury (ALI)/acute respiratory distress syndrome (ARDS) patients reduced in-hospital mortality.

2. Low tidal volume ventilation was also associated with an increase in ventilator-free days and a decrease in the number of days with systemic organ failure. There was no significant difference in the incidence of barotrauma between the low and high tidal volume groups.

3. Patients assigned to lower tidal volume ventilator settings initially required a higher positive end-expiratory pressure (PEEP) to maintain arterial oxygenation and were more likely to develop respiratory acidosis, although the difference disappeared by day 7.

Original Date of Publication: May 2000

Study Rundown: In an effort to maintain normal partial pressure of carbon dioxide and arterial pH, patients with ALI or ARDS requiring mechanical ventilation traditionally received higher tidal volumes (10-15 mL/kg) compared to healthy individuals. However, studies in animals showed that higher tidal volumes were associated with increased lung inflammation and injury. This multi-center, randomized, controlled trial compared traditional tidal volume therapy (12 mL/kg) to low tidal volume therapy (6 mL/kg) in mechanically ventilated patients with ALI/ARDS for 28 days. Results revealed that the traditional tidal volume group had significantly increased in-hospital mortality compared to the low tidal volume group. There was no difference in barotrauma between the groups. In summary, this study demonstrated that lower tidal volumes in ALI/ARDS patients reduced in-hospital mortality and the number of days that patients required mechanical ventilation. Of note, patients in the lower tidal volume group required higher PEEP and had a slight, but significant, respiratory acidosis, both of which resolved after 7 days. This suggested that although lower tidal volumes required a higher respiratory rate to maintain adequate ventilation, its benefits on mortality outweighed the transient acid/base and oxygenation imbalances that were effectively managed with higher PEEP and sodium bicarbonate infusion, respectively.

In-Depth [randomized controlled trial]: This trial was conducted at 10 university centers across the United States from 1996-1999. Eligible patients were above the age of 18, intubated, mechanically ventilated, and had an acute decrease to a P/F ratio (i.e., partial pressure of arterial oxygen to fraction of inspired oxygen) of 300 or less with evidence of bilateral lung edema on recent chest radiograph. Patients with chronic lung disease, high pulmonary capillary wedge pressure or evidence of left atrial hypertension, less than 6 months of estimated survival, and other medical problems that would cause poor respiration or oxygenation were excluded. The authors randomized patients to traditional tidal volume therapy of 12 mL/kg or low tidal volume therapy of 6 mL/kg for 28 days. The investigators tracked patients weekly for a total of 180 days. The primary endpoint was in-hospital mortality, with a significant reduction from 39.8% in the traditional group to 31.0% in the low tidal volume group (p = 0.007, 95%CI 2.4-15.3%). There was also a significant decrease in the number of ventilator-free days in the low tidal volume group (p = 0.007) and in the number of days free from organ failure (p = 0.006).

The Acute Respiratory Distress Syndrome Network. Ventilation with Lower Tidal Volumes as Compared with Traditional Tidal Volumes for Acute Lung Injury and the Acute Respiratory Distress Syndrome. New England Journal of Medicine. 2000 May 4;342(18):1301–8.

The CAPRICORN trial: Carvedilol reduces mortality after acute myocardial infarction

1. Carvedilol reduced mortality from cardiovascular causes and recurrent non-fatal infarction after acute myocardial infarction (MI).

2. While carvedilol treatment was associated with a 23% relative risk reduction in all-cause mortality, this did not reach statistical significance.

3. These findings were consistent with previous trials exploring the benefits of beta-blockers in managing acute myocardial infarction.

Original Date of Publication: May 2001

Study Rundown: While previous studies had established the benefits of beta-blockade in managing MI, these trials were conducted prior to widespread use of thrombolysis or angioplasty for reperfusion as well as prior to the introduction of angiotensin converting enzyme (ACE) inhibitors. Thus, the CAPRICORN trial explored the long-term efficacy of carvedilol in patients suffering from acute MI, taking into account recent advances in management. The trial demonstrated that beta-blockers conferred considerable benefits in patients suffering from acute MI. While carvedilol was associated with a relative risk reduction in all-cause mortality of 23%, this did not reach statistical significance due to statistical adjustment partway through the study. However, carvedilol significantly reduced mortality from cardiovascular causes and recurrent non-fatal MI. While previous studies examined beta-blockade prior to the widespread use of reperfusion and ACE inhibitors in managing MIs, the findings from the CAPRICORN trial are consistent with the older data.

In-Depth [randomized controlled trial]: Patients were included if they were 18 years of age, had suffered a definite MI 3-21 days before randomization, had a left ventricular ejection fraction (LVEF) <40%, and had concurrent treatment with ACE inhibitors for at least 48 hours, unless there was a proven intolerance to ACE inhibitors. They were randomized to either the carvedilol group (maximum dose of 25 mg PO BID) or to placebo. The co-primary endpoints were 1) all-cause mortality and 2) all-cause mortality and cardiovascular hospital admissions. Secondary endpoints were sudden death and hospital admission for heart failure, while other endpoints were recurrent non-fatal MI and all-cause mortality or recurrent non-fatal MI. A total of 1959 patients were recruited from 163 centers in 17 different countries and followed for a mean of 1.3 years. Approximately 46% of patients required reperfusion therapy, largely through thrombolysis, though some did undergo primary angioplasty. Notably, about 98% of patients were taking ACE inhibitors at the time of randomization. While all-cause mortality was reduced by 23% in the carvedilol group, this did not reach statistical significance. There were also no significant differences between the groups in terms of secondary endpoints. Patients in the carvedilol group, however, experienced significantly lower rates of cardiovascular-caused mortality and non-fatal MI.

Dargie HJ. Effect of carvedilol on outcome after myocardial infarction in patients with left-ventricular dysfunction: the CAPRICORN randomised trial. Lancet. 2001 May 5;357(9266):1385–90.

The CURE trial: Clopidogrel reduces mortality after acute coronary syndrome

1. The addition of clopidogrel reduced the risk of death from cardiovascular causes, nonfatal myocardial infarction, or other ischemic events in patients with acute coronary syndrome (ACS) without ST elevation.

2. Adding clopidogrel increased the risk of major and minor bleeding, but not life-threatening bleeding.

Original Date of Publication: August 2001

Study Rundown: ACS refers to symptoms attributed to the occlusion of coronary arteries. ST-segment changes help classify ACS, with ST-elevation suggesting a transmural infarct, which typically requires immediate revascularization. Patients suffering ACS without ST-elevation typically do not undergo urgent revascularization. Prior to the Clopidogrel in Unstable Angina to Prevent Recurrent Events (CURE) trial, therapy for ACS without ST-elevation consisted mainly of aspirin and heparin. The purpose of the CURE trial was to explore whether the addition of clopidogrel, a thienopyridine class antiplatelet agent, could further reduce the risk of recurrent ischemic events in patients suffering from ACS without ST-elevation.

Treatment with clopidogrel resulted in a significantly lower risk of death from cardiovascular causes, nonfatal myocardial infarction, or stroke compared to placebo. Of note, the addition of clopidogrel resulted in significantly higher rates of major and minor bleeding complications, though not life-threatening bleeds. Based on the findings of this study, clopidogrel has become widely used in current ACS practice, in addition to aspirin, heparin, and other medications.

In-Depth [randomized controlled trial]: This randomized, controlled trial compared clopidogrel with placebo in addition to aspirin in patients presenting with acute coronary syndromes without ST-segment elevation. Patients were eligible for the trial if they were hospitalized within 24 hours of symptom onset and did not have ST-segment elevation. Patients with contraindications to antithrombotic or antiplatelet therapy, at high risk of bleeding or severe heart failure, taking oral anticoagulants, and those who had revascularization in the past three months or glycoprotein IIb/IIIa inhibitors in the past 3 days were excluded. The first primary outcome was the composite of death from cardiovascular causes, nonfatal myocardial infarction, or stroke. The second primary outcome was the composite of the first primary outcome with refractory ischemia. Severe ischemia, heart failure and need for revascularization were secondary outcomes and other outcomes were bleeding complications categorized as life threatening, major, or minor.

A total of 12 562 patients from 482 centers in 28 countries were enrolled in the trial. Patients in the clopidogrel group experienced significantly lower rates of the first primary outcome, when compared with patients receiving placebo (RR 0.80; 95%CI 0.72-0.90). The rate of the second primary outcome was also significantly lower in patients treated with clopidogrel (RR 0.86; 95%CI 0.79-0.94). Significantly fewer patients in the clopidogrel group experienced severe ischemia (RR 0.74; 95%CI 0.61-0.90) or recurrent angina (RR 0.91; 95%CI 0.85-0.98). Major bleeding, defined as bleeding requiring transfusion of 2 or more units of blood, was significantly more common in the clopidogrel group (RR 1.38; 95%CI 1.13-1.67).

Yusuf S, Zhao F, Mehta SR, Chrolavicius S, Tognoni G, Fox KK, et al. Effects of clopidogrel in addition to aspirin in patients with acute coronary syndromes without ST-segment elevation. New England Journal of Medicine. 2001 Aug 16;345(7):494–502.

The Rivers trial: Early goal-directed therapy reduces mortality in severe sepsis and septic shock

1. Early goal-directed therapy (EGDT) in patients with severe sepsis and septic shock prior to admission to the intensive care unit was associated with significantly reduced organ dysfunction and mortality rates compared to standard therapy to achieve parameters for hemodynamic support.

Original Date of Publication: November 2001

Study Rundown: Thee systemic inflammatory response syndrome (SIRS) is diagnosed when 2 of the following criteria are present: 1) body temperature <36°C or >38°C, 2) heart rate >90 beats/min, 3) respiratory rate >20 breaths/minute or $PaCO_2 <32$ mmHg, 4) WBC $<4x10^9$/L, WBC $>12x10^9$/L, or $>10\%$ bands. Sepsis refers to SIRS that results from infection and this can progress to severe sepsis (i.e., sepsis with organ dysfunction, hypoperfusion, or hypotension) or septic shock (i.e., severe sepsis with hypotension despite adequate fluid resuscitation). In this spectrum of conditions, circulatory changes may arise, resulting in insufficient oxygen delivery to meet metabolic demands. These changes lead to global tissue hypoxia, which may foreshadow multiorgan failure and death. The onset of global tissue hypoxia represents a turning point in the development of sepsis, where intervention may help to avoid poor outcomes.

Commonly referred to as the Rivers trial, this study sought to explore whether EGDT before admission to the intensive care unit (ICU) could reduce the incidence of multiorgan dysfunction, mortality, and the use of health care resources compared to standard therapy in patients with severe sepsis and septic shock. In summary, patients in the standard therapy group had significantly higher APACHE II, SAPS II, and MODS mortality prediction scores compared to patients receiving EGDT. Moreover, the EGDT group experienced significantly lower in-hospital, 28-day, and 60-day mortality rates when compared to patients undergoing standard therapy. The Rivers trial was criticized for being conducted at a single center. Since the trial, numerous multicenter, randomized, controlled trials have been completed comparing EGDT with usual care and have demonstrated no significant difference between the approaches in terms of outcomes.

In-Depth [randomized controlled trial]: This study, conducted at a single tertiary care center in Detroit, randomized 263 patients to either standard therapy or EGDT for 6 hours prior to ICU admission. Patients were included in the trial if they met SIRS criteria and had a systolic blood pressure ≤90 mmHg or a serum lactate ≥4 mmol/L. Exclusion criteria included age <18 years, pregnancy, or the presence of an acute cerebral vascular event, acute coronary syndrome, acute pulmonary edema, status asthmaticus, cardiac dysrhythmias, contraindication to central venous catheterization, and burn injury, amongst others. Outcome measures included vital signs, resuscitation endpoints, measures of organ dysfunction, and mortality prediction scores (i.e., APACHE II, SAPS II, MODS), and mortality. In the EGDT group, all patients received arterial lines and central venous lines with the ability to monitor central venous oxygen saturation (ScvO2). EGDT involved targeting a series of treatment goals for patients:

1.   Central venous pressure (CVP) ≥8-12 mmHg (through crystalloid boluses)
2.   Mean arterial pressure (MAP) ≥65 mmHg (through vasopressor administration)
3.   Urine output ≥0.5 mL/kg/hour
4.   ScvO2 ≥70% (through transfusion of red cells and dobutamine)

After the initial 6-hour period, patients receiving standard therapy had significantly higher APACHE II, SAPS II, and MODS compared to those receiving EGDT ($p < 0.001$ for all comparisons), suggesting higher levels of organ dysfunction in the standard therapy group. Moreover, in-hospital mortality rates (RR 0.58; 95%CI 0.38-0.87), 28-day mortality (RR 0.58; 95%CI 0.39-0.87), and 60-day mortality (RR 0.67; 95%CI 0.46-0.96) were all significantly lower in the EGDT group. There were no significant differences between the groups in terms of measures of health care resource consumption (i.e., mean duration of vasopressor therapy, mechanical ventilation, hospital stay).

Rivers E, Nguyen B, Havstad S, Ressler J, Muzzin A, Knoblich B, et al. Early Goal-Directed Therapy in the Treatment of Severe Sepsis and Septic Shock. New England Journal of Medicine. 2001 Nov 8;345(19):1368–77.

Mild hypothermia improves neurological outcome after cardiac arrest

1. Initiation of a hypothermia protocol for 24 hours after a cardiac arrest significantly improved neurological outcome in surviving patients compared to the normothermia group.

2. Patients who underwent the hypothermia protocol had a significantly lower mortality rate at 6 months.

3. There were no significant differences in adverse outcomes between the groups.

Original Date of Publication: February 2002

Study Rundown: This landmark trial demonstrated that inducing mild hypothermia early in patients who suffered a cardiac arrest reduced permanent neurological damage secondary to global cerebral ischemia. The subjects who underwent cooling within 4 hours of cardiac arrest experienced superior neurological outcomes (according to the Pittsburgh cerebral performance scale) as well as a lower mortality rate 6 months out from the event. There was no difference in adverse outcomes between the groups in the first 7 days after the event, although data showed a trend toward susceptibility to infections in the hypothermia group. The subjects in the normothermia group had a higher prevalence of diabetes mellitus and coronary artery disease compared to the hypothermia group; however, controlling for these baseline differences did not alter the study findings. While the study was not blinded, neurological assessment 6 months after therapy was blinded. The time to initiation of the hypothermia protocol also varied within the group, ranging from 61 to 192 minutes, with a median of 105 minutes. In summary, patients who underwent cooling within 4 hours after a cardiac arrest from ventricular fibrillation experienced a significantly higher rate of favorable neurological outcomes compared to the patients who underwent standard normothermia treatment.

In-Depth [randomized controlled trial]: The trial assigned 275 patients arriving to the ED with a cardiac arrest due to ventricular fibrillation to either standard normothermia or to a mild hypothermia protocol. Eligible subjects were patients between 18-75 years of age who had suffered a cardiac arrest from ventricular fibrillation and had an estimated 5-15 minute delay before cardiac resuscitation was started. Patients with coagulopathies, pregnancy, terminal illness, other causes of cardiac arrest, in a coma state at baseline, or hypotensive or hypoxic for 30 minutes or 15 minutes, respectively, prior to randomization were excluded. The group assigned to mild hypothermia treatment was cooled to a target temperature between 32°C to 34°C with the use of an external cooling device and ice packs, if necessary. Investigators maintained the temperature at 32°C to 34°C for 24 hours, and followed with passive rewarming, which averaged out to an 8-hour period.

The study demonstrated that the group assigned to mild hypothermia treatment experienced a significantly higher rate of favorable neurological outcomes (as assessed blindly 6 months later via the Pittsburgh cerebral performance scale) compared to the group that underwent standard normothermia treatment (55% vs. 39%, RR 1.40; 95%CI 1.08-1.81). The hypothermia group also had a significantly lower 6-month mortality rate compared to the normothermia group (RR 0.74; 95%CI 0.58-0.95). There were no significant differences in complication rates in the first 7 days after randomization between the groups.

Hypothermia after Cardiac Arrest Study Group. Mild Therapeutic Hypothermia to Improve the Neurologic Outcome after Cardiac Arrest. New England Journal of Medicine. 2002 Feb 21;346(8):549–56.

The SAFE trial: Normal saline vs. albumin for fluid resuscitation

1. There was no significant difference in 28-day mortality when comparing albumin and normal saline for fluid resuscitation in the intensive care unit (ICU) setting.

2. Compared to normal saline, fluid resuscitation with albumin did not yield any significant benefits in terms of secondary outcomes (i.e., length of ICU/hospital stay, duration of supportive treatment measures).

Original Date of Publication: May 2004

Study Rundown: In various types of shock, resuscitation with intravenous fluids helps to maintain circulating pressure and tissue perfusion. A myriad of options are available for fluid resuscitation, including blood products, non-blood products, or a combination. Crystalloid and colloid solutions are classes of fluids that may be used. Crystalloid solutions are composed of sterile water and electrolytes, in concentrations that are similar to human serum. Colloids contain an additional colloidal substance (e.g., albumin, dextran) that does not cross semi-permeable membranes. As a result, colloids are more effective at maintaining intravascular volume. While studies have demonstrated that crystalloids and colloids have different effects on physiological measures, it remains uncertain which may be more beneficial in reducing mortality. This is an important consideration because colloid solutions are more expensive than crystalloids. Moreover, previous systematic reviews reached conflicting conclusions, with studies suggesting albumin-containing solutions were linked with increased mortality and others suggesting there was no significant difference when compared to crystalloids.

The Saline versus Albumin Fluid Evaluation (SAFE) trial was a randomized, controlled trial designed to explore whether the use of 4% albumin led to any significant difference in mortality when compared with 0.9% sodium chloride (i.e., normal saline) in intensive care settings. The trial found no significant difference between the groups in 28-day mortality. Moreover, there were no differences between the groups in length of ICU/hospital stay, duration of mechanical ventilation, or duration of renal replacement therapy.

In-Depth [randomized controlled trial]: This study was conducted in 16 tertiary intensive care units in Australia and New Zealand. Patients were eligible if they were ≥18 years of age, were admitted to intensive care, and required fluid administration. Patients were excluded if they were admitted after cardiac surgery, liver transplantation, or for burns treatment. A total of 6997 patients were randomized to receive either 4 percent albumin or normal saline. Fluids were provided in identical 500 mL bottles. The primary outcome measure was death from any cause in the first 28 days after randomization, while secondary outcomes included the duration of mechanical ventilation, the duration of renal replacement therapy, and the duration of ICU/hospital stay. There was no significant difference between the albumin and saline groups in 28-day mortality (RR 0.99; 95%CI 0.91-1.09). Moreover, there were no significant differences between the groups in terms of length of ICU stay (p = 0.44), length of hospital stay (p = 0.30), duration of mechanical ventilation (p = 0.74), or duration of renal replacement therapy (p = 0.41).

Finfer S, Bellomo R, Boyce N, French J, Myburgh J, Norton R, et al. A comparison of albumin and saline for fluid resuscitation in the intensive care unit. New England Journal of Medicine. 2004 May 27;350(22):2247–56.

The ICTUS trial: Early invasive vs selectively invasive management for acute coronary syndrome

1. There was no significant difference in the composite rate of death, nonfatal myocardial infarction (MI), or rehospitalization for angina in patients with acute coronary syndrome (ACS) treated with early invasive or selectively invasive strategies.

2. Myocardial infarction was significantly more frequent in the early invasive management group but rehospitalization was significantly less frequent in this group.

Original Date of Publication: September 2005

Study Rundown: Guidelines of the American College of Cardiology-American Heart Association and European Society of Cardiology recommend an early invasive strategy for the treatment of ACS without ST-segment elevation. The Invasive versus Conservative Treatment in Unstable Coronary Syndromes (ICTUS) trial suggested that selectively invasive management may be an acceptable alternative approach to treatment. With advances in medical therapy and higher rates of revascularization, patients treated with the selectively invasive strategy showed no difference in the cumulative rate of death, nonfatal MI, or rehospitalization for angina 1 year after randomization. These results suggest that an early invasive strategy may not be superior to a selectively invasive strategy for the treatment of ACS without ST-segment elevation and with elevated cardiac troponin T levels.

In-Depth [randomized controlled trial]: The authors assigned 1200 patients with ACS without ST-segment elevation and with elevated cardiac troponin T levels to management with early invasive strategy or selectively invasive strategies. Both treatment groups received optimized medical therapy. The early invasive strategy involved angiography within 24 to 48 hours of randomization and percutaneous coronary intervention when appropriate. Patients assigned to selectively invasive management were scheduled for angiography and revascularization only if symptoms persisted despite medical therapy or if patients showed hemodynamic or rhythmic instability. A composite of death, recurrent MI or rehospitalization for angina within 1 year was measured as the primary endpoint. There was no significant difference in the cumulative event rate at 1 year between the groups (RR 1.07; 95%CI 0.87-1.33; p = 0.33).

Mortality 1 year after randomization was 2.5% in both groups. The risk of MI was significantly higher in the early invasive strategy group (p = 0.005), while rehospitalization was significantly less frequent in this group (p = 0.04).

De Winter RJ, Windhausen F, Cornel JH, Dunselman PHJM, Janus CL, Bendermacher PEF, et al. Early Invasive versus Selectively Invasive Management for Acute Coronary Syndromes. New England Journal of Medicine. 2005 Sep 15;353(11):1095–104.

The TORCH trial: Combination of salmeterol and fluticasone in COPD

1. The combination of salmeterol and fluticasone did not significantly reduce all-cause mortality in patients with chronic obstructive pulmonary disease (COPD).

2. When compared with salmeterol alone, fluticasone alone, and placebo, combination therapy significantly reduced the risk of exacerbations and the need for systemic corticosteroids during exacerbations.

Original Date of Publication: February 2007

Study Rundown: The Towards a Revolution in COPD Health (TORCH) trial explored whether combination therapy with salmeterol (a long-acting beta-agonist) and fluticasone propionate (an inhaled corticosteroid) would significantly reduce mortality in patients with COPD as compared with placebo. This landmark study determined that combination therapy was not significantly associated with a reduced all-cause mortality when compared with placebo. Treatment with combination therapy, however, significantly reduced the risk of moderate or severe COPD exacerbations, as well as the likelihood that patients would require systemic corticosteroids during their exacerbations when compared with placebo.

In-Depth [randomized controlled trial]: A total of 6184 COPD patients were randomized to 4 different treatment arms: 1) 1545 were randomized to the placebo group, 2) 1542 were randomized to the salmeterol-only group, 3) 1551 were randomized to the fluticasone-only group, and 4) 1546 were randomized to the combination therapy group (i.e., salmeterol and fluticasone). Eligible patients had at least a 10 pack-year smoking history, were between 40-80 years old, diagnosed with COPD, exhibited a pre-bronchodilator forced expiratory volume in 1 second (FEV1) of less than 60% of the predicted value, showed an increase in FEV1 with use of 400 mcg of albuterol of less than 10% of the predicted value, and had a ratio of pre-bronchodilator FEV1 to forced vital capacity (FVC) of equal to or less than 0.70. Patients were excluded if they had a non-COPD pulmonary condition (e.g., lung cancer, sarcoidosis, asthma), prior lung-volume-reduction surgery or lung transplant, long term supplemental oxygen (i.e., greater than or equal to 12 hours/day), less than 6 weeks of oral corticosteroids, serious uncontrolled disease, received any investigational drugs in the 4 weeks prior to entry, evidence of alcohol or drug abuse, known hypersensitivity to inhaled corticosteroids, bronchodilators, or lactose, or known deficiency of alpha-1 anti-trypsin.

There was no significant difference in all-cause mortality between patients in the combination therapy group compared to the placebo group (HR 0.825; 95%CI 0.681-1.002). While there was no significant difference in all-cause mortality when comparing combination therapy with salmeterol-only therapy (HR 0.932, 95%CI 0.765-1.134), combination therapy was linked to significant reduction in all-cause mortality when compared with fluticasone alone (HR 0.774; 95%CI 0.641-0.934). Combination therapy was also associated with a significantly reduced risk of moderate or severe exacerbation as compared with salmeterol-only (HR 0.88; 95%CI 0.81-0.95), fluticasone-only (HR 0.91; 95%CI 0.84-0.99), and placebo (HR 0.75; 95%CI 0.69-0.81). Moreover, combination therapy was linked to a significant reduction in the risk of exacerbations requiring systemic corticosteroids compared to salmeterol-only (HR 0.71; 95%CI 0.63-0.79), fluticasone-only (HR 0.87; 95%CI 0.78-0.98), and placebo (HR 0.57; 95%CI 0.51-0.64).

Calverley PMA, Anderson JA, Celli B, Ferguson GT, Jenkins C, Jones PW, et al. Salmeterol and Fluticasone Propionate and Survival in Chronic Obstructive Pulmonary Disease. New England Journal of Medicine. 2007 Feb 22;356(8):775–89.

The **CORTICUS** trial: Hydrocortisone does not reduce mortality in septic shock

1. In patients with septic shock, there was no significant difference in mortality between groups receiving low-dose hydrocortisone compared to placebo.

2. Hydrocortisone therapy was linked to a quicker reversal of shock, but an increased frequency of superinfection.

Original Date of Publication: January 2008

Study Rundown: Recommendations that patients with septic shock be treated with low-dose corticosteroids were based on a limited set of evidence and largely dependent on a single trial. Although insufficiently powered, the Corticosteroid Therapy of Septic Shock (CORTICUS) study was the largest trial to date investigating the use of hydrocortisone in patients with septic shock. The results of the study pointed to a lack of benefit of hydrocortisone therapy in patients with septic shock. It also suggested that response to a corticotropin test is not a useful prognostic factor for response to hydrocortisone. In summary, hydrocortisone therapy did not reduce mortality in this group of patients with septic shock and therapy may be associated with increased incidence of superinfection.

In-Depth [randomized controlled trial]: The authors randomly assigned 499 patients with septic shock to receive low-dose hydrocortisone therapy or placebo. All patients were assessed for a response to a corticotropin test. The primary end point was the rate of death at 28 days in patients without a response to corticotropin. There was no significant difference in the primary outcome between the hydrocortisone and placebo groups (39.2% vs. 36.1%, respectively; $p = 0.69$). There was also no significant difference in the rate of death at 28 days in patients who responded to corticotropin, nor was there a significant difference in overall deaths between the study groups (34.3% vs. 31.5%; $p = 0.51$). Time to reversal of shock was shorter in the hydrocortisone group than the placebo group (3.3 days vs. 5.8 days for all patients). There was a higher incidence of superinfections in the hydrocortisone group, including new episodes of sepsis and septic shock (OR 1.37; 95%CI 1.05-1.79).

Sprung CL, Annane D, Keh D, Moreno R, Singer M, Freivogel K, et al. Hydrocortisone Therapy for Patients with Septic Shock. New England Journal of Medicine. 2008 Jan 10;358(2):111–24.

The ACCORD trial: Intensive glucose control associated with increased mortality

1. Previous studies linked intensive blood glucose control to a reduced risk of microvascular complications. However, questions remained regarding the impact on macrovascular complications and mortality.

2. This study found that targeting HbA1c <6.0% resulted in a higher risk of cardiovascular and all-cause mortality as compared with standard therapy (i.e., targeting HbA1c between 7.0-7.9%).

Original Date of Publication: June 2008

Study Rundown: The Action to Control Cardiovascular Risk in Diabetes (ACCORD) trial sought to explore whether more intensive glucose control regimens were associated with better outcomes in patients with type 2 diabetes mellitus. Prior to the ACCORD trial, several randomized controlled trials examined blood sugar control in type 2 diabetics. The University Group Diabetes Program (UGDP) study, a randomized controlled trial conducted in 1970, suggested that there was no benefit of glycemic control in new-onset type 2 diabetics. Subsequently, a second randomized trial conducted in Japan demonstrated a reduction in the incidence of microvascular complications with better blood sugar control, while a third demonstrated no significant reduction in cardiovascular events in patients with better blood sugar control. Perhaps the most notable study, however, was the UK Prospective Diabetes Study (UKPDS), a randomized, controlled trial involving 5102 patients with newly diagnosed type 2 diabetes. The study was conducted over a 20-year period (1977-1997) and conclusively demonstrated that microvascular complications were reduced by intensively controlling blood glucose. Despite these studies, however, there was no sufficiently powered, randomized trial explicitly examining the effect of intensive glucose control on cardiovascular outcomes. Thus, the aim of the ACCORD trial was to determine whether intensive therapy to control blood glucose levels (targeting HbA1c <6.0%) in type 2 diabetics would reduce cardiovascular events, compared to standard therapy (targeting HbA1c from 7.0-7.9%). In summary, this trial demonstrated that intensive glucose lowering significantly increases the risk of cardiovascular and all-cause mortality as compared with standard therapy.

In-Depth [randomized controlled trial]: The study spanned 77 centers across Canada and the United States. Patients were eligible for the trial if they had type 2 diabetes and an HbA1c ≥7.5%. Moreover, eligible patients were either between 40-79 years of age with cardiovascular disease or 55-79 years of age with anatomical evidence of atherosclerosis, albuminuria, left ventricular hypertrophy, or ≥2 additional risk factors for cardiovascular disease (i.e., dyslipidemia, hypertension, current smoker, or obesity). Investigators randomized patients to two different treatment arms: 1) intensive therapy targeting HbA1c <6.0% or 2) standard therapy targeting HbA1c between 7.0-7.9%. The primary outcome was nonfatal myocardial infarction (MI), nonfatal stroke, or death from cardiovascular causes. Secondary outcomes included all-cause mortality. A total of 10,251 participants were involved in the final analyses. There was no significant difference in the composite primary outcome between the study groups (HR 0.90; 95%CI 0.78-1.04), though the intensive group experienced significantly fewer nonfatal MIs (HR 0.76; 95%CI 0.62-0.92) and significantly more deaths from cardiovascular causes (HR 1.35; 95%CI 1.04-1.76). All-cause mortality was significantly higher in the intensive group (HR 1.22; 95%CI 1.01-1.46). Notably, there were significantly more instances of hypoglycemia in the intensive therapy group as compared with standard therapy (16.2% vs. 5.1%, $p < 0.001$).

Action to Control Cardiovascular Risk in Diabetes Study Group, Gerstein HC, Miller ME, Byington RP, Goff DC, Bigger JT, et al. Effects of intensive glucose lowering in type 2 diabetes. New England Journal of Medicine. 2008 Jun 12;358(24):2545–59.

The ECASS III trial: Administering alteplase up to 4.5 hours after onset of acute ischemic stroke improves neurological outcomes

1. Alteplase administered between 3 to 4.5 hours after the onset of acute ischemic stroke was associated with improved functional outcomes at 90 days, compared to placebo.

Original Date of Publication: September 2008

Study Rundown: Previously, the National Institute of Neurological Disorders and Stroke (NINDS) trial demonstrated that, compared to placebo, treatment of acute ischemic stroke with tissue plasminogen activator (t-PA) within 3 hours of symptom onset significantly improved functional outcomes 3 months after the incident. However, there remained uncertainty regarding the efficacy and safety of administering t-PA more than 3 hours after the onset of acute ischemic stroke. Two previous European trials (i.e., ECASS I and II) had investigated the use of alteplase up to 6 hours after the onset of stroke, but these studies did not demonstrate any benefits. The ECASS III trial was a randomized, controlled trial designed to explore the efficacy and safety of utilizing alteplase, a recombinant t-PA, 3 to 4.5 hours after the onset of stroke.

Treating acute ischemic stroke patients with intravenous alteplase 3 to 4.5 hours after the onset of symptoms significantly improved neurological outcomes at 3 months compared to placebo. While patients in the alteplase group experienced a significantly higher risk of intracranial hemorrhage, mortality was not significantly different between the groups. Some clinicians criticized the trial for excluding patients with severe stroke signs and for a change of protocol during the trial. Regardless, its findings have informed practice as current recommendations suggest administering recombinant t-PA up to 4.5 hours after the onset of acute ischemic stroke.

In-Depth [randomized controlled trial]: This double-blind, placebo-controlled trial examined the use of alteplase at a dose of 0.9 mg/kg. Patients were eligible for the trial if they had a stroke with a clearly defined time of onset, a measurable deficit, and a computed tomographic scan of the brain that demonstrated no evidence of intracranial hemorrhage at baseline. Exclusion criteria included stroke or serious head trauma in the preceding 3 months, major surgery in the past 14 days, history of intracranial hemorrhage, rapidly improving or minor symptoms, and seizure at the onset of stroke. The study involved 821 patients and had a primary outcome measure of disability at 90 days, as assessed using the modified Rankin Scale. The secondary outcome measure was a global measure at 90 days as determined using the modified Rankin Scale, Barthel Index, NIHSS, and Glasgow Outcome Scale. Safety outcomes included mortality at 90 days, intracranial hemorrhage (any, symptomatic), symptomatic edema, or other events. Patients in the alteplase group were significantly more likely to have favorable outcomes of both the primary and secondary outcomes when compared to the placebo group. Patients in the alteplase group, however, experienced a significantly higher risk of intracranial hemorrhage, including symptomatic intracranial hemorrhage, in the first 36 hours after treatment ($p < 0.001$). There were no significant differences between the groups in terms of mortality.

Hacke W, Kaste M, Bluhmki E, Brozman M, Dávalos A, Guidetti D, et al. Thrombolysis with Alteplase 3 to 4.5 Hours after Acute Ischemic Stroke. New England Journal of Medicine. 2008 Sep 25;359(13):1317–29.

The UPLIFT trial: Tiotropium improves quality of life in chronic obstructive pulmonary disease

1. Tiotropium did not reduce the mean rate of decline in forced expiratory volume in 1 second (FEV1), a common metric of chronic obstructive pulmonary disease (COPD) progression.

2. Tiotropium significantly improved patient quality of life, mean FEV1, and decreased the incidence of disease exacerbation.

Original Date of Publication: October 2008

Study Rundown: Clinicians can assess COPD by measuring the rate of decline in a patient's FEV1. Previous studies found that at 1 year after initiation, tiotropium, a once-daily, inhaled anticholinergic drug, reduced the decline in FEV1 in contrast to shorter-acting anticholinergic drugs, inhaled corticosteroids, or the mucolytic agent N-acetylcysteine. The Understanding Potential Long-Term Impacts on Function with Tiotropium (UPLIFT) trial assessed the longer-term effects of tiotropium by extending its treatment period to 4 years. The study revealed that in patients with COPD who were permitted to use any respiratory medication concomitantly except other anticholinergic drugs, tiotropium was associated with improved lung function, improved quality of life, and a decreased incidence of disease exacerbation, but ultimately did not slow the rate of decline in FEV1. Study limitations included a relatively high drop-out rate in both the placebo group (44.6%) and tiotropium group (36.2%). Additionally, the study's subjects were predominantly male (75%), limiting generalizability. Tiotropium's main disadvantage is that it is more costly than other alternatives. Given that tiotropium did not affect the rate of disease progression, its use may be better suited to preventing disease exacerbation in patients with moderate or severe cases of COPD. Finally, since patients could not use other inhaled anticholinergics during the study, the study could not compare the efficacy of tiotropium with that of other anticholinergics.

In-Depth [randomized controlled trial]: UPLIFT was a 4-year, randomized, double-blinded trial involving 5993 patients recruited from 490 centers in 37 countries. Of the recruited patients, only 3535 completed the study. Patients with a diagnosis of COPD, age ≥ 40 years, a smoking history of >10 pack-years, a post-bronchodilator FEV1 $\leq 70\%$, and an FEV1 $\leq 70\%$ of the forced vital capacity (FVC) were eligible for the study. Exclusion criteria included a history of asthma, COPD exacerbation, or pulmonary infection. The investigators randomized patients to receive either tiotropium or placebo. All other respiratory medications except inhaled anticholinergic drugs were permitted. The primary endpoint was the rate of decline in the mean FEV1 before and after bronchodilation at day 30. Secondary endpoints include changes in quality of life (as measured by St. George's Respiratory Questionnaire), exacerbations of COPD, and death from any cause. The mean FEV1 values were significantly improved in the tiotropium group at all time points compared to the control, although the mean decline in FEV1 was not significantly different before bronchodilation (p = 0.95) or after bronchodilation (p = 0.21). The incidence of COPD exacerbation decreased significantly with tiotropium treatment compared to placebo (HR 0.96, p < 0.001), while the difference in quality of life also favored tiotropium (p < 0.001). However, the incidence of death from any cause was not significantly different between the groups (HR=0.89, p = 0.09).

Tashkin DP, Celli B, Senn S, Burkhart D, Kesten S, Menjoge S, et al. A 4-Year Trial of Tiotropium in Chronic Obstructive Pulmonary Disease. New England Journal of Medicine. 2008 Oct 9;359(15):1543–54.

The NICE-SUGAR trial: Intensive glycemic control harmful in the intensive care unit

1. Intensive glycemic control in critically ill patients significantly increased 90-day mortality when compared to conventional glycemic control.

2. The incidence of severe hypoglycemia was significantly higher in patients receiving intensive glycemic control.

Original Date of Publication: March 2009

Study Rundown: In the intensive care unit (ICU), hyperglycemia is a common problem that is associated with increased morbidity and mortality. Previously conducted trials, systematic reviews, and meta-analyses reached conflicting conclusions on the effects of intensive glycemic control. Different groups, however, recommended intensive control for critically ill patients. The Normoglycemia in Intensive Care Evaluation-Survival Using Glucose Algorithm Regulation (NICE-SUGAR) trial sought to determine the impacts of intensive glycemic control on mortality in ICU patients. The trial demonstrated that intensive glucose control to target 81-108 mg/dL (4.5-6.0 mmol/L) was associated with a significantly increased 90-day mortality when compared to conventional glucose control to target ≤180 mg/dL (10.0 mmol/L). Moreover, the risk of severe hypoglycemia was significantly higher in the intensive control group. Based on the findings of this study, intensive glucose control was not recommended for patients in the ICU.

In-Depth [randomized controlled trial]: The study involved 6104 participants recruited from 42 hospitals from across Australia, New Zealand, and Canada. Patients were eligible if they stayed a minimum of 3 consecutive days in the ICU. Investigators randomly assigned patients to either intensive glucose control (target blood glucose between 81-108 mg/dL, or 4.5-6.0 mmol/L) or conventional glucose control (target blood glucose ≤180 mg/dL, or ≤10 mmol/L). Glucose control was achieved through insulin infusion as needed. The intervention was stopped when the patient was eating or discharged from the ICU. The primary outcome was death from any cause within 90 days after randomization. Secondary outcomes included survival time in the first 90 days, cause-specific death, and durations of mechanical ventilation/renal replacement therapy/ICU stay/hospital stay. Intensive glucose control was associated with significantly increased risk of mortality at day 90 when compared to conventional control (OR 1.14; 95%CI 1.02-1.28; ARI 2.6%, NNH 38). The incidence of severe hypoglycemia was significantly higher in patients undergoing intensive glucose control (OR 14.7; 95%CI 9.0-25.9). There were no significant differences between the groups in mechanical ventilation (p = 0.56) or renal replacement therapy requirements (p = 0.39). Moreover, there were no differences between the groups in terms of duration of ICU (p = 0.84) or hospital stay (p = 0.86).

NICE-SUGAR Study Investigators, Finfer S, Chittock DR, Su SY-S, Blair D, Foster D, et al. Intensive versus conventional glucose control in critically ill patients. New England Journal of Medicine. 2009 Mar 26;360(13):1283–97.

The SOAP-II trial: First-line vasopressor for shock management

1. There was no significant difference in 28-day, 6-month, or 12-month mortality when comparing dopamine and norepinephrine as first-line vasopressors in managing shock.

2. Dopamine was associated with a significantly higher rate of arrhythmias and severe arrhythmias when compared to norepinephrine.

Original Date of Publication: March 2010

Study Rundown: The Sepsis Occurrence in Acutely Ill Patients II (SOAP-II) trial compared the use of norepinephrine and dopamine as first-line agents in treating patients suffering from circulatory shock. At the time, guidelines and recommendations suggested that either agent may be used as the first-line vasopressor. Some studies, however, had suggested that dopamine use was a predictor of mortality in shock. The SOAP-II trial demonstrated that there were no significant differences in mortality when comparing dopamine and norepinephrine as first-line vasopressors. Dopamine, however, was associated with a significantly higher rate of arrhythmias, as well as severe arrhythmias that led to withholding of the study drug. Moreover, the study demonstrated significantly increased 28-day mortality with dopamine use in a pre-specified subgroup of patients who had cardiogenic shock. These findings challenged the American College of Cardiology-American Heart Association recommendation at the time, which suggested using dopamine as the first-line agent in patients suffering from acute myocardial infarction and hypotension.

In-Depth [randomized controlled trial]: A total of 1679 patients were enrolled from 8 centers in Belgium, Austria, and Spain and randomized to receive dopamine or norepinephrine dosed by body weight. Patients were eligible if they were $\geq$18 years of age and required a vasopressor for treatment of shock. Shock was defined as a mean arterial pressure <70 mmHg or systolic blood pressure <100 mmHg, despite adequate fluid resuscitation, and clinical signs of tissue hypoperfusion (e.g., altered mental state, mottled skin, urine output <0.5 mL/kg/hour). The primary outcome was 28-day mortality, while secondary outcomes included mortality in the intensive care unit (ICU), in hospital mortality, 6- and 12-month mortality, and days requiring ICU care or organ support. There were no significant differences between the groups in terms of 28-day mortality, mortality in the ICU, or mortality in hospital at 6 and 12 months. There were no significant differences between the groups in terms of number of days requiring ICU care or organ support. The study demonstrated a significantly higher incidence of arrhythmias in the dopamine group compared to the norepinephrine group (24.1% vs. 12.4%, p < 0.001). The dopamine group also experienced a significantly higher incidence of severe arrhythmia, which necessitated stopping the study drug (6.1% vs. 1.6%, p < 0.001). In the pre-specified subgroup of patients suffering cardiogenic shock, 28-day mortality was significantly higher in the dopamine group compared to the norepinephrine group (p = 0.03).

De Backer D, Biston P, Devriendt J, Madl C, Chochrad D, Aldecoa C, et al. Comparison of Dopamine and Norepinephrine in the Treatment of Shock. New England Journal of Medicine. 2010 Mar 4;362(9):779–89.

The CRASH-2 trial: Tranexamic acid reduces mortality in trauma patients

1. Tranexamic acid significantly reduced all-cause mortality in trauma patients with significant hemorrhage, compared to placebo.

2. There were no significant differences in the incidence of vascular occlusive events or the need for transfusion or surgery between the tranexamic acid and placebo groups.

Original Date of Publication: July 2010

Study Rundown: While prior studies demonstrated the benefit of tranexamic acid to manage surgical bleeding, no randomized trials had explored its use in managing trauma patients. The Clinical Randomisation of an Antifibrinolytic in Significant Hemorrhage (CRASH)-2 trial demonstrated that using tranexamic acid in trauma patients suffering from significant hemorrhage reduced all-cause mortality without any significant increase in the incidence of fatal or non-fatal vascular occlusive events. Subsequent analyses of the CRASH-2 trial data demonstrated that tranexamic acid should be delivered as soon as possible, as it is much less effective when given more than 3 hours following the injury. Given its effectiveness and cost-effectiveness, authors of the CRASH-2 trial successfully petitioned for tranexamic acid to be added to the World Health Organization's List of Essential Medicines.

In-Depth [randomized controlled trial]: A total of 20 211 patients were drawn from 274 hospitals in 40 countries and randomized as part of the study. Patients were eligible if they suffered, or were at risk of, significant hemorrhage (i.e., systolic blood pressure <90 mmHg, or heart rate >110 beats per minute, or both) within 8 hours of injury. Only patients in which the responsible physician was uncertain about whether to treat with tranexamic acid were eligible; patients with clear indications or contraindications were excluded. Patients were randomized to placebo or tranexamic acid. Those in the tranexamic acid group received a loading dose of 1 g infused intravenously over 10 minutes, followed by 1 g over 8 hours. The primary outcome was death in hospital within 4 weeks of injury, while secondary outcomes included vascular occlusive events, surgical intervention, receipt of blood transfusion, and the number of units of blood products transfused. Tranexamic acid significantly reduced all-cause mortality compared to placebo (RR 0.91; 95%CI 0.85-0.97). In particular, patients in the tranexamic group had a significantly lower risk of death secondary to bleeding (RR 0.85; 95%CI 0.76-0.96). There were no significant differences between the groups in the risk of fatal or non-fatal vascular occlusive events or need for transfusion of blood products or surgery.

CRASH-2 trial collaborators, Shakur H, Roberts I, Bautista R, Caballero J, Coats T, et al. Effects of tranexamic acid on death, vascular occlusive events, and blood transfusion in trauma patients with significant haemorrhage (CRASH-2): a randomised, placebo-controlled trial. Lancet. 2010 Jul 3;376(9734):23–32.

The ACURASYS trial:
Neuromuscular blockade in early acute respiratory distress syndrome

1. In patients with severe acute respiratory distress syndrome (ARDS), treatment with neuromuscular blockade in the first 48 hours significantly reduced 90-day and 28-day mortality, compared to placebo.

2. The treatment group experienced significantly lower rates of barotrauma.

3. There were no differences between the groups in the rate of intensive care unit (ICU)-acquired paresis.

Original Date of Publication: September 2010

Study Rundown: ARDS is characterized by hypoxemic respiratory failure, bilateral chest infiltrates, and high mortality. While the ARMA trial had demonstrated that lung-protective mechanical ventilation was effective, no other measures had convincingly reduced mortality from ARDS at the time of this study. The ARDS et Curarisation Systematique (ACURASYS) trial was conducted to evaluate if early treatment of ARDS with cisatracurium besylate, a neuromuscular blocker, would significantly improve outcomes. In summary, treating patients with severe ARDS with neuromuscular blockade in the first 48 hours of onset significantly reduced 90- and 28-day mortality. Patients receiving neuromuscular blockade also experienced significantly lower rates of barotrauma, while there were no significant differences between the groups in the rate of ICU-acquired paresis. One criticism of the study is that the authors did not use train-of-four stimulation to assess the extent of neuromuscular blockade, and based their dosing solely on a previous smaller study.

In-Depth [randomized controlled trial]: A total of 340 patients from 40 ICUs across France enrolled in the trial. Patients were eligible for the trial if they were receiving invasive mechanical ventilation, had acute hypoxemic respiratory failure, and met severe ARDS criteria (i.e., $PaO_2:FiO_2$ ratio <150 with positive end-expiratory pressure ≥ 5 cm H_2O, tidal volumes between 6-8 mL/kg, bilateral pulmonary infiltrates, non-cardiogenic edema) for ≤ 48 hours. Exclusion criteria included age <18 years, treatment with neuromuscular blockade at enrollment, known pregnancy, increased intracranial pressure, severe chronic liver disease, bone-marrow transplantation or chemotherapy-induced neutropenia, and pneumothorax, amongst others. Investigators randomized patients to receive cisatracurium besylate (15 mg rapid infusion, followed by continuous infusion of 37.5 mg/hour) or a placebo infusion. The primary outcomes were in-hospital and 90-day mortality. The secondary outcomes included 28-day mortality, the rate of barotrauma, and the rate of ICU-acquired paresis.

The only baseline difference between the groups was a significantly lower $PaO_2:FiO_2$ ratio in the cisatracurium group compared to the placebo group (p = 0.03). After adjusting for baseline $PaO_2:FiO_2$, treatment with cisatracurium significantly reduced 90-day mortality compared to placebo (HR 0.68; 95%CI 0.48-0.98). Moreover, 28-day mortality was also significantly lower in the cisatracurium group (ARR -9.6%; 95%CI -19.2 to -0.2%). Patients in the cisatracurium group also had significantly lower rates of barotrauma (RR 0.43; 95%CI 0.20-0.93) and ICU-acquired paresis (p = 0.51) compared to patients receiving placebo.

Papazian L, Forel J-M, Gacouin A, Penot-Ragon C, Perrin G, Loundou A, et al. Neuromuscular Blockers in Early Acute Respiratory Distress Syndrome. New England Journal of Medicine. 2010 Sep 16;363(12):1107–16.

The LACTATE trial: Early lactate-guided therapy in intensive care patients

1. Therapy aimed at reducing lactate levels by 20% every 2 hours during the first 8 hours of intensive care unit (ICU) admission reduced in-hospital mortality and decreased ICU stays.

2. Patients in the early lactate-guided therapy group received more fluids and started on vasopressors earlier than in the control group, but did not have a faster reduction rate of lactate levels.

Original Date of Publication: September 2010

Study Rundown: Elevated blood lactate levels are a known prognostic factor for morbidity and mortality in the ICU. This multi-center, open-label, randomized controlled trial compared standard early goal-directed therapy (EGDT) to EGDT combined with early lactate-guided therapy in patients admitted to the ICU with increased lactate levels. The goal of early lactate-guided therapy was to reduce the lactate level by at least 20% every 2 hours during the first 8 hours of admission in hopes of reducing end-organ damage and improving outcomes in the ICU. The trial found that lactate-guided therapy significantly reduced in-hospital mortality, mechanical ventilation, and ICU stay. There was no difference in the time to stopping vasopressors or in the initiation of renal replacement therapy. In summary, this study demonstrated that frequent monitoring of lactate levels (every 2 hours), with the goal of reducing levels by 20% per 2 hours, during the initial 8 hours of admission to the ICU was beneficial to patients. Of note, there was no significant difference in the rate of lactate reduction between the groups, despite more aggressive fluid and vasopressor resuscitation in the lactate group. This suggested that trending lactate levels early on may be useful as an indicator of improvement, or lack thereof, in a patient undergoing aggressive resuscitation in the ICU.

In-Depth [randomized controlled trial]: This trial was conducted at 4 ICUs across the Netherlands between 2006 and 2008. Eligible patients were all ICU patients above the age of 18 with a lactate level at or above 3.0 mEq/L on admission. The study excluded patients with liver failure or post-liver surgery, recent epileptic seizures, a contraindication for a central venous catheterization, an evident aerobic cause of hyperlactatemia, or those with a do-not-resuscitate status. Patients were randomized into 2 groups: 1) the experimental group where therapy was aimed to decrease lactate levels by at least 20% every 2 hours or 2) the control group with standard therapy, where the team only had the admission lactate level. Treatment period was first 8 hours of ICU admission. Patients were followed to hospital discharge or death. The primary endpoint was in-hospital mortality, with significant reduction in-hospital mortality observed in the lactate-guided therapy group after adjustment for age, sex, and initial assessment of organ failure by APACHE and SOFA scores (HR 0.61; 95%CI 0.43-0.87). There was also a decrease in ICU stay in the lactate-guided therapy group (HR 0.65; 95%CI 0.50-0.85) compared to the standard therapy group.

Jansen TC, van Bommel J, Schoonderbeek FJ, Sleeswijk Visser SJ, van der Klooster JM, Lima AP, et al. Early Lactate-Guided Therapy in Intensive Care Unit Patients. Am J Respir Crit Care Med. 2010 Sep 15;182(6):752–61.

The PROSEVA trial: Proning in severe ARDS

1. In patients with severe acute respiratory distress syndrome (ARDS), prone-positioning significantly reduced 28- and 90-day mortality when compared to patients who remained in supine position only.

2. Proned patients were also successfully extubated at higher rates and required fewer days of ventilation when compared to supine patients.

Original Date of Publication: June 2013

Study Rundown: ARDS is characterized by the 4 following criteria: 1) lung injury of acute onset (i.e., within 1 week of a clinical insult), 2) bilateral opacities on chest imaging, 3) lung infiltrates not cardiogenic in nature, and 4) $PaO_2:FiO_2$ ratio <300. ARDS can be caused by pneumonia, sepsis, blood transfusions, trauma, aspiration, pancreatitis, medications, and chemical inhalation. Previously, the ARMA trial demonstrated that lower tidal volume ventilation significantly reduced in-hospital mortality, while the ACURASYS trial revealed that neuromuscular blockade early in severe ARDS also led to reduced mortality. In the Proning Severe ARDS Patients (PROSEVA) trial, patients with severe ARDS were randomized to either prone-positioning for 16 hours or left in supine position. In summary, proning significantly reduced 28- and 90-day mortality compared to leaving patients in the supine position. Proned patients also experienced significantly higher rates of successful extubation and fewer days requiring ventilation compared to those in the supine group. Notably, all of the centers involved in this study had considerable experience with proning patients.

In-Depth [randomized controlled trial]: This trial was conducted at 27 intensive care units (ICUs) across France and Spain, all of which had at least 5 years of experience with prone positioning. Of the 3449 patients admitted with ARDS, 474 patients were randomized as part of this trial to either sessions consisting of 16 consecutive hours of prone positioning or remaining in the supine position. The inclusion criteria were ARDS (i.e., as defined using the American-European Consensus Conference criteria), endotracheal intubation and mechanical ventilation for ARDS <36 hours, and severe ARDS (i.e., PF ratio <150 mmHg, FiO2 >0.60, PEEP >5 cm H2O, tidal volume 6 mL/kg). The primary endpoint was 28-day mortality, while the secondary endpoints included 90-day mortality, rate of successful extubation, and the number of ventilator-free days.

In the majority of patients, the cause of ARDS was pneumonia. The average number of proning sessions per patient was 4±4, while the mean duration per session was 17±3 hours. All patients in the prone positioning group underwent at least 1 session. The risk of 28-day mortality was significantly lower in patients who underwent proning compared to those who remained in the supine position (aHR 0.42; 95%CI 0.26-0.66). This difference remained significant at 90 days (aHR 0.48; 95%CI 0.32-0.72). Moreover, patients in the prone group experienced significantly higher rates of successful extubation at day 90 (HR 0.45; 95%CI 0.29-0.70) and significantly higher numbers of ventilation-free days at day 28 and 90 (p < 0.001 at both time points). With regards to complications, patients in the supine group experienced significantly more cardiac arrests compared to the prone group (p = 0.02).

Guérin C, Reignier J, Richard J-C, Beuret P, Gacouin A, Boulain T, et al. Prone Positioning in Severe Acute Respiratory Distress Syndrome. New England Journal of Medicine. 2013 Jun 6;368(23):2159–68.

IV. Gastroenterology

The Child-Pugh score: Prognosis in chronic liver disease and cirrhosis

1. The Child-Pugh score was developed in 1973 to predict surgical outcomes in patients presenting with bleeding esophageal varices.

3. Presently, the score is used with the Model for End-Stage Liver Disease (MELD) to determine priority for liver transplantation.

Original Date of Publication: August 1973

Study Rundown: Originally developed in 1973, the Child-Pugh score estimated the risk of operative mortality in patients with bleeding esophageal varices. It has since been modified, refined, and become a widely used tool to assess prognosis in patients with chronic liver disease and cirrhosis. The score considers 5 factors, 3 of which assess the synthetic function of the liver (i.e., total bilirubin level, serum albumin, and international normalized ratio, or INR) and 2 of which are based on clinical assessment (i.e., degree of ascites and degree of hepatic encephalopathy). Critics of the Child-Pugh score have noted its reliance on clinical assessment, which may result in inconsistency in scoring. Others have suggested that its broad classifications of disease are impractical when determining priority for liver transplantation; nevertheless, it remains widely used. The MELD is a newer scoring system that has been developed to address some of the concerns with the Child-Pugh score, and both systems are often used in conjunction to determine liver transplantation priority.

In-Depth [case series study]: Thirty-eight consecutive cases of bleeding esophageal varices requiring surgery were included in the study. The severity of liver disease was assessed in each patient based on five clinical features: 1) total bilirubin level, 2) serum albumin, 3) prothrombin time (now measured as the INR), 4) the degree of ascites, and 5) the grade of hepatic encephalopathy. The total point score was used to determine the patient's Child-Pugh class (Figure). Class A patients (n = 7) experienced a 29% operative mortality rate, while Class B (n = 13) and Class C (n = 18) patients had operative mortality rates of 38% and 88%, respectively. Since its publication, the Child-Pugh score has undergone modifications and is currently used to assess the severity and prognosis of chronic liver disease and cirrhosis. It is often used together with the MELD to determine the priority for liver transplantation. The current Child-Pugh scoring system is outlined below.

Factor	1 point	2 points	3 points
Total bilirubin (μmol/L)	<34	34-50	>50
Serum albumin (g/L)	>35	28-35	<28
PT INR	<1.7	1.71-2.30	>2.30
Ascites	None	Mild	Moderate to Severe
Hepatic encephalopathy	None	Grade I-II (or suppressed with medication)	Grade III-IV (or refractory)

	Class A	Class B	Class C
Total points	5-6	7-9	10-15
1-year survival	100%	80%	45%

Pugh RNH, Murray-Lyon IM, Dawson JI , Pietroni MC, Williams R. Transection of the oesophagus for bleeding oesophageal varices. Br J Surg. 1973 Aug 1;60(8):646–9.

Endoscopic biliary drainage in acute cholangitis

1. For patients with severe acute cholangitis due to choledocholithiasis, endoscopic biliary drainage reduced hospital mortality compared to surgical decompression.

2. Endoscopic biliary drainage was associated with fewer post-treatment complications, although the decrease was not statistically significant for all types of complications.

Original Date of Publication: June 1992

Study Rundown: At the time of this study, surgical decompression was the conventional treatment for severe acute cholangitis arising from choledocholithiasis. Surgery, however, was associated with significant morbidity and mortality. Several uncontrolled studies had shown that endoscopic biliary drainage was a safe therapeutic alternative for acute cholangitis that reduced the rate of mortality. This study was the first randomized, controlled trial that sought to determine the benefits of endoscopic biliary drainage compared to surgical decompression for patients with severe acute cholangitis. Results demonstrated that endoscopic biliary drainage was associated with significantly lowered hospital mortality rates compared to surgical decompression. Endoscopic intervention also significantly reduced the rates of certain complications, including the rates of ventilator support and residual stones after procedure.

A potential study limitation is that patients randomized to receive surgical decompression experienced longer wait times before undergoing treatment compared to patients randomized to receive endoscopic biliary drainage. The treatment delay for the surgery group, on the order of a couple hours, was due in part to the limited number of immediately available operating rooms. This delay could have resulted in worsened cholangitis in the surgery group specifically, and may have potentially biased the study's results in favor of endoscopic biliary drainage. However, these delays reflect the challenges in arranging emergent surgery that occur in practice. In summary, the findings of this study support the use of endoscopic biliary drainage as a safe and effective treatment for severe acute cholangitis due to choledocholithiasis.

In-Depth [randomized controlled trial]: This trial enrolled 82 patients from the Queen Mary Hospital in Hong Kong. Eligible patients included those diagnosed with acute cholangitis due to choledocholithiasis based on the presence of septic shock or progressive biliary sepsis manifesting as mental confusion or antibiotic-refractory fever. All patients underwent emergency diagnostic endoscopic retrograde cholangio-pancreatography (ERCP) prior to randomization for endoscopic biliary drainage or surgical decompression. A total of 41 patients were randomized to each treatment group. All patients received definitive therapy following biliary drainage. Mortality was defined as death within 48 hours after biliary drainage, in the absence of other contributory causes. Morbidity included any complications that arose after treatment. Cholangitis was considered to have resolved once body temperature and blood pressure were normalized for at least 8 hours.

The mortality rate was significantly lower for patients undergoing endoscopic biliary drainage compared to patients undergoing surgical decompression (10% vs. 32%; p < 0.03). The rate of complications was not significantly different between the groups (34% vs. 66%; p > 0.05). Only the rates of residual calculi and ventilator support were significantly lower for patients receiving endoscopic drainage compared to surgery. The time needed to normalize body temperature and blood pressure was not different between patients receiving endoscopic biliary drainage and surgical decompression.

Lai ECS, Mok FPT, Tan ESY, Lo C, Fan S, You K, et al. Endoscopic Biliary Drainage for Severe Acute Cholangitis. New England Journal of Medicine. 1992 Jun 11;326(24):1582–6.

Omeprazole vs placebo for bleeding peptic ulcer

1. Patients presenting with upper gastrointestinal bleeds experienced a significantly lower risk of continued bleeding and need for surgery when treated with omeprazole compared to placebo.

2. There was no significant difference in mortality between the groups, though the omeprazole group had significantly lower red cell transfusion requirements.

Original Date of Publication: April 1997

Study Rundown: Upper gastrointestinal bleeding is a common cause of hospitalization. While endoscopy has long been an important component of managing upper gastrointestinal bleeds, there were no well-studied medical therapies at the time this trial was conducted. It had been shown that platelet function is poorer in low pH, thus, it was thought that reducing gastric acidity would help control bleeding. Prior studies with H2-receptor antagonists demonstrated mixed results, as intravenous famotidine was not shown to be effective. The purpose of this trial was to explore whether treatment with a proton pump inhibitor would improve mortality and need for surgery in patients presenting with upper gastrointestinal bleeds. In summary, patients treated with omeprazole had significantly lower rates of continued bleeding and surgery for ongoing bleeding compared to those being treated with placebo. There was no significant difference between the groups in bleeding-related mortality 30 days after admission.

In-Depth [randomized controlled trial]: This trial was conducted at a single tertiary care center in India. A total of 220 patients were randomized to either treatment with oral omeprazole 40 mg every 12 hours for 5 days or matching placebo. After appropriate resuscitation, all patients underwent upper endoscopy within 12 hours after admission. Patients with duodenal, gastric or stomal ulcers and stigmata of recent hemorrhage (i.e., arterial spurting, visible vessel, oozing from ulcer, adherent clot to ulcer) were considered eligible for the trial. Exclusion criteria were severe terminal illness that made endoscopy dangerous or undesirable, profuse hemorrhage with persistent shock necessitating emergent surgical intervention, or bleeding from a Mallory-Weiss tear/varices/erosion/tumors/unknown source. Endpoints studied were continued bleeding, recurrent bleeding, surgery, and mortality within 30 days after admission from causes related to bleeding or treatment. The risk of continued bleeding was significantly higher in the placebo group compared to the omeprazole group (OR 4.7; 95%CI 2.7-7.4). The risk of surgery to control bleeding was also significantly higher in the placebo group (OR 3.9; 95%CI 1.7-8.5). There was no significant difference between the 2 groups in terms of the risk of mortality. Patients in the omeprazole group required significantly fewer units of blood transfused per patient (p < 0.001).

Khuroo MS, Yattoo GN, Javid G, Khan BA, Shah AA, Gulzar GM, et al. A Comparison of Omeprazole and Placebo for Bleeding Peptic Ulcer. New England Journal of Medicine. 1997 Apr 10;336(15):1054–8.

Intravenous omeprazole after endoscopy reduces rebleeding in patients with peptic ulcers

1. After endoscopic treatment, intravenous omeprazole significantly reduced the risk of rebleeding in patients with peptic ulcers at 3, 7, and 30 days when compared with placebo.

Original Date of Publication: August 2000

Study Rundown: Previous research had demonstrated that proton pump inhibitors in upper gastrointestinal bleeding prior to upper endoscopy significantly reduced the risk of rebleeding and need for surgery to control bleeding. The purpose of this trial was to explore whether continuing proton pump inhibitors after endoscopy would provide any benefits. The findings of this trial demonstrated the value of intravenous proton pump inhibitor after endoscopy in reducing the risk of rebleeding in patients with peptic ulcers. The fact that this study was carried out at a single center in a predominantly Chinese population may limit the generalizability of the study. Moreover, the use of intravenous omeprazole is another concern, as it may not be available in certain other practice settings. Other studies, however, have demonstrated similar benefits with using orally administered proton pump inhibitors. In summary, intravenous omeprazole is associated with reduction in the risk of rebleeding in patients with bleeding peptic ulcers after endoscopic treatment.

In-Depth [randomized controlled trial]: The trial was conducted at the Chinese University of Hong Kong. Patients were eligible for the trial if they were >16 years of age and if endoscopic treatment of ulcers was successful. A total of 240 patients were randomized to receive either intravenous omeprazole (i.e., 80 mg bolus, then 8 mg/hour for 72 hours) or placebo after endoscopic treatment for bleeding peptic ulcers. Patients receiving placebo had significantly higher risk of recurrent bleeding at 3 days (RR 4.80; 95%CI 1.89-12.2; $p < 0.001$), 7 days (RR 3.71; 95%CI 1.68-8.23), and 30 days (RR 3.38; 95%CI 1.60-7.13) compared to those receiving omeprazole. Moreover, omeprazole significantly reduced the length of hospitalization ($p = 0.006$) and blood transfusion requirements ($p = 0.04$), though there were no significant differences in mortality between the 2 groups at 30 days (RR 2.40; 95%CI 0.87-6.60).

Lau JYW, Sung JJY, Lee KKC, Yung M, Wong SKH, Wu JCY, et al. *Effect of Intravenous Omeprazole on Recurrent Bleeding after Endoscopic Treatment of Bleeding Peptic Ulcers. New England Journal of Medicine. 2000 Aug 3;343(5):310–6.*

Decrease in symptom severity linked to infliximab Crohn's treatment

1. The severity of Crohn's disease as assessed by the Pediatric Crohn's Disease Activity Index (PCDAI) in patients recruited from 3 pediatric specialty centers decreased significantly over the course of a 12-week treatment regimen with infliximab.

2. All patients were on corticosteroids at the start of the study; however, steroid administration decreased significantly over the course of the investigation.

Original Date of Publication: August 2000

Study Rundown: Crohn's disease is an inflammatory bowel disease (IBD) often diagnosed in adolescence and young adulthood and results from an immune-mediated, inflammatory process with the potential to affect any portion of the gastrointestinal tract. Knowing that tumor necrosis factor $-\alpha$ (TNF-α), a cytokine involved in the modulation of the inflammatory responses, is increased in patients with Crohn's and that the drug infliximab (Remicade) acts to neutralize TNF-α, this study built upon encouraging research in adult patients in investigating the potential utility of infliximab in the pediatric population. In this study, 19 patients with poor response to other therapies were started on varying infliximab dosing schedules. All patients were on daily prednisone at baseline. Crohn's disease symptom status was assessed at baseline, 1 month, and 3 months into the study through physician assessment and use of the PCDAI.

Over the study period, the severity of Crohn's symptoms by PCDAI score and the doses of steroids used to treat disease decreased significantly. This study was limited by the variation in infliximab dosing schedules, lack of a control group, and small sample size. However, it stands as one of the first studies to investigate the use of infliximab in a pediatric population with Crohn's and indicated many potential positive outcomes. Following Food and Drug Administration approval in 2006, infliximab was, and still is, used in pediatric patients with moderate to severe Crohn's who have not responded adequately to other therapies. While only 3 of the 19 patients in this study experienced any type of adverse reactions, adverse effects from long-term use, including lymphoma, are of major concern in patients. The risk of malignancy along with other severe reactions continues to be investigated. In addition, many patients with Crohn's are on combined therapies, the efficacy and adverse effects of these regimens are also under investigation.

In-Depth [prospective cohort]: Pediatric patients with Crohn's disease, treated at 3 IBD specialty centers, and who had responded poorly or not at all to previously treatment strategies or depended entirely on corticosteroids, were eligible to participate. A total of 19 patients were recruited (average age 14.4 years, with a mean 3.5 years since diagnosis) to receive infliximab administered intravenously at a dose of 5 mg/kg over 2 hours. The number of treatments varied among participants. Treatment outcomes were assessed by physician assessment and the PCDAI, a physician-completed health evaluation, filled out prior to infliximab treatment and then 4 and 12 weeks after initiation. Patients were followed for an additional 3 to 9 months following the 12-week evaluation. At the time of treatment initiation, all patients had moderate to severe disease as measured by the evaluation tool and all were on daily corticosteroids with 14 participants on an additional agent.

Over the course of treatment, all patients experienced symptomatic improvement. After 4 weeks of therapy, 9 patients were asymptomatic and PCDAI values significantly decreased from 42.1 ± 13.7 to 10.0 ± 5.6 ($p < 0.0001$). Over the 12-week study period, patients became increasingly symptomatic, but the 12-week PCDAI still remained significantly lower than the score at the time of treatment initiation at 26.8 ± 16.4 ($p < 0.01$). Prednisone dosing decreased over the course of the study with doses at both 4 weeks and 12 weeks significantly lower than at baseline (28 ± 14 mg at baseline vs. 20 ± 12 mg at 4 weeks and 8 ± 12 mg at 12 weeks, $p < 0.01$) and 9 participants on no corticosteroids at the study's conclusion. At final follow-up, 3 patients had inactive disease, 9 had mild disease, and 4 had moderate disease. Three patients experienced adverse reactions such as dyspnea and rash which were controlled in 2 who received pretreatment with diphenhydramine prior to administration of infliximab.

Hyams JS, Markowitz J, Wyllie R. Use of infliximab in the treatment of Crohn's disease in children and adolescents. The Journal of Pediatrics. 2000 Aug 1;137(2):192–6.

The MELD score: Predicting survival in end-stage liver disease

1. The Model for End-Stage Liver Disease (MELD) is a reliable tool for predicting short-term survival in patients with advanced liver disease.

2. The score is generalizable to diverse etiologies and a wide range of disease severity.

Original Date of Publication: February 2001

Study Rundown: The MELD was originally developed to predict outcomes in patients after a transjugular intrahepatic portosystemic shunt (TIPS) procedure. This study assessed whether the model could reliably predict short-term survival in patients with chronic liver disease. The investigators found that MELD scores were a good predictor of 1-week, 3-month and 1-year survival, which had important implications for the model's use in the allocation of donor livers. Previously, the Child-Turcotte-Pugh (CTP) system was used to rank patients according to urgency and medical need, however the broad classifications made it difficult to rank patients according to severity of disease. Another issue with CTP scores was the subjectivity involved in some of the criteria (e.g., assessment of ascites and encephalopathy). The MELD criteria were an improvement on these aspects of CTP scores as patients were assigned a numerical score based on objective measures.

In-Depth [cohort study]: This study evaluated the validity of the MELD score for predicting survival in patients with end-stage liver disease. The model used measures of serum creatinine, total serum bilirubin, International Normalized Ratio (INR) for prothrombin time and etiology of cirrhosis to assess disease severity. The model was assessed in 4 independent samples, which included patients hospitalized with advanced end-stage liver disease, ambulatory patients with noncholestatic cirrhosis, ambulatory patients with primary biliary cirrhosis (PBC) and a historical group of cirrhotic patients from a period when liver transplantation was not widely available. The primary outcome measure was 3-month survival and validity was also assessed for predicting 1-week and 1-year survival. The C statistics for 3-month mortality in the hospitalized, ambulatory noncholestatic, ambulatory PBC and historical groups respectively were 0.87, 0.80, 0.87 and 0.78. These values changed minimally when etiology of disease was excluded from the model. The MELD score was found to be a reliable tool to predict survival in patients with chronic liver disease.

Kamath PS, Wiesner RH, Malinchoc M, Kremers W, Therneau TM, Kosberg CL, et al. A model to predict survival in patients with end-stage liver disease. Hepatology. 2001 Feb 1;33(2):464–70.

Omeprazole before endoscopy in patients with gastrointestinal bleeding

1. Compared to placebo, treating patients with omeprazole bolus and infusion prior to endoscopy significantly reduced the need for endoscopic therapy, reduced the rate of post-endoscopy active bleeding, and reduced the length of hospitalization.

2. Treating patients with omeprazole pre-endoscopy did not significantly reduce the need for emergency surgery and did not reduce 30-day mortality as compared with placebo.

Original Date of Publication: April 2007

Study Rundown: In patients with upper gastrointestinal bleeding, infusion of a high-dose proton-pump inhibitor (PPI) after hemostasis via endoscopy was known to reduce recurrent bleeding and improved clinical outcomes. The adjuvant use of high-dose PPIs in endoscopic therapy has also been endorsed and confirmed in 2 meta-analyses. Clot formation over arteries is a pH-dependent process; a gastric pH > 6 is thought to be critical for platelet aggregation. Prior to this study, treatment with PPIs was often initiated before endoscopy in patients presenting with upper gastrointestinal bleeding. However, there was a lack of evidence to support such an approach. This trial demonstrated that omeprazole bolus and infusion before endoscopy accelerated the resolution of bleeding in ulcers and reduced the need for endoscopic therapy. Moreover, omeprazole treatment prior to endoscopy was associated with reduced active bleeding post-endoscopy and led to shorter hospital stays. There were no significant differences between the groups in the rate of recurrent bleeding within 30 days, need for emergency surgery, or 30-day mortality.

In-Depth [randomized controlled trial]: Participants in the trial were randomized to 2 treatment groups: 1) patients received an intravenous infusion of omeprazole or 2) a placebo. Each patient received an 80-mg intravenous bolus injection followed by continuous infusion of 8 mg per hour until endoscopic examination the following morning. Patients were eligible for the trial if they had hypotensive shock with a systolic blood pressure ≤90 mmHg or pulse ≥110 beats per minute was stabilized after their initial resuscitation. Exclusion criteria included long-term aspirin use, unstable condition requiring urgent endoscopy, a moribund state, and a known PPI allergy. A total of 188 of those evaluated were excluded for other reasons that were not mentioned. The primary study endpoint was the need for endoscopic therapy at the first endoscopic examination. Secondary endpoints included signs of bleeding, need for urgent endoscopy, duration of hospital stay, need for transfusion, need for emergency surgery to achieve hemostasis, and rates of recurrent bleeding and death from any cause within 30 days after randomization.

A total of 638 patients underwent randomization. Compared to patients treated with placebo, patients in the omeprazole group required significantly less endoscopic treatment (RR 0.67; 95%CI 0.51-0.90). Moreover, patients treated with omeprazole also required less endoscopic therapy for bleeding peptic ulcers (RR 0.61; 95%CI 0.44-0.84) and had less post-endoscopy active bleeding (RR 0.44; 95%CI 0.23-0.83) compared to those treated with placebo. Notably, a larger proportion of omeprazole-treated patients had hospital stays <3 days compared to those on placebo (RR 1.23; 95%CI 1.07-1.42). There were no significant differences between the groups in the rate of recurrent bleeding within 30 days, need for emergency surgery, or 30-day mortality.

Lau JY, Leung WK, Wu JCY, Chan FKL, Wong VWS, Chiu PWY, et al. Omeprazole before Endoscopy in Patients with Gastrointestinal Bleeding. New England Journal of Medicine. 2007 Apr 19;356(16):1631–40.

Early transjugular intrahepatic portosystemic shunt in cirrhosis and variceal bleeding

1. In patients with severe liver disease and variceal bleeding, early transjugular intrahepatic portosystemic shunt (TIPS) significantly reduced rates of treatment failure, length of hospitalization, and mortality compared to control.

2. There were no significant differences between the two groups in the rates of adverse events.

Original Date of Publication: June 2010

Study Rundown: Variceal bleeding is a major cause of death for patients with liver cirrhosis and portal hypertension. Guidelines at the time of this study recommended treatment consisting of vasoactive drugs (e.g., octreotide), prophylactic antibiotics, and endoscopic techniques such as variceal ligation for dealing with variceal bleeding. When standard treatment failed, TIPS had been shown to be effective, though associated with substantial mortality due in large part to hepatic encephalopathy. Previous studies suggested that the earlier use of TIPS can decrease mortality for patients with severe liver disease who are at a high risk of treatment failure. This trial was the first trial to compare the use of early TIPS with the current standard of care for acute variceal bleeding.

Results showed that early use of TIPS was associated with a significant decrease in the rate of rebleeding and failure to control bleeding. Early TIPS also significantly reduced mortality and led to shorter stays in the intensive care unit (ICU). Notably, early TIPS use was not associated with a significantly higher rate of adverse events, such as hepatic encephalopathy. A major limitation of the study was its small size (only 63 patients were randomized), meaning it was insufficiently powered for subgroup analyses. Thus, for example, the study could not determine whether early TIPS had greater benefit for the study's more severe cases of liver disease (those classified as Child-Pugh class C) in comparison to the study's less severe cases (those classified as Child-Pugh class B). In summary, results of this study supported the early use of TIPS for the treatment of patients with severe liver disease and variceal bleeding. Importantly, the results suggested that use of early TIPS was not associated with an increased risk of hepatic encephalopathy.

In-Depth [randomized controlled trial]: Sixty-three patients from 9 centers in Europe were enrolled in this trial. Eligible patients had liver disease classified as Child-Pugh class B (i.e., moderately severe) or class C (i.e., most severe), had liver cirrhosis with acute bleeding of esophageal varices, and were already receiving treatment in the form of vasoactive drugs (e.g., octreotide), antibiotics, and endoscopic band ligation (EBL). Patients who were older than 75 years, were pregnant, had hepatocellular carcinoma, had previous TIPS, had portal-vein thrombosis, or had heart failure were excluded. Within 24 hours of admission, 31 patients were randomized to the "early-TIPS" group, where they received treatment with a polytetrafluoroethylene-covered stent within 72 hours after randomization. The remaining 32 patients were randomized to the "pharmocotherapy-EBL" group, where they continued to receive vasoactive drug therapy followed treatment with nonspecific beta-blockers (e.g., propranolol and nadolol) and EBL-TIPS was provided as a rescue therapy. The primary endpoint was the composite outcome of failure to control bleeding and the failure to prevent rebleeding in the next year. Secondary endpoints included mortality at 6 weeks and 1 year, the development of sequelae associated with portal hypertension, and the number of days spent in the ICU.

Results demonstrated that 97% of the early-TIPS group avoided occurrence of the primary endpoint, compared to 50% in the pharmacotherapy-EBL group ($p < 0.001$). At 1 year, the survival rate was 86% in the early-TIPS group compared to 61% in the pharmacotherapy-EBL group ($p < 0.001$). Patients in the pharmacotherapy-EBL group spent a higher proportion of their follow-up time in the ICU ($p = 0.01$). There was no difference in the rate of adverse rates for both treatment groups, including for hepatic encephalopathy ($p=0.13$), and development of ascites ($p = 0.11$).

García-Pagán JC, Caca K, Bureau C, Laleman W, Appenrodt B, Luca A, et al. Early Use of TIPS in Patients with Cirrhosis and Variceal Bleeding. New England Journal of Medicine. 2010 Jun 24;362(25):2370–9.

The COGENT: Omeprazole with antiplatelet therapy in upper gastrointestinal bleeding

1. In patients treated with dual antiplatelet therapy, the addition of omeprazole significantly reduced the rate of gastrointestinal events compared to placebo.

2. The addition of omeprazole to clopidogrel and aspirin did not significantly change the rate of cardiovascular events compared to placebo.

Original Date of Publication: November 2010

Study Rundown: Antiplatelet therapy is commonly prescribed to people who suffer from cardiovascular disease, including myocardial infarctions, transient ischemic attacks, and stroke. A common complication of antiplatelet therapy, however, is gastrointestinal bleeding and this risk is increased when patients are being treated with dual antiplatelet agents. Moreover, evidence from observational studies were inconsistent with regards to a potential interaction between clopidogrel, a commonly prescribed antiplatelet agent, and proton pump inhibitors (PPIs). Thus, the purpose of the Clopidogrel and Optimization of Gastrointestinal Events Trial (COGENT) was to assess the efficacy and safety of clopidogrel and PPIs in patients with coronary artery disease. The trial revealed that treatment with omeprazole in patients on dual antiplatelet therapy reduced the rate of gastrointestinal events without a significant difference in the rate of cardiovascular events. Notably, this trial was stopped prematurely, as there was an unexpected loss of funding. As a result, the intended study enrollment and event rates were not achieved. Nevertheless, this study provided evidence in support of the use of proton pump inhibitors in patients on dual antiplatelet therapy to reduce the rate of gastrointestinal events.

In-Depth [randomized controlled trial]: Originally published in NEJM in 2010, this randomized, controlled trial assessed the risk of gastrointestinal bleeding in patients receiving dual antiplatelet therapy with and without concomitant omeprazole. A pharmaceutical company was involved in the design of the study. A total of 3761 patients from 393 sites in 15 countries being treated with aspirin (75-325 mg daily) and clopidogrel (75 mg daily) were randomized to receive either omeprazole (20 mg daily) or placebo in addition. Patients were eligible for the study if they were ≥21 years of age and it was anticipated that they would require clopidogrel and aspirin therapy for the next 12 months. The primary endpoint was a composite of upper gastrointestinal events, including upper gastrointestinal bleeding, symptomatic uncomplicated gastroduodenal ulcers, obstruction, and perforation. The primary cardiovascular safety endpoint was a composite of death from cardiovascular causes, nonfatal myocardial infarction, coronary revascularization, or ischemic stroke. The trial was stopped prematurely when the sponsor suddenly lost financial backing. At 180 days, the omeprazole group had a significantly lower rate of gastrointestinal events when compared to the placebo group (HR 0.34; 95%CI 0.18-0.63). The omeprazole group also experienced significantly less overall gastrointestinal bleeding as compared with placebo (HR 0.30; 95%CI 0.13-0.66). There was no significant difference between the 2 groups in terms of the rate of cardiovascular events (HR 0.99; 95%CI 0.68-1.44).

Bhatt DL, Cryer BL, Contant CF, Cohen M, Lanas A, Schnitzer TJ, et al. Clopidogrel with or without Omeprazole in Coronary Artery Disease. New England Journal of Medicine. 2010 Nov 11;363(20):1909–17.

V. Hematology/Oncology

Vena caval filters in pulmonary embolism prophylaxis

1. Permanent vena caval filter placement in addition to anticoagulant therapy reduced the short-term occurrence of pulmonary embolism (PE), but increased the long-term risk of recurrent deep vein thrombosis (DVT).

2. There was no significant difference in efficacy between low molecular-weight heparin (LMWH) and unfractionated heparin (UFH) as early anticoagulant therapy for PE prophylaxis.

Original Date of Publication: February 1998

Study Rundown: In patients who are at high-risk for PE and have a contraindication to anticoagulation, a vena caval filter is a potential option to reduce the risk of PE. This multicenter study in France is the only randomized, controlled trial that evaluated whether filter placement decreases the incidence of PE, as well as DVT both in short-term and long-term follow-up. The study demonstrated that the use of a permanent vena caval filter in addition to heparin therapy reduced the occurrence of a PE in the short-term. The data, however, also showed that in long-term follow-up of 2 years, there was a significant increase in recurrent DVTs in patients who received a filter. This most likely relates to thrombosis at the filter site, but it may counteract the benefits gained earlier with the reduction in PE occurrence. In summary, this study showed that filters lower the risk of PE in the short-term, but later increase the risk of recurrent DVT. It also confirmed the results of previous studies that showed no difference in effectiveness between LMWH and UFH for early anticoagulant therapy. Overall, the evidence in this study does not support the use of inferior vena cava (IVC) filters in addition to anticoagulant therapy to prevent PE's and recurrent DVT's. Of note, this study excluded patients with DVT who had a contraindication to anticoagulation, which is one of the commonly cited indications for filter placement.

In-Depth [randomized controlled trial]: This study was a multicenter, non-blinded, 2x2, randomized-controlled trial that randomized 400 patients to vena caval filter placement or no placement, and to receive LMWH or UFH as a bridge to warfarin. Patients over 18 years of age with confirmed DVT with or without concomitant symptomatic PE, and whose physicians believed they were at high risk for a PE, were eligible for the study. Patients with history of IVC filter placement, contraindication to anticoagulant therapy, or likelihood of noncompliance were excluded. Two hundred patients were assigned to receive vena caval filters. One hundred ninety-five of the 400 patients were assigned to LMWH while the other 205 were assigned to UFH for the first 8-12 days of anticoagulant therapy. The subjects underwent a baseline V/Q scan and/or pulmonary angiography to evaluate for a PE. All subjects were transitioned to warfarin therapy after 8-12 days for a duration of 3 months or maintained on UFH if oral anticoagulation was not possible. Patients were followed for 2 years. The primary outcome was occurrence of a symptomatic PE within the first 12 days of anticoagulant therapy. The secondary outcome was occurrence of symptomatic PE, DVT, major filter complication, and/or major bleeding during the follow-up period.

Filter vs. No Filter

The study demonstrated that there were significantly fewer patients (2 vs. 9 patients) in the filter group compared to the non-filter group who had had a PE in the first 12 days of anticoagulation therapy (OR 0.22; 95%CI 0.05-0.90). Results were similar when analysis was adjusted for heparin therapy and presence of PE at enrollment. In the 2-year follow-up, there was a significantly higher number of recurrent DVTs in the filter group compared to the no-filter group (OR 1.87; 95%CI 1.10-3.20). There was no significant difference in PE incidence, mortality, or major bleeding between the groups at the 2-year mark.

LMWH vs. UFH

There was no significant difference in incidence of PE or DVT between the anticoagulant groups during the first 12 days as well as at the 2-year mark. There was also no statistical significance in mortality or adverse effects between the groups. There was no evidence of statistically significant interaction between filter and heparin anticoagulant therapy for both primary and secondary outcome events.

Decousus H, Leizorovicz A, Parent F, Page Y, Tardy B, Girard P, et al. A Clinical Trial of Vena Caval Filters in the Prevention of Pulmonary Embolism in Patients with Proximal Deep-Vein Thrombosis. New England Journal of Medicine. 1998 Feb 12;338(7):409–16.

No survival difference in lumpectomy and mastectomy for breast cancer

1. In women with stage I or II breast cancer, there was no significant difference in overall survival in women treated with total mastectomy compared to breast-conserving surgery.

2. Adjuvant radiation therapy was associated with reduced ipsilateral recurrence in lumpectomy-treated women.

Original Date of Publication: October 2002

Study Rundown: Breast cancer is the most common type of cancer affecting women. These cancers arise from tissues in the breast, with the 2 most common types being ductal and lobular carcinomas. Risk factors for developing breast cancer include increasing age, being female, having a family history of breast cancer, certain genetic defects (i.e., BRCA1 and BRCA2), and early menarche/late menopause. While the incidence of breast cancer has increased steadily over the past decades, mortality rates have declined significantly since the 1980s. This may be attributed to increased screening, more effective screening programs, and better treatment amongst numerous other factors. Breast cancer treatment consists of a combination of local and systemic therapy, depending on the cancer characteristics and staging. In the 1970s, several studies were conducted to address lingering questions regarding the surgical management of breast cancer. Several randomized controlled trials were conducted to assess the efficacy of breast-conserving therapy.

One particular study explored whether lumpectomy, a procedure where the tumor was resected with clean margins, with or without radiation therapy was comparable to radical mastectomy. Previous analyses suggested that there were no significant differences in survival between the study groups. This study reported the 20-year findings of this randomized controlled trial. Lumpectomy followed by radiation therapy was not associated with not reduced survival or reduced recurrence of breast cancer in the ipsilateral breast when compared to radical mastectomy and lumpectomy alone, respectively. Currently, systemic therapy is used routinely as adjuvant treatment after surgery to reduce the risk of distant micrometastases.

In-Depth [randomized controlled trial]: This trial followed 1851 women diagnosed with invasive breast tumors with positive or negative axillary lymph nodes (i.e., stage I or II). Participants were randomized to treatment total mastectomy, lumpectomy or lumpectomy followed by breast irradiation. These findings were reported after 20 years of follow-up. Breast irradiation was associated with reduced recurrence in the ipsilateral breast in women treated with lumpectomy and who had tumor-free margins on surgical specimens. The benefit of radiation therapy was independent of nodal status. At 20-year follow-up after surgery, 14.3% of women who underwent lumpectomy with radiation had a recurrence in the ipsilateral breast compared to 39.2% in women who underwent lumpectomy alone (p < 0.001). No significant difference was found in disease-free survival or overall survival among the 3 treatment groups.

Fisher B, Anderson S, Bryant J, Margolese RG, Deutsch M, Fisher ER, et al. Twenty-Year Follow-up of a Randomized Trial Comparing Total Mastectomy, Lumpectomy, and Lumpectomy plus Irradiation for the Treatment of Invasive Breast Cancer. New England Journal of Medicine. 2002 Oct 17;347(16):1233–41.

The CLOT trial: Dalteparin vs warfarin for venous thromboembolism in malignancy

1. Dalteparin, a low-molecular-weight heparin (LMWH), was superior to warfarin in preventing recurrent venous thromboembolism (VTE) in the setting of malignancy.

2. There was no significant difference in risk of major bleeding with dalteparin as compared to warfarin.

Original Date of Publication: July 2003

Study Rundown: Prior to the Randomized Comparison of Low-Molecular-Weight Heparin versus Oral Anticoagulant Therapy for the Prevention of Recurrent Venous Thromboembolism in Patients with Cancer (CLOT) trial, patients with VTE in the setting of malignancy were treated similarly to patients with other high-risk hypercoagulable states. That is, these patients were treated with long-term oral anticoagulation, like warfarin, with initial bridging with subcutaneous heparin or LMWH. There were questions as to whether the more predictable pharmacokinetics and drug interactions of LMWH could offer benefits compared to oral anticoagulants in the setting of cancer, given that these patients are often undergoing complex treatment regimens and are frequently further burdened with degrees of liver dysfunction and malnutrition. The CLOT trial sought to address whether long-term anticoagulation with subcutaneous dalteparin offered benefit compared to oral anticoagulation in the cancer population in preventing recurrent VTE. The study demonstrated that dalteparin was superior in preventing recurrent VTEs in the setting of malignancy when compared to oral anticoagulation with warfarin. There was no significant difference between the therapies in terms of bleeding risk. Given these results, in the setting of acute VTE associated with malignancy without active bleeding, it is reasonable to initiate treatment with a LMWH as opposed to oral vitamin K antagonists for up to 6 months to prevent recurrent VTEs.

In-Depth [randomized controlled trial]: The study included 676 patients from 48 clinical centers in 8 countries. Patients were eligible for the trial if they were adult patients with active cancer and newly diagnosed, symptomatic proximal deep vein thrombosis, pulmonary embolism, or both. Patients were excluded from the trial if they weighed ≤40 kg, had an Eastern Cooperative Oncology Group performance status of 3 or 4, had been treated with therapeutic heparin for >48 hours before randomization, had active or serious bleeding in the 2 weeks prior, had platelet count <75,000/mm³, had contraindications to heparin treatment or contrast medium, had creatinine ≥3 times the upper limit of normal, were pregnant, or could not return for follow-up. Patients were randomized to 2 groups: 1) warfarin with initial bridging using dalteparin and 2) dalteparin only. The study lasted for 6 months. The primary outcome was the first episode of objectively documented, symptomatic recurrent DVT and/or PE during the study period. Secondary outcomes studied included any bleeding event. The incidence of recurrent thromboembolism in the dalteparin only group was significantly lower than the oral anticoagulation group (HR 0.48; 95%CI 0.30-0.77). There was no significant difference in bleeding detected between the groups, with 6% of patients in the dalteparin group and 4% in the oral anticoagulation group experiencing bleeding (p = 0.27). The mortality rates were 39% and 41% in the dalteparin and oral anticoagulation groups (p = 0.53), respectively, and it was noted that 90% of these deaths were attributed to progression of malignancy.

Lee AYY, Levine MN, Baker RI, Bowden C, Kakkar AK, Prins M, et al. Low-Molecular-Weight Heparin versus a Coumarin for the Prevention of Recurrent Venous Thromboembolism in Patients with Cancer. New England Journal of Medicine. 2003 Jul 10;349(2):146–53.

Finasteride significantly reduces the incidence of prostate cancer

1. Finasteride therapy significantly reduced the incidence of prostate cancer compared to placebo.

2. Patients treated with finasteride were significantly more likely to have high-grade prostate cancers in a sample healthy population.

3. Patients treated with finasteride experienced significantly higher rates of sexual side effects, including erectile dysfunction, loss of libido, and gynecomastia.

Original Date of Publication: July 2003

Study Rundown: While some evidence at the time suggested that finasteride, which inhibits the conversion of testosterone to dihydrotestosterone, reduced the risk of prostate cancer, there were no large, randomized, controlled trials to support this observation. In this landmark study, patients with a prostate-specific antigen (PSA) of ≤3.0 ng/mL and normal rectal examination were randomized into 2 groups. In the first group patients received finasteride 5 mg daily and in the second group patients were given placebo. Over the 7-year trial period, this study demonstrated that patients treated with finasteride experienced a significantly lower incidence of prostate cancer than those in the placebo group. Patients in the finasteride group also had significantly higher likelihood of developing high-grade prostate cancer. The finasteride group experienced increased sexual side effects such as decreased potency, libido, and ejaculate volumes, but also decreased urinary problems such as incontinence, frequency, and urinary tract infections. Nevertheless, in the final analysis, mortality from prostate cancer was low in both groups (5 prostate cancer-related deaths in each group).

In-Depth [randomized controlled trial]: This double-blinded, randomized, controlled trial included participants ≥55 years of age, who had a normal rectal examination, and had a PSA level of ≤3.0 ng/mL. A total of 18 882 men were randomized to receive either finasteride 5 mg daily or placebo and followed for 7 years. The primary outcome measured was prevalence of prostate cancer over the course of the study. Secondary outcomes were prostate cancer mortality and tumor grade (specifically, Gleason grade ≥7) based on prostate biopsies. At the end of the study, all participants not diagnosed with prostate cancer were offered a prostate biopsy at 7 years ±90 days after randomization. The study was terminated 15 months prior to its anticipated completion - at this time, 81.3% of participants had completed the 7-year follow-up.

In the final analysis of 9060 participants, the rate of prostate cancer diagnosis was significantly lower in the finasteride group compared to placebo (RRR 24.8%; 95%CI 18.6-30.6; $p < 0.001$). A total of 48.4% of prostate cancer diagnoses were made based on end-of-study prostate biopsies, while the others were made based on cause-driven biopsies or interim procedures. Finasteride treatment was associated with higher rates of high-grade prostate cancer, defined as tumors of Gleason grade 7 or higher (37.0% vs. 22.2%, $p < 0.001$). The use of finasteride was also associated with higher rates of various sexual side effects, including reduced ejaculate volume (60.4% vs. 47.3%), erectile dysfunction (67.4% vs. 61.5%), loss of libido (65.4% vs. 59.6%), and gynecomastia (4.5% vs. 2.8%, $p < 0.001$ for all comparisons). Urinary urgency/frequency (12.9% vs. 15.6%), urinary retention (4.2% vs. 6.3%), and prostatitis (4.4% vs. 6.1%) rates were all significantly higher in the placebo group ($p < 0.001$ for all comparisons). There was no significant difference in mortality from prostate cancer in the two groups (5 deaths per group).

Thompson IM, Goodman PJ, Tangen CM, Lucia MS, Miller GJ, Ford LG, et al. The Influence of Finasteride on the Development of Prostate Cancer. New England Journal of Medicine. 2003 Jul 17;349(3):215–24.

Dexamethasone effective as an initial therapy for immune thrombocytopenic purpura

1. Of 125 patients with newly diagnosed immune thrombocytopenic purpura (ITP), 106 (85%) had an initial response to high-dose dexamethasone therapy.

2. Half of the 106 patients with an initial response to high-dose dexamethasone had a sustained response after 6 months of follow-up.

Original Date of Publication: August 2003

Study Rundown: This study assessed the effectiveness of high-dose dexamethasone as an initial therapy for newly diagnosed ITP. The results were promising as 85% of patients showed an initial response to therapy and half of these patients had a sustained response after six months of follow-up. This demonstrated that a short course (i.e., four days) of high-dose glucocorticoids could be effective as an initial treatment for ITP, avoiding the numerous and potentially severe complications associated with longer courses of prednisone, which was the standard therapy at the time. The high-dose dexamethasone was well-tolerated. No patients discontinued treatment due to side effects in this study. This prospective case-series involved a relatively large sample of patients; however, the study lacked a control group to compare its performance to a placebo or treatment with prednisone.

In-Depth [case series study]: This study recruited consecutive adult patients who presented with a new diagnosis of ITP. Of 157 consecutive patients, 125 met eligibility criteria – a platelet count of less than 20 000 per mm^3, or a platelet count of less than 50 000 per mm^3 and clinically significant bleeding. The exclusion criteria were relapsed ITP, treatment with corticosteroids in the previous 6 months, a history of clinically significant adverse effects from previous corticosteroid treatment (e.g., psychosis, avascular necrosis), uncontrolled hypertension or diabetes mellitus, and pregnancy. Patients were treated with 40 mg daily of oral dexamethasone for 4 days. Initial treatment response was defined as an increase in platelet count of at least 30 000 per mm^3, a platelet count greater than 50 000 per mm^3 by day 10 after treatment was started, and bleeding cessation. A sustained response was defined as a platelet count above 50 000 per mm^3 after 6 months of follow-up. Of the 125 patients included, 106 (85%) had an initial response to high-dose dexamethasone. Of the

19 patients who did not have a treatment response, 14 responded to either intravenous immune globulin or anti-D immune globulin. The remaining patients underwent splenectomy or received cytotoxic therapy. The median follow-up period was 30.5 months. Of the 106 patients with an initial response to dexamethasone therapy, 53 (50%) had a sustained response and required no further treatment. The remaining 53 patients had a relapse but responded to a second course of high-dose dexamethasone. No patient discontinued treatment due to adverse effects.

Cheng Y, Wong RSM, Soo YOY, Chui CH, Lau FY, Chan NPH, et al. Initial Treatment of Immune Thrombocytopenic Purpura with High-Dose Dexamethasone. New England Journal of Medicine. 2003 Aug 28;349(9):831–6.

The Wells DVT criteria: A clinical prediction model for deep vein thrombosis

1. The Wells DVT criteria estimated the pre-test probability of deep vein thrombosis (DVT).

2. D-dimer testing in outpatients informed the need for venous ultrasonography in the diagnosis of DVT.

Original Date of Publication: September 2003

Study Rundown: DVT is a condition where blood clots form in the deep venous system. While DVTs most frequently occur in the lower extremities, they may also develop in the upper extremities and other deep veins, such as the portal vein. Patients with DVT often present with pain, swelling, and erythema in the affected extremity. Pulmonary embolism is a concerning and potentially life-threatening complication of DVT, as pieces of thrombus may embolize to the lungs. As a result, patients with DVT are often treated with anticoagulants or, in certain circumstances, mechanical vena caval filters. Originally developed in 1995, the Wells DVT criteria help determine a patient's pre-test probability of having a DVT. These criteria have been subsequently refined and included in an algorithm to guide diagnostic evaluation for DVT using D-dimer testing and venous ultrasonography. This study was published in 2003 and helped elucidate the role of D-dimer in evaluating patients with suspected DVT. The trial found that the D-dimer test had a negative predictive value of 99.1% (95%CI 96.7-99.9) in patients with low pre-test probability of DVT. In patients likely to have a DVT, its negative predictive value was 89.0% (95%CI 80.7-94.6). Thus, D-dimer testing was deemed useful to rule out DVT in patients with low likelihood of thrombus based on clinical assessment.

In-Depth [randomized controlled trial]: In this study, 1096 outpatients who presented with a suspected DVT were first assessed using the clinical model to determine their pre-test probability of DVT (i.e., likely or unlikely). Investigators then randomized patients to the control group (i.e., ultrasonography) or to the intervention group (i.e., D-dimer and ultrasonography). There were no significant differences between the groups in terms of thromboembolic events encountered in follow-up at 3 months. The D-dimer group was associated with significantly lower use of venous ultrasonography, compared to the control group. In patients unlikely to have DVT, the D-dimer test had a negative predictive value of 99.1% (95%CI 96.7-99.9). In patients likely to have DVT, the D-dimer test had a negative predictive value of 89.0% (95%CI 80.7-94.6).

The Wells DVT criteria (Figure)

≥2 indicates that the probability of DVT is likely; <2 indicates that the probability of DVT is unlikely.

Criteria	Points
Active cancer	1
Bedridden recently >3 days or major surgery within 4 weeks	1
Calf swelling >3 cm compared to the other leg (measured 10 cm below tibial tuberosity)	1
Collateral (nonvaricose) superficial veins present	1
Entire leg swollen	1
Localized tenderness along deep venous system	1
Pitting edema, greater in symptomatic leg	1
Paralysis, paresis, or recent plaster immobilization of the lower extremity	1
Previously documented DVT	1
Alternative diagnosis to DVT as likely or more likely	-2

Wells PS, Anderson DR, Rodger M, Forgie M, Kearon C, Dreyer J, et al. Evaluation of D-Dimer in the Diagnosis of Suspected Deep-Vein Thrombosis. New England Journal of Medicine. 2003 Sep 25;349(13):1227–35.

Hepatocellular carcinoma screening reduces mortality in high risk patients

1. Patients at a high risk for hepatocellular carcinoma (HCC) who underwent biannual screening with serum alpha-fetal protein (AFP) levels and liver ultrasound were much more likely to be diagnosed with cancer in the earlier stages and receive curative treatment.

2. Biannual screening for hepatocellular carcinoma led to a significant reduction in 5-year mortality.

Original Date of Publication: July 2004

Study Rundown: Since the 1970s, it has been common practice to screen for HCC in high-risk patients with AFP levels and ultrasound. However, this trial was the first randomized controlled trial to demonstrate a reduction in mortality with biannual combined screening. Compared to the control group, the group who received screening (at least once) during the course of the study had HCC diagnosed at earlier stages than the control group. More subjects in the screening group were able to undergo resectable surgery than in the control group. Five-year survival was 46.4% in the screening group and 0.00% in the control group. In summary, biannual screening with AFP levels and ultrasound significantly improved survival in patients with hepatitis B virus (HBV) who were found to have HCC. Biannual screening was shown to detect cancers at an earlier stage that allowed for more effective and curative therapy. Of note, the study only included patients with known chronic hepatitis infections. In addition, the majority of the participants was male and under the age of 50. Currently, the HCC screening guidelines do not discriminate by age, but it is important to know that these results may not be as accurate for an older population.

In-Depth [randomized controlled trial]: This study was conducted in primary care centers across Shanghai, China from 1993 to 1997. Eligible patients were all patients 35-59 years of age who either had a history of chronic hepatitis or serum evidence of a hepatitis B infection. Patients with a known history of HCC, other malignant diseases, or serious illnesses were excluded. Investigators randomized patients to screening vs no screening groups. Screening included a biannual serum AFP level and liver ultrasound. A subject's participation at least once in the screening was required for inclusion in the screening group. The median number of screenings a subject participated in was 5. Serum AFP levels above 20 mcg/L were considered abnormal. Any abnormality found on screening was re-evaluated by screening a 2nd time to reduce false-positives. Patients were followed for 5 years.

The primary end-point was mortality from HCC, with a significant reduction observed in the screening group (83.2 per 100 000) compared to the no-screening group (131.5 per 100 000 with a rate ratio of 0.63, 95%CI 0.41-0.98). Patients in the screening group were also more likely to be diagnosed with HCC at earlier stages (60.5% were diagnosed with Stage I HCC in the screening group compared to 0.0% in the no-screening group). Forty-six percent of HCC patients in the screening group were able to undergo surgical resection while 50.7% in the no-screening group were treated conservatively. Five-year survival was 46.4% in the screening group and 0.00% in the control group (X^2 35.50, p < 0.01).

Zhang B-H, Yang B-H, Tang Z-Y. Randomized controlled trial of screening for hepatocellular carcinoma. J Cancer Res Clin Oncol. 2004 Mar 20;130(7):417–22.

The PLCO trial 1: PSA and digital rectal examination in prostate cancer screening

1. Subjects who underwent annual prostate-specific antigen (PSA) testing for 6 years and annual digital rectal examination (DRE) for 4 years had a significantly increased incidence of prostate cancer compared to usual care.

2. Screening with PSA testing and DRE did not significantly reduce mortality from prostate cancer compared to usual care.

Original Date of Publication: March 2009

The Prostate, Lung, Colorectal, and Ovarian (PLCO) Cancer Screening Trial is a large population-based randomized trial sponsored by the National Cancer Institute (NCI) to explore the effects of screening on cancer mortality. The trial has been conducted at 10 different centers across the U.S. Participants randomized to the intervention group receive active screening for PLCO cancers (i.e., chest x-ray, flexible sigmoidoscopy, CA-125, transvaginal ultrasound, PSA, digital rectal examination) in the first 6 years of the trial and are subsequently followed for another 7 years. Participants randomized to the usual care group are managed with usual medical care and are followed for 13 years. The trial began in 1993 and the screening phase of the trial was completed in 2006, though follow-up will continue until 2015. We report below on the findings regarding prostate cancer screening using PSA testing and digital rectal examination.

Study Rundown: The combination of PSA testing and DRE was been the standard screening approach for prostate cancer for several decades. While many clinicians used this approach, there was significant uncertainty regarding the benefits and harms of prostate cancer screening. This led to the release of conflicting guidelines from different organizations, such as the American Cancer Society and the U.S. Preventative Task Force (USPSTF). The prostate component of the PLCO trial assessed the effect of annual PSA testing for 6 years and annual DRE for 4 years on mortality rates from prostate cancer. The study revealed that screening with PSA testing and DRE was associated with an increased incidence of prostate cancer, but not with a significant reduction in mortality when compared with usual care. Thus, the concern was that prostate cancer screening may expose patients to the risks of overdiagnosis and overtreatment of prostate cancer, with no actual benefit in survival.

The limitations of this study included a relatively high PSA testing and DRE rate in the control group, ranging from 40%-52% for PSA testing and 41%-46% for DRE. This rate of screening in the control group may have reduced the relative difference in prostate cancer mortality between the control and screening groups. Secondly, about 44% of subjects in both groups had undergone 1 or more PSA tests at baseline, which may have excluded more easily detectable cancers prior to the enrollment in the study, thereby also potentially leading to a reduction in the observed difference in prostate cancer mortality. Finally, it is possible that improvements in prostate cancer therapy equally reduced death from prostate cancer in both experimental groups, thereby dampening the survival benefits of early cancer detection from screening. In summary, the prostate component of the PLCO trial found that screening with PSA testing and DRE was not associated with significant decreases in prostate cancer mortality.

In-Depth [randomized controlled trial]: The PLCO trial was a randomized, controlled trial that enrolled 154 900 participants between 55-74 years of age from 10 study centers in the U.S. The exclusion criteria were a history of PLCO cancer, current cancer treatment, and more than one instance of PSA testing in the 3 years prior to enrollment. Of the enrolled participants, 38 343 were assigned to the screening group that received annual PSA testing for 6 years and annual DRE for 4 years, while 38 350 were assigned to the control group. Follow-up remains planned for all subjects for at least 13 years, but the results of this study were released with at least 7 years of follow-up for all patients and 10 years of follow-up for 67% of the patients due to public health considerations raised by the study's results. At 7 years, more subjects in the screening group were diagnosed with prostate cancer than in the control group (rate ratio 1.22; 95%CI 1.16-1.29). This difference persisted for patients with 10 years of follow-up (rate ratio 1.17; 95%CI 1.11-1.22). There was, however, no significant difference in mortality from prostate cancer between the screening and control groups at 7 years (rate ratio 1.16; 95%CI 0.76-1.76) or 10 years of follow-up (rate ratio 1.09; 95%CI 0.76-1.76).

Andriole GL, Crawford ED, Grubb RL, Buys SS, Chia D, Church TR, et al. Mortality Results from a Randomized Prostate-Cancer Screening Trial. New England Journal of Medicine. 2009 Mar 26;360(13):1310–9.

The RE-COVER trial: Dabigatran non-inferior to warfarin in treating acute venous thromboembolism

1. The RE-COVER trial demonstrated that treating acute venous thromboembolism (VTE) with 6 months of dabigatran 150 mg twice daily was non-inferior to dose-adjusted warfarin to an INR of 2-3.

2. Though dabigatran therapy does not require international normalized ratio (INR) monitoring, it is considerably more expensive than warfarin.

Original Date of Publication: December 2009

Study Rundown: Prior to the publication of the RE-COVER trial, dabigatran, an oral, direct thrombin inhibitor, had been shown to be as effective as enoxaparin in the prevention of venous thromboembolism after elective hip and knee arthroplasty. Another study had demonstrated that dabigatran was as effective as warfarin when used for stroke prophylaxis in patients with atrial fibrillation, while also having a similar safety profile and not requiring periodic INR monitoring. The purpose of the RE-COVER trial was to determine whether or not dabigatran could be used as an alternative to warfarin in the treatment of acute VTE. The findings demonstrated that in patients with acute VTE, dabigatran was non-inferior to warfarin in preventing symptomatic VTE or death associated with VTE. A larger number of patients in the dabigatran group discontinued their medication due to an adverse effect, and the incidence of dyspepsia was also higher in the dabigatran group. One common criticism of the study is that a pharmaceutical company played a large part in designing and conducting the trial. It is also important to note that treatment with dabigatran is considerably more expensive than warfarin, and that dabigatran should only be considered in patients with sufficient renal function.

In-Depth [randomized controlled trial]: The RE-COVER trial, published in NEJM in 2009, was a randomized, double-blind, non-inferiority trial comparing dabigatran with warfarin in the treatment of acute VTE. A total of 2564 patients were randomized to receive either 6 months of dabigatran 150 mg twice daily or dose-adjusted warfarin with a target INR of 2-3. Patients in both groups were treated with at least 5 days of parenteral anticoagulation prior to starting on their oral anticoagulants. Notably, the study was funded, designed, and conducted by the manufacturer of dabigatran in conjunction with the study steering committee. The primary efficacy endpoint was a composite of symptomatic VTE or death associated with VTE in the 6 month period after randomization. Patients were assessed at 7 days after randomization, and then monthly for 6 months. Patients were recruited from 228 different centers in 29 countries. Parenteral anticoagulation was given for a mean of 10 days in both groups.

Dabigatran was demonstrated to be to be non-inferior to warfarin in the primary efficacy outcome. There were no significant differences between the groups in terms of the incidence of major bleeding, though patients in the warfarin group experienced a significantly higher rate of any bleeding event. Significantly more patients in the dabigatran group experienced an adverse event that led to discontinuation of the study drug (HR 1.33; 95%CI 1.01-1.76). Patients in the dabigatran group also experienced significantly higher incidence of dyspepsia compared to the warfarin group (2.9% in dabigatran group, 0.6% in warfarin group).

Schulman S, Kearon C, Kakkar AK, Mismetti P, Schellong S, Eriksson H, et al. Dabigatran versus Warfarin in the Treatment of Acute Venous Thromboembolism. New England Journal of Medicine. 2009 Dec 10;361(24):2342–52.

The EINSTEIN-DVT trial: Rivaroxaban in acute deep vein thrombosis

1. Rivaroxaban was non-inferior to standard therapy of enoxaparin and vitamin K antagonist (VKA) in treating acute, symptomatic deep vein thrombosis (DVT).

2. The risk of major and clinically relevant nonmajor bleeding was not significantly different when comparing rivaroxaban with standard therapy.

Original Date of Publication: December 2010

Study Rundown: The EINSTEN-DVT trial demonstrated that rivaroxaban is non-inferior to standard therapy (i.e., enoxaparin and warfarin) in treating acute, symptomatic DVT and preventing the recurrence of symptomatic venous thromboembolism (VTE). Moreover, this study demonstrated that there was no significant increase in the risk of bleeding with rivaroxaban, when compared to standard therapy. The new oral anticoagulants have shown much promise in randomized controlled trials thus far, particularly in treating acute VTE, VTE prophylaxis, and stroke prophylaxis in atrial fibrillation. Compared with low molecular weight heparins and VKA, these new oral agents are much easier to administer and also far less cumbersome with regards to monitoring. Concerns remain, however, regarding the lack of effective reversal agents for these medications, as numerous studies have demonstrated increased risk of clinically relevant bleeding. In summary, rivaroxaban was non-inferior to standard therapy, consisting of enoxaparin and warfarin, in treating acute, symptomatic DVT. Given the lack of a reversal agent, however, physicians should exercise caution in selecting the appropriate patients for treatment with the new oral anticoagulants.

In-Depth [randomized controlled trial]: The EINSTEN-DVT trial consisted of two studies carried out in parallel. The first was an open-label, non-inferiority study that compared the effects of rivaroxaban with standard therapy (i.e., subcutaneous enoxaparin followed by a VKA) in treating acute, symptomatic DVT (the Acute DVT study). In the rivaroxaban group, patients received 15 mg BID for 3 weeks, followed by 20 mg OD for the remainder of the treatment time (3, 6, or 12 months). Patients in the standard therapy group were managed with enoxaparin until international normalized ratios (INR) exceeded 2, and their VKA dose was titrated to an INR of 2-3. The second was a double-blind, superiority study that compared 6-12 months of treatment with rivaroxaban with placebo after patients had completed 6-12 months of treatment for venous thromboembolism (the Extension study). Patients in the rivaroxaban group received 20 mg OD. In both studies, the primary outcome was the recurrence of symptomatic venous thromboembolism (i.e., DVT, non-fatal or fatal pulmonary embolism). Notably, patients were excluded from both studies if they had creatinine clearance <30 mL/min. or clinically significant liver disease (i.e., acute hepatitis, chronic active hepatitis, cirrhosis).

A total of 3449 patients were randomized to as part of the Acute DVT study, while 1197 were enrolled in the Extension study. In the Acute DVT study, there were no significant differences between the two groups in terms of the primary outcome (HR 0.68; 95%CI 0.44-1.04). Moreover, there were no significant differences in terms of major bleeding (HR 0.63; 95%CI 0.33-1.30). In the Extension study, the rivaroxaban group experienced significantly lower rates of the primary outcome, as compared to the placebo group (HR 0.18; 95%CI 0.09-0.39). Patients in the rivaroxaban group, however, did experience significantly higher rates of major and clinically relevant nonmajor bleeding (HR 5.19; 95%CI 2.3-11.7).

EINSTEIN Investigators, Bauersachs R, Berkowitz SD, Brenner B, Buller HR, Decousus H, et al. Oral rivaroxaban for symptomatic venous thromboembolism. New England Journal of Medicine. 2010 Dec 23;363(26):2499–510.

The EINSTEIN-PE trial: Rivaroxaban to treat pulmonary embolism

1. Rivaroxaban, an oral factor Xa inhibitor, was non-inferior to standard anticoagulation therapy (i.e., low-molecular weight heparin [LMWH] and a vitamin K antagonist) in the prevention of recurrent thromboembolism following a pulmonary embolism (PE).

2. The rate of major bleeding was significantly lower with rivaroxaban than with standard anticoagulant therapy.

Original Date of Publication: April 2012

Study Rundown: For many years, standard therapy for PE consisted of LMWH followed by a vitamin K antagonist, such as warfarin. Although effective, treatment with warfarin requires frequent blood tests and is thus burdensome for patients. The EINSTEIN-PE trial found that treatment with rivaroxaban alone was non-inferior to standard therapy in preventing recurrent thromboembolism. It also demonstrated that rivaroxaban, an oral factor Xa inhibitor, did not require laboratory monitoring for the prevention of recurrent thromboembolism following an acute PE. The rivaroxaban group also had significantly fewer major bleeding events when compared with standard therapy. A major limitation of the EINSTEIN-PE trial was its open-label design, which increased the risk of bias. Notably, 5% of patients participating in the study had cancer. Previous studies, including the CLOT trial, have helped establish guidelines recommending the use of LMWH in treating thromboembolism in the context of malignancy, and this recommendation has not changed in light of the findings of the EINSTEIN-PE trial. The study was funded by 2 pharmaceutical companies.

In-Depth [randomized controlled trial]: Originally published in 2012, the EINSTEIN-PE trial was a randomized, open-label, non-inferiority trial involving 4832 patients. Eligible patients were those who had an acute, symptomatic PE with or without symptomatic deep vein thrombosis (DVT). Investigators randomized patients to receive rivaroxaban or standard therapy (i.e., enoxaparin with either warfarin or acenocoumarol). The primary efficacy outcome was recurrent venous thromboembolism (i.e., PE and/or DVT), and the primary safety outcome was clinically relevant nonmajor bleeding or major bleeding (defined as bleeding in critical sites). Rivaroxaban was non-inferior to standard therapy in preventing recurrent venous thromboembolism post-PE (HR 1.12; 95%CI 0.75-1.68). The rate of major bleeding was also lower in the rivaroxaban group, as compared to standard therapy (HR 0.49; 95%CI 0.31-0.79).

EINSTEIN–PE Investigators, Büller HR, Prins MH, Lensin AWA, Decousus H, Jacobson BF, et al. Oral rivaroxaban for the treatment of symptomatic pulmonary embolism. New England Journal of Medicine. 2012 Apr 5;366(14):1287–97.

The PLCO trial 2: Flexible sigmoidoscopy in colon cancer screening

1. Compared to usual care, screening with flexible sigmoidoscopy significantly reduced the incidence of colon cancer in the distal and proximal colon.

2. Screening with flexible sigmoidoscopy significantly reduced mortality cancers of the distal colon only when compared with usual care.

Original Date of Publication: June 2012

The Prostate, Lung, Colorectal, and Ovarian (PLCO) Cancer Screening Trial is a large population-based randomized trial sponsored by the National Cancer Institute (NCI) to explore the effects of screening on cancer mortality. The trial has been conducted at 10 different centers across the U.S. Participants randomized to the intervention group receive active screening for PLCO cancers (i.e., chest x-ray, flexible sigmoidoscopy, CA-125, transvaginal ultrasound, PSA, digital rectal examination) in the first 6 years of the trial and are subsequently followed for another 7 years. Participants randomized to the usual care group are managed with usual medical care and are followed for 13 years. The trial began in 1993 and the screening phase of the trial was completed in 2006, though follow-up will continue until 2015. Here, we report on the findings regarding colorectal cancer screening using flexible sigmoidoscopy.

Study Rundown: Colon cancer screening with fecal occult blood testing (FOBT) was previously reported to reduce colon cancer incidence and mortality. Flexible sigmoidoscopy is an endoscopic procedure where the most distal segment of the colon is examined. Previous studies conducted in Europe suggested that sigmoidoscopy was associated with reductions in both colon cancer incidence and mortality. The colorectal component of the PLCO trial assessed the effect of screening with two flexible sigmoidoscopies, spaced 3 or 5 years apart, on the incidence of and mortality from colon cancer in patients from the U.S. This study demonstrated that screening with flexible sigmoidoscopy was associated with a significant reduction in incidence of both distal and proximal colon cancer, regardless of the stage of the cancer, when compared to the usual-care group. Screening was also associated with a significant reduction in mortality independent of cancer stage, but only for distal colon cancer. For proximal colon cancer, screening resulted in reduced mortality for cancers staged I, II, or III, but not IV.

Study limitations included a substantial rate of endoscopy use in the usual-care group during the time the intervention group was undergoing screening - 46.5% of the usual-care group underwent either a flexible sigmoidoscopy or colonoscopy. This use may have dampened the difference in incidence and mortality between the usual-care and screening groups. In summary, the colorectal component of the PLCO trial found that screening with flexible sigmoidoscopy was associated with decreased colon cancer mortality and incidence. The study results support routine screening with flexible sigmoidoscopy followed by colonoscopy for cases of abnormal screening results.

In-Depth [randomized controlled trial]: The PLCO cancer trial was a randomized, controlled trial that enrolled 154 900 participants between 55-74 years of age from 10 study centers in the U.S. The primary exclusion criteria were a history of PLCO cancer, ongoing cancer treatment, and lower endoscopy (i.e., flexible sigmoidoscopy, colonoscopy, or barium enema) in the previous 3 years. Of the enrolled participants, 77 445 were randomized to receive flexible sigmoidoscopy at baseline and again after 3 or 5 years, while the other 77 455 were assigned to receive usual care. The primary endpoint was death from colon cancer, while secondary endpoints included colorectal cancer incidence, cancer stage, survival, harms of screening, and all-cause mortality. The primary analysis was an intention-to-screen comparison of mortality between the two experimental groups.

At a median follow-up of 11.9 years, the intervention group experienced a significant 21% reduction in colon cancer incidence compared to the usual care group (RR 0.79; 95%CI 0.72-0.85). This reduction was observed for both distal colon cancer (RR 0.71, 95%CI 0.64-0.80) and proximal colon cancer (RR 0.86; 95%CI 0.76-0.97). Additionally, there was a 26% reduction in colon cancer mortality due to screening (RR 0.74; 95%CI 0.63-0.87). This reduction was only significant for distal colon cancer (RR 0.50; 95%CI 0.38-0.64), but not proximal colon cancer (RR 0.97; 95%CI 0.77-1.22).

Schoen RE, Pinsky PF, Weissfeld JL, Yokochi LA, Church T, Laiyemo AO, et al. Colorectal-Cancer Incidence and Mortality with Screening Flexible Sigmoidoscopy. New England Journal of Medicine. 2012 Jun 21;366(25):2345–57.

The ATLAS trial: Duration of adjuvant tamoxifen in estrogen receptor-positive breast cancer

1. Among women with early estrogen receptor (ER)-positive breast cancer, continuing adjuvant tamoxifen for 10 years significantly reduced breast cancer recurrence, breast cancer mortality, and overall mortality when compared with stopping at 5 years after diagnosis.

2. Patients treated with adjuvant tamoxifen for 10 years had significantly higher risk of endometrial cancer and pulmonary embolism.

Original Date of Publication: March 2013

Study Rundown: In women with ER-positive breast cancer, previous trials had demonstrated that treatment with adjuvant tamoxifen for 5 years significantly reduced the risk of recurrence both during the treatment time and for 10 years after. During this 15-year period, mortality from breast cancer was also significantly reduced. Tamoxifen treatment, however, is linked with significantly increased risk of certain side effects, including endometrial cancer and thromboembolic disease. The Adjuvant Tamoxifen: Longer Against Shorter (ATLAS) trial compared the effects of 10 years of adjuvant tamoxifen treatment with 5 years of adjuvant tamoxifen treatment on outcomes in patients with ER-positive breast cancer. Over the duration of follow up, 10-year treatment significantly reduced breast cancer recurrence, breast cancer mortality, and overall mortality compared to the standard 5-year course of tamoxifen. However, this increased benefit came at the expense of significantly increased rates of endometrial cancer and pulmonary embolism. The study remains ongoing and future data will help elucidate the longer-term effects of prolonged tamoxifen treatment in patients with early ER-positive breast cancer.

In-Depth [randomized controlled trial]: This multinational study included 12 894 women with early breast cancer, 6454 of whom were randomized to continue tamoxifen for 10 years (i.e., the intervention group) after diagnosis and 6440 of whom were randomized to stop tamoxifen use at 5 years (i.e., the control group). While all 12 894 were included in the analysis for side effects, only women with ER-positive disease were included in the main analysis for breast cancer recurrence and mortality - 6846 women. Patients were eligible for inclusion if they had early breast cancer (i.e., completely resectable disease), they had subsequently received tamoxifen and were still on it (or had stopped in the past year and could resume treatment quickly), they were clinically free of disease (i.e., local recurrence resected, no distant recurrence), follow-up was practicable, and there was uncertainty between the patient and her physician regarding whether to continue tamoxifen treatment. There were no restrictions based on patient age, the type of initial surgery or histology, hormone receptor status, nodal status, or other treatments. Patients were not eligible if they had any contraindications to continuing tamoxifen (e.g., pregnancy, breastfeeding, retinopathy, endometrial hyperplasia).

In women with ER-positive disease, continuing tamoxifen treatment for 10 years significantly reduced the risk of breast cancer recurrence (RR 0.84; 95%CI 0.76-0.94), breast cancer mortality (RR 0.83; 95%CI 0.72-0.96), and overall mortality (RR 0.87; 95%CI 0.78-0.97) when compared to 5 years of treatment. Notably, during years 5-14 after diagnosis, the absolute recurrence reduction was 3.7% with extended tamoxifen treatment (21.4% vs. 25.1%). The relative risk of pulmonary embolus (RR 1.87; 95%CI 1.13-3.07) and endometrial cancer (RR 1.74; 95%CI 1.30-2.34) were significantly higher in women who continued tamoxifen compared to the control group, while the risk of ischemic heart disease was significantly reduced (RR 0.76; 95%CI 0.60-0.95).

Davies C, Pan H, Godwin J, Gray R, Arriagada R, Raina V, et al. Long-term effects of continuing adjuvant tamoxifen to 10 years versus stopping at 5 years after diagnosis of oestrogen receptor-positive breast cancer: ATLAS, a randomised trial. Lancet. 2013 Mar 9;381(9869):805–16.

The AMPLIFY trial: Apixaban for treatment of venous thromboembolism

1. Apixaban was found to be non-inferior to conventional therapy (i.e., enoxaparin followed by warfarin) in the treatment of acute venous thromboembolism (VTE).

2. Major bleeding was found to be significantly less common in patients treated with apixaban as compared with conventional therapy.

Original Date of Publication: August 2013

Study Rundown: New oral anticoagulants are being increasingly used for a number of different indications, including stroke prophylaxis in patients with atrial fibrillation and treatment of venous thromboembolic disease. The purpose of the Apixaban for the Initial Management of Pulmonary Embolism and Deep vein thrombosis as First-Line Therapy (AMPLIFY) trial was to determine if apixaban, an oral factor Xa inhibitor, was non-inferior to conventional therapy (i.e., enoxaparin followed by warfarin) for the treatment of acute VTE disease. In summary, apixaban was found to be non-inferior to conventional therapy in preventing recurrent venous thromboembolism or death from venous thromboembolism. The rate of major bleeding was significantly lower in patients treated with apixaban as compared with conventional therapy. Of note, the study was funded and partially designed by two pharmaceutical companies.

In-Depth [randomized controlled trial]: This randomized, non-inferiority trial was conducted at 358 centers in 28 countries. A total of 5400 patients were enrolled and randomized to treatment with apixaban or conventional therapy (i.e., enoxaparin for 5 days and warfarin for 6 months with target INR between 2-3). Patients were included in the trial if they were >18 years of age, had objectively confirmed proximal deep vein thrombosis (DVT) and/or pulmonary embolism. Exclusion criteria included active bleeding, a high risk of bleeding, other contraindications to anticoagulation, cancer, provoked venous thromboembolic disease, dual antiplatelet therapy, and creatinine clearance <25 mL/min. The primary efficacy outcome was a composite of recurrent symptomatic venous thromboembolism or death from venous thromboembolism. Secondary outcomes included each component of the primary outcome, in addition to cardiovascular mortality and all-cause mortality. The primary safety outcome was major bleeding. There was no difference in the rate of the primary outcome in the two groups (RR 0.84; 95%CI 0.60-1.18) and the findings met criteria for non-inferiority. Moreover, there were no significant differences between the groups in terms of the risk of cardiovascular or all-cause mortality. Major bleeding occurred significantly less frequently in patients treated with apixaban compared to those on conventional therapy (RR 0.31; 95%CI 0.17-0.55).

Agnelli G, Buller HR, Cohen A, Curto M, Gallus AS, Johnson M, et al. Oral Apixaban for the Treatment of Acute Venous Thromboembolism. New England Journal of Medicine. 2013 Aug 29;369(9):799–808.

VI. Imaging and Intervention

Ultrasound sensitive for appendicitis, improves outcomes

1. Among patients with signs and symptoms consistent with acute appendicitis (AA), ultrasound demonstrated a sensitivity and specificity of 80% and 100%, respectively.

2. The use of ultrasound led to an appropriate change in patient management in 26.1% of cases.

Original Date of Publication: September 1987

Study Rundown: AA is a common cause of abdominal pain in both children and adults, and can be challenging to diagnose by physical examination alone. By the mid-1980s a number of small, retrospective studies had been performed suggesting a diagnostic role for graded-compression ultrasound (GCUS), a technique that involves the application of pressure to abdominal wall with the ultrasound probe to minimize obscuring bowel gas. However, the results were felt to be equivocal, and GCUS was not widely adopted. In the present trial, the question of GCUS as a diagnostic tool in the evaluation of patients with suspected AA was addressed prospectively in a large cohort of patients at a single academic medical center. All enrolled patients were imaged after initial assessment by a surgeon, and changes in planned patient management were recorded alongside the diagnostic performance of GCUS. Results showed a high sensitivity and specificity for AA as well as a favorable trend toward improved patient care, with changes in management made for over one-quarter of patients. Notably, GCUS was not able to visualize the appendix in a significant minority of cases, in part reflecting limitations in ultrasound technology at the time of the study's publication.

In-Depth [prospective cohort]: A total of 111 consecutive patients (mean age 29 years, range 8-86 years) with a clinical presentation concerning for AA were prospectively enrolled at a single academic medical center over a 5 month period. All enrolled patients were first clinically evaluated by a member of the surgical staff using a combination of physical examination, laboratory studies, and plain x-ray images. Immediately following this, patients then received comprehensive abdominal ultrasound using graded compression for optimization of bowel visualization. All ultrasound studies were performed by radiologists and evaluated on several parameters, including appendiceal visualization, certainty of appendiceal visualization, and the presence imaging findings consistent with complications such as appendiceal perforation. After a maximum period of 6 hours of patient observation and prior to being informed of ultrasound findings, the evaluating surgeon was then asked to provide recommendations for operative or non-operative management. Imaging findings were then provided alongside an opportunity to alter management plans. The final diagnosis was determined using surgical pathology, intraoperative findings, or clinical diagnosis in combination with radiology and other supporting data.

An unequivocal ultrasound diagnosis was rendered in 83 (74.8%) patients. Among these patients, the overall sensitivity and specificity for the diagnosis of AA were 80% and 100%, respectively. When considering only those patients with non-perforated AA, the sensitivity remained essentially unchanged at 80.5% but decreased to 28.5% for patients with perforated AA. This was felt to be related to obscuration of the bowel wall by free intra-abdominal fluid and difficult patient examination secondary to peritonitis. In 29 (26.1%) patients, GCUS led to an appropriate change in management, including 16 (14.4%) patients originally triaged to conservative management who instead underwent surgical intervention. Among 4 of the 28 (14.3%) patients without a definitive final diagnosis, the appendix was unequivocally visualized but the patients did not undergo surgery because of symptom resolution.

Puylaert JBCM, Rutgers PH, Lalisang RI, de Vries BC, van der Werf SDJ, Dörr JPJ, et al. A Prospective Study of Ultrasonography in the Diagnosis of Appendicitis. New England Journal of Medicine. 1987 Sep 10;317(11):666–9.

CT evaluation in pancreatitis strongly correlates with patient outcomes

1. Among patients with acute pancreatitis, the presence and degree of pancreatic necrosis correlated with average hospital length of stay, complications, and mortality.

2. By combining existing an existing acute pancreatitis grading system with computed tomography (CT) evaluation of pancreatic necrosis, the authors generated a CT Severity Index that strongly correlated with patient outcomes.

Original Date of Publication: February 1990

Study Rundown: Acute pancreatitis is a common condition involving inflammation of the pancreas. Though most patients have a benign course without associated complications, some develop severe disease associated with high rates of morbidity and mortality. Numerous attempts have been made to estimate patient prognosis in acute pancreatitis, including attempts to correlate imaging findings with patient outcomes using CT. Due to limitations in early CT technology, however, pancreatitis grading scales suffered from poor sensitivity and specificity and were not widely used. In this trial, the study authors attempted to build on these prior works by using contrast-enhanced CT to evaluate the presence and degree of pancreatic necrosis as a prognostic indicator in acute pancreatitis. Using a prospective patient cohort at a single institution, the study authors demonstrated a strong, positive relationship between pancreatic necrosis and patient outcomes. Compared to those with a normal-appearing pancreas by CT, patients with necrosis had significantly longer hospital lengths of stay and higher rates of complications. All deaths in the study cohort were in patients with pancreatic necrosis. Combining this information with previously-described rating scales, the authors were then able to generate the CT Severity Index (CTIS), a numeric scale to predict the risk of complications and death. Applying this scale to the study cohort, morbidity and mortality strongly correlated with CTIS score. Primary limitations of this study included modest sample size and the associated low mortality rate. Subsequent work in pancreatitis imaging has expanded upon this landmark trial, the results of which remain in modern clinical practice as the modified CTIS.

In-Depth [prospective cohort]: Eighty-eight patients (mean age, 52 years) with signs and symptoms of acute pancreatitis were enrolled. All patients were initially managed with standard medical therapy, including nasogastric suction, analgesia, and intravenous fluids. Surgical intervention was pursued in patients with sepsis refractory to medical management. All patients underwent CT imaging of the abdomen with intravenous and oral contrast for evaluation of pancreatic necrosis at the time of admission, and a subset of patients received additional, subsequent CT imaging (mean number of CTs/patients, 2.9). Scans were interpreted blindly and assessed for two specific features: the patient's five-point pancreatitis grade, based on previously published data; and the qualitative degree of decreased pancreatic parenchymal enhancement. This latter variable was taken to represent the presence of pancreatic necrosis, and was reported as one of four possible severities. Additional collected data included Ranson's score, hospital length of stay, morbidity—defined as pancreatic abscess or pseudocyst formation—and mortality.

At the end of the trial, 66 (75.0%) patients had uncomplicated courses and recovered with medical therapy alone, while 22 (25.0%) patients required surgical intervention. Five (5.7%) patients died. In total, pancreatic necrosis was detected in 18 (20.5%) patients. Average length of stay was 109 days among patients with >50% necrosis, as compared to 25 days among those without evidence of necrosis at presentation. The average Ranson's score (a marker of severity, maximum score 11) was 1.9 among those without necrosis and 5.5 among those with >50% necrosis. Patients with CT evidence of necrosis had morbidity and mortality rates of 82% and 23%, respectively, as compared with respective rates of 6% and 0% among those without necrosis. The positive predictive value for abscess formation of 77% among patients with necrosis, and the negative predictive value of abscess formation among those without necrosis was 97%. By combining pancreatitis grade and CT extent of pancreatic necrosis, a CT Severity Index was created with a maximum score of 10 (highest severity). Among study patients with a CTSI 0-3, there was 3% mortality and 8% morbidity; among patients with CTSI 7-10, mortality and morbidity were 17% and 92%, respectively.

Puylaert JBCM, Rutgers PH, Lalisang RI, de Vries BC, van der Werf SDJ, Dörr JPJ, et al. A Prospective Study of Ultrasonography in the Diagnosis of Appendicitis. New England Journal of Medicine. 1987 Sep 10;317(11):666–9.

Breast ultrasound sensitive for cancer, carries a low false positive rate

1. In a large cohort of women referred for evaluation of one or more solid breast lesions, ultrasound (US) showed a sensitivity of 98.4% for malignancy and was associated with a negative predictive value of 99.5%.

Original Date of Publication: July 1995

Study Rundown: US is a powerful medical imaging tool. It is portable, quickly generates clinically-relevant data, and is not associated with ionizing radiation exposure. The technology has found applications in nearly every area of medicine, and has been particularly beneficial in the area of breast imaging. At the time of this study, US was used to help identify simple breast cysts, a common and benign finding that can generate initial concern when identified on mammography. Given the success of US in this area, numerous attempts were made to expand the technology's use to include other indeterminate breast lesions, particularly solid masses. Initial studies were unsupportive, however, and multiple guideline sets were published explicitly recommending against the use of US for solid breast mass evaluation.

Given dramatic improvements in the resolution and functional capabilities of US, however, this issue was revisited in 1995 with publication of this prospective trial. A large cohort of women with suspicious breast lesions referred for breast US were evaluated over several years. Only women with solid lesions were considered. All women underwent biopsy following their US, and biopsy and imaging results were compared to determine the diagnostic performance of US. Results revealed that, contrary to prior data, US was highly sensitive for malignancy in solid breast masses. Conversely, in the absence of concerning imaging features, US appropriately excluded malignancy with few diagnostic errors. Strengths of the trial included its prospective methodology, the large number of patients successfully enrolled, and the low attrition rate. The primary limitations of the trial included heterogeneous biopsy methods and the inherent variability associated with subjective rating scales. Today, breast US remains a substantial component of the breast imager's toolkit, and is routinely used for solid breast mass evaluation.

In-Depth [prospective cohort]: A total of 662 patients (mean age 47 years) with suspicious breast lesions were prospectively enrolled over an approximately

4-year period following referral for breast US. The most common reason for referral was an antecedent abnormal mammogram. A total of 750 solid nodules were evaluated by US. Studies were blindly interpreted by 5 breast radiologists and findings were classified as "benign" or "malignant" based on the presence or absence of several previously-published imaging features. When no features were present, a classification of "indeterminate" was made. When available, initial mammograms and their interpretations were also reviewed. All enrolled patients subsequently underwent either core needle or excisional biopsy for definitive pathologic diagnosis. These final diagnoses were compared with imaging results to determine the diagnostic performance of US in the evaluation of suspicious solid breast lesions.

Pathologic examination revealed 625 (83%) benign nodules and 125 (17%) malignant nodules. The most common malignant lesion was infiltrating ductal adenocarcinoma, and the most common benign lesion was fibroadenoma. One hundred (73%) of the 137 malignant nodules were correctly diagnosed by US. The overall sensitivity and specificity for breast US in the detection of malignancy were 98.4% and 67.8%, respectively. Due to a high false positive rate, the positive predictive value was 38%, while the negative predictive value was 99.5%, with only 2 false positive examinations. Twenty-seven nodules that were interpreted as malignant or indeterminate by US had been previously interpreted as definitively or probably benign by mammography. An additional 44 nodules accurately interpreted as malignant by US were interpreted as indeterminate by mammography. The US features most strongly associated with malignancy were speculation (OR 5.5), taller-than-wider shape (OR 4.9), and angular margins (OR 4.0).

Stavros AT, Thickman D, Rapp CL, Dennis MA, Parker SH, Sisney GA. Solid breast nodules: use of sonography to distinguish between benign and malignant lesions. Radiology. 1995 Jul 1;196(1):123–34.

Percutaneous ethanol injection safe and effective in hepatocellular carcinoma

1. In a large prospective cohort of patients with hepatocellular carcinoma (HCC) and contraindications to surgical management, the use of percutaneous ethanol injection (PEI) was associated with favorable survival outcomes and few adverse events at five years.

Original Date of Publication: October 1995

Study Rundown: First described in the mid-1980s, the use of PEI for the treatment of HCC generated significant interest in the oncology community. Though surgical resection or liver transplant have historically been the preferred means of managing HCC patients, PEI was among the first in a subset of minimally-invasive treatment modalities to show promise for patients with contraindications to surgical treatment. Advantages of PEI over surgery include the low cost, short treatment time, lack of need for general endotracheal anesthesia, and the ability to perform the procedure in the outpatient setting. The majority of early PEI trials suggested treatment efficacy and improved patient survival; however, these trials were generally small in size and tracked patient outcomes for only short post-treatment intervals, and thus their validity remained uncertain.

This trial was the first to enroll a large, prospective cohort and follow them over several years after PEI with the goal of more definitively defining the procedure's outcomes among HCC patients. Conducted at multiple clinical sites in Italy, the trial included patients with absolute or relative contraindications to surgical management and followed them for an average of three years following PEI. Given the large but highly heterogeneous population within the trial, the authors were able to generate survival data stratified according to discrete clinical factors such as tumor size, multiplicity, and Child class. The results showed overall survival trends comparable to surgical resection, and outlined in particular how survival after PEI varied as a function of patient-specific factors, most notably Child class. The rate of major complications was low, and only one death was attributable to the procedure. With these data published, PEI became the de facto standard of care for patients with contraindications to surgery and ushered in, alongside transarterial chemoembolization, the modern era of minimally-invasive HCC therapies.

In-Depth [case series study]: A total of 746 patients (76% men; mean age 64 years) were prospectively enrolled from nine academic medical centers in Italy. Primary enrollment criteria included a pre-enrollment diagnosis of HCC and either tumor inoperability (as defined by factors such as multiple tumor foci and advanced patients age), patient refusal of surgical intervention, or referral for non-operative management at the request of the primary treating physician. Prior to PEI, all enrolled patients underwent ultrasound and contrast-enhanced computed tomography (CT) to assess disease burden. PEI was performed without general anesthesia in the outpatient setting under ultrasound guidance in one or more sessions. Treatment efficacy was assessed at one month by ultrasound, CT, and serum alpha fetoprotein, and then by imaging at 3-6 month intervals thereafter. Kaplan-Meier survival curves were generated and stratified according to factors such as tumor size, tumor number, and Child class.

The mean follow-up time was 36 months (range 12-90 months). Cumulative five-year survival varied from 26-40% among patients with one or more HCC lesions without extrahepatic involvement, and was 47% and 29% for Child class A and B patients, respectively. Among those patients with extrahepatic disease or Child class C cirrhosis, cumulative five-year survival was 0%. Local recurrence at the site of prior PEI was noted in 17% of lesions, the majority of which were treated with repeat PEI. The 30-day mortality rate was 0%, and the overall procedure-specific mortality rate was 0.1%. Major complications such as significant bleeding occurred in 1.3% of patients. Though not formally evaluated, the average cost of PEI at the participating centers was approximately $1,000 USD, as compared to $30,000 USD for surgical resection.

Livraghi T, Giorgio A, Marin G, Salmi A, de Sio I, Bolondi L, et al. Hepatocellular carcinoma and cirrhosis in 746 patients: long-term results of percutaneous ethanol injection. Radiology. 1995 Oct 1;197(1):101–8.

Non-contrast CT sensitive and specific for kidney stones

1. Among patients with acute flank pain, non-contrast computed tomography (CT) of the abdomen and pelvis demonstrated a sensitivity of 97% and a specificity of 96% for the diagnosis of kidney stones.

2. Non-contrast CT was associated with a low false negative rate and was able to suggest alternative diagnoses in a significant number of patients without evidence of kidney stones, thus increasing the overall diagnostic yield.

Original Date of Publication: January 1996

Study Rundown: Kidney stones, or nephrolithiasis, are a common cause of pain among patients presenting to the emergency department. Historically, the evaluation of patients with suspected nephrolithiasis consisted of plain radiographs together with clinical history, physical examination, and laboratory data. However, this combination was associated with a high false negative rate. The diagnostic yield was improved with the widespread adoption of intravenous pyelography (IP), a fluoroscopic technique in which dye is introduced into the urinary tract and imaged by x-rays in real-time. The use of IP improved stone detection but was associated with higher radiation exposure and the need for contrast administration, and the false negative rate remained high. There remained a significant need for a fast, accurate diagnostic technique among patients with suspected stone disease. With the introduction of CT into standard practice, there was a strong push towards its adoption as the standard for evaluation of nephrolithiasis given its high spatial and contrast resolution.

In the present study, patients with symptoms concerning for nephrolithiasis were imaged with non-contrast CT of the abdomen and pelvis to determine the presence or absence of stones within the urinary tract. These patients then underwent a combination of repeat imaging, surgery, or close clinical follow-up to determine the final diagnosis. The results suggested that non-contrast CT was highly sensitive and specific for the nephrolithiasis, as well as associated with few false negative findings. Moreover, because of the ability to imaging other structures within the abdomen and pelvis in high resolution, CT was able to identify possible alternative diagnosis, such as appendicitis or infection, in nearly 33% of patients without evidence of stones. The study was limited by the use of a composite reference standard and the lack of outcome data. Today, non-contrast CT in conjunction with ultrasonography remains the diagnostic gold standard among patients with suspected kidney stones.

In-Depth [prospective cohort]: A total of 292 consecutive patients referred for evaluation of possible nephrolithiasis at a single center underwent non-contrast CT of the abdomen and pelvis by standard protocol. Images were blindly reviewed by 2 radiologists with expertise in CT interpretation, and imaging diagnoses were made by consensus. Findings considered positive for nephrolithiasis included direct visualization of a stone within the ureters or bladder, or unilateral collecting system dilation and perinephric stranding without direct stone visualization. Of the original cohort that underwent imaging, 210 patients (98 male, 112 female; age range 18-85 years) went on to have diagnostic confirmation in the form of surgery, repeat imaging, or clinical follow-up. The results of the study suggested a sensitivity and negative predictive value of 97%, and a specificity and positive predictive value of 96%. The overall diagnostic accuracy of non-contrast CT in the evaluation of patients with suspected nephrolithiasis was 97%. Thirty-one patients without evidence of stone disease on CT (27.6%) were found to have unsuspected extra-renal abnormalities, the most common of which was symptomatic adnexal masses.

Smith RC, Verga M, McCarthy S, Rosenfield AT. Diagnosis of acute flank pain: value of unenhanced helical CT. American Journal of Roentgenology. 1996 Jan 1;166(1):97–101.

The Canadian CT Head Rule

1. The Canadian CT Head Rule consists of 7 predictor variables to assess the need for computed tomography (CT) imaging in patients with minor head injuries.

2. This study demonstrated that the rule is highly sensitive and may help to reduce the number of CT scans ordered.

Original Date of Publication: May 2001

Study Rundown: First published in The Lancet in 2001, the Canadian CT Head Rule was designed to identify patients who required CT after suffering minor head injuries. The definition of a minor head injury is a history of loss of consciousness, amnesia, or disorientation and a Glasgow Coma Scale (GCS) score of 13-15. At the time, there were conflicting guidelines regarding the use of CT in patients suffering these injuries, and the Canadian CT Head Rule sought to standardize the management of patients while reducing the number of unnecessary CT scans. This study developed the Rule and found it to be a highly sensitive clinical decision rule for patients with minor head injuries. Moreover, the findings suggested that the Rule may help reduce the number of CT scans ordered in assessing patients with minor head injuries.

In-Depth [prospective cohort]: This trial was carried out in 10 Canadian community and academic centers. The primary outcome was the need for neurological intervention (i.e., death within 7 days due to head injury, or need for craniotomy, elevation of skull fracture, intracranial pressure monitoring, or intubation for head injury within 7 days), while the secondary outcome was the presence of clinically important brain injury identified on CT. Patients requiring a CT were identified by standardized physician assessments, which included assessing for pre-determined predictor variables. Patients not requiring a CT were followed-up with a phone call 14 days after their assessment. A total of 3121 patients were enrolled, and 2078 of these patients received CT scans. Logistic regression was carried out to develop a model for identifying cases with clinically important brain injury, and the model was used to generate the 7 predictors in the Canadian CT Head Rule (Figure).

CT head is only required for minor head injury patients with any of these findings:

High risk (for neurological intervention)

1. GCS score <15 at 2 hours after injury
2. Suspected open or depressed skull fracture
3. Any sign of basal skull fracture (i.e., hemotympanum, "racoon" eyes, CSF otorrhea/rhinorrhea, Battle's sign)
4. Vomiting ≥2 episodes
5. Age ≥65 years

Medium risk (for brain injury on CT)

1. Amnesia before impact ≥30 minutes
2. Dangerous mechanism (i.e., pedestrian struck by motor vehicle, occupant ejected from motor vehicle, fall from elevation ≥3 feet/5 stairs)

Subsequent analyses demonstrated that the 5 "high risk" factors had a sensitivity of 100% (95%CI 92-100%) and specificity of 68.7% (95%CI 67-70%) for neurological intervention, while CT scans would have been ordered in 32.2% of patients. When all 7 factors were considered, the sensitivity was 98.4% (95%CI 96-99%) and specificity was 49.6% (95%CI 48-51%) for clinically-important brain injury on CT, while CT scans would have been ordered in 54.3% of patients.

Stiell IG, Wells GA, Vandemheen K, Clement C, Lesiuk H, Laupacis A, et al. The Canadian CT Head Rule for patients with minor head injury. Lancet. 2001 May 5;357(9266):1391–6.

Diffusion-weighted MRI highly sensitive for acute stroke

1. Among patients with acute neurologic deficits presenting within 6 hours of symptom onset, diffusion-weighted magnetic resonance imaging (DWI) was significantly more sensitive and specific for the diagnosis of ischemic stroke compared non-contrast computed tomography (NCCT).

Original Date of Publication: September 2002

Study Rundown: Thrombolysis is a widely accepted method for the management of acute ischemic stroke, with the goal of opening blocked vessels to restore blood flow to at-risk brain tissue. One of the primary requirements for the administration of intravenous thrombolytic drugs is the exclusion of intracranial hemorrhage as an explanation for a patient's acute neurologic symptoms. NCCT is the method of choice for fast and accurate detection of intracranial bleeding. Its performance in the detection of early acute ischemic stroke, however, is generally poor, with a reported sensitivity of approximately 40-60% within the first 6 hours from symptom onset. DWI is an attractive alternative imaging technique that allows for the high-resolution depiction of areas of reduced blood flow in the brain much earlier than is generally possible with NCCT.

In this comparative trial, patients presenting to the emergency department with symptoms concerning for acute ischemic stroke were assigned to undergo both NCCT and DWI in a randomized order. For each patient and for each imaging study, the presence or absence of stroke was determined alongside other parameters to determine the diagnostic utility of both methods. The results suggested that DWI is significantly more sensitive and specific than NCCT for the diagnosis of acute ischemic stroke. Additionally, researchers found that inter-reader reliability differed greatly between the two imaging modalities, with almost perfect agreement when using DWI and only modest agreement when using NCCT, suggesting that DWI is less susceptible to interpretive errors than NCCT. This was the first trial to provide a head-to-head comparison of the two diagnostic imaging methods for stroke, and it served to significantly strengthen the evidence base in support of DWI that had been built in prior trials.

In-Depth [prospective cohort]: In this study, 54 consecutive patients presenting to a single academic medical center emergency department with symptoms concerning for acute ischemic stroke were prospectively enrolled to undergo both NCCT and DWI in a randomized order. Primary inclusion criteria included presentation for evaluation within six hours of symptom onset and a National Institute of Health Stroke Scale (NIHSS) greater than 3, with higher values indicating greater stroke severity. All images were read by expert neuroradiologists and stroke neurologists and categorized according to the presence or absence of ischemic stroke, the vascular distribution of the stroke, the stroke subtype (none, lacunar, territorial, or hemodynamic), and other parameters. Readers were blinded to the specific details of each case.

Overall, NCCT demonstrated a sensitivity and specificity of 61% and 65%, respectively, for the diagnosis of acute ischemic stroke, and inter-reader reliability was moderate. DWI significantly outperformed NCCT, with a sensitivity and specificity of 91% and 95%, respectively, and almost perfect inter-reader reliability. Notably, no acute lacunar infarcts were visible on NCCT while four were diagnosed using DWI, suggesting that DWI may also be superior for the identification of specific stroke subtypes. All infarcts in this study were within the middle cerebral artery distribution, and the mean NIHSS of enrolled patients was 11 (range 3-27). The mean time from initial evaluation to the receipt of diagnostic imaging was comparable for both modalities (NCCT = 180 minutes, DWI = 189 minutes).

Fiebach JB, Schellinger PD, Jansen O, Meyer M, Wilde P, Bender J, et al. CT and Diffusion-Weighted MR Imaging in Randomized Order Diffusion-Weighted Imaging Results in Higher Accuracy and Lower Interrater Variability in the Diagnosis of Hyperacute Ischemic. Stroke. 2002 Sep 1;33(9):2206–10.

The PIOPED II trial: CT sensitive and specific for pulmonary embolism

1. Multidetector computed tomographic angiography (CTA) was highly sensitive and specific for the diagnosis of pulmonary embolism (PE) when compared to a composite reference standard.

2. When combined with computed tomographic venography (CTV), sensitivity was increased without a significant increase in the specificity, positive predictive value, or negative predictive value.

Original Date of Publication: June 2006

Study Rundown: PE refers to the blockage of one or more arteries within the lung by a blood clot or other substance that originated within another part of the body. It is a commonly considered diagnosis among patients presenting to the emergency department with shortness of breath and chest pain, and failure to diagnose PE is associated with significant mortality. Historically, the diagnosis was made by the introduction of contrast material directly into the pulmonary arteries by a catheter. This technique was replaced by ventilation-perfusion (VQ) scanning, which compares patterns of blood flow and oxygenation in the lung using a radioactive tracer. Though significantly less invasive, VQ scanning was often difficult to interpret and was itself replaced by CTA beginning in the 1980s and 1990s.

Early reports of the diagnostic performance of CTA were generally positive but mixed, and the optimal method for evaluating patients with suspected PE initially remained uncertain. In the second Prospective Investigation of Pulmonary Embolism Diagnosis (PIOPED II) trial, CTA with and without concomitant lower extremity CTV was compared with a composite reference standard including both VQ scanning and conventional angiography. The results of this trial showed that both CTA and combined CTA-CTV were highly sensitive and specific for the diagnosis of PE, and that the combination of clinical judgment with the results from CTA or CTA-CTV evaluation was sufficient to accurately rule-in and rule-out PE in the vast majority of patients.

In-Depth [prospective cohort]: This prospective trial was conducted at 8 clinic sites throughout North America. All adult patients with signs and symptoms concerning for acute PE who were referred for evaluation were consecutively screened for enrollment (n = 7284). Both inpatients and outpatients were considered. Key exclusion criteria included anticoagulant use, hemodialysis, critical illness, patients on ventilators, and recent myocardial infarction. Following screening and consent, all enrolled patients (n = 1090) underwent combined CTA-CTV, as well as one or more of the components that together formed the composite reference standard. This included VQ scanning, lower extremity venous ultrasonography with Doppler imaging, and, when necessary, digital subtraction angiography (DSA) of the pulmonary arteries. All imaging studies were reviewed by 2 blinded radiologists unaffiliated with the clinical sites, with additional radiologists serving as arbiters in the event of discordant interpretations. Patients were considered to have a positive CTA if there was any partial or complete filling defect identified within one or more pulmonary arteries, and a positive CTV if there was any partial or complete filling defect identified within one of the lower extremity veins. Using the composite reference standard, patients were diagnosed with PE if any of the following conditions were met: high probability VQ scan in a patient without a history of PE; filling defect on pulmonary DSA; or visualized lower extremity clot by ultrasound.

A total of 824 patients (mean age 51.7 ± 17.1 years; 62% women; 89% outpatient) successfully completed both CTA-CTV and the composite reference standard. Among this cohort, 192 PEs were diagnosed. For those with diagnostic-quality CTA alone (773 patients, 94%), the sensitivity was 83% and the specificity was 96%, while the positive and negative predictive values were 86% and 95%, respectively. Considering those patients with diagnostic-quality combined CTA-CTV (737 patients, 89%) separately, the sensitivity was 90% and the specificity was 95%, while the positive and negative predictive values were 85% and 97%, respectively. The results varied substantially by clinical suspicion, with a positive predictive value of 96% among those with a high pre-test probability of PE and a positive predictive value of 58% among those with a low-pretest probability. Complications associated with CTA-CTV were rare and included mild allergic reactions and transiently increased creatinine.

Stein PD, Fowler SE, Goodman LR, Gottschalk A, Hales CA, Hull RD, et al. Multidetector Computed Tomography for Acute Pulmonary Embolism. New England Journal of Medicine. 2006 Jun 1;354(22):2317–27.

The NLST trial: CT screening reduces lung cancer mortality

1. Low-dose computed tomography (CT) screening significantly reduced lung cancer mortality when compared to screening with chest radiography.

2. Screening for lung cancer with either modality resulted in very high false positive rates.

Original Date of Publication: August 2011

Study Rundown: Prior studies have shown that lung cancer screening using chest radiography does not decrease lung cancer mortality. The use of molecular markers in screening is also under study, but currently unsuitable for clinical application. In contrast, observational studies have suggested that low-dose helical CT may be superior to chest radiography in detecting early-stage lung cancer. The National Lung Screening Trial (NLST) was a randomized, controlled study that compared 3 annual low-dose CTs with chest radiography in lung cancer screening. In summary, this study demonstrated that low-dose CT screening significantly reduced lung cancer-related mortality when compared with chest radiography. Additionally, low-dose CT screening detected more lower-stage cancers than chest radiography and low-dose CT significantly decreased all-cause mortality.

Strengths of the study include the participants' high adherence rate. Approximately 95% of participants adhered to the three rounds of screening in the low-dose CT group, while 93% adhered in the radiography group. Advancements in CT scanners since the time of the study may lead to further reductions in lung cancer mortality, though may also contribute to higher rates of false positives. The major limitations of this study are the limited follow-up and the very high false-positive rates in both the CT and radiography groups. Recently, the United States Preventive Services Task Force issued a draft statement recommending screening high-risk individuals with low-dose CT on an annual basis based on the results of the NLST trial, though there remains controversy in this area. The American Cancer Society, for example, recommends discussing screening with low-dose CT, while cautioning patients about the high likelihood of false positives and potential further investigation.

In-Depth [randomized controlled trial]: The NLST was a randomized trial that enrolled 53 454 patients. Eligible patients were between 55-74 years of age, had at least a 30 pack-year smoking history, and, if former smokers, had stopped smoking within the last 15 years. The exclusion criteria were a previous diagnosis of lung cancer, having a chest CT in the previous 18 months, hemoptysis, or unexplained weight loss in the previous year. In the end, 26 722 patients were randomized to screening through 3 annual low-dose CTs and 26 732 to 3 annual chest radiographs. Chest radiography, rather than community care, was chosen for the control group because the concomitant Pancreatic, Lung, Colorectal, and Ovarian (PLCO) cancer trial was evaluating the effect of chest radiography versus community care for lung cancer. Data analysis was conducted according to the intention-to-screen principle. For low-dose CT, any non-calcified nodule larger than 4 mm in diameter was classified as a positive finding. For chest radiography, any non-calcified nodule was classified as a positive finding. Results showed that low-dose CT was associated with a significant 20.0% relative reduction in lung cancer mortality (95%CI 6.8-26.7%, p = 0.004). Low-dose CT was also associated with significantly higher incidence of lung cancer (RR 1.13; 95%CI 1.03-1.23). All-cause mortality was significantly lower in the low-dose CT group by 6.7% (95%CI 1.2-13.6%, p = 0.02).

National Lung Screening Trial Research Team, Aberle DR, Adams AM, Berg CD, Black WC, Clapp JD, et al. Reduced lung-cancer mortality with low-dose computed tomographic screening. New England Journal of Medicine. 2011 Aug 4;365(5):395–409.

CT scans increase the risk of malignancy in children and young adults

1. In this retrospective cohort analysis of children and young adults without previous malignancy, patients exposed to multiple computed tomography (CT) scans had over 3 times the risk of developing leukemia and brain tumors.

Original Date of Publication: August 2012

Study Rundown: While the connection between radiation exposure and malignancy was previously identified, research on the subject matter drew from high-dose radiation exposure secondary to atomic bombs in Japan. At the time of its publication, this study was the first to use a cohort to examine the malignancy risk associated with low-dose radiation from CT scans. Through retrospective analysis, researchers investigated the relationship between CT-induced radiation exposure during childhood and young adulthood and development of leukemia and brain cancer, as these malignancies occur in particularly radiosensitive tissue. Children under the age of 15 who received 5-10 head CTs were exposed to around 50 milligrays (mGy) of radiation to their marrow, while 2-3 head CTs exposed these children to about 60 mGy of brain radiation. For comparison, the average chest radiograph exposes a child to 0.05 to 0.3 mGy.

Investigators reported an over 3 times increased risk of developing leukemia with exposure to $\geq$30 mGy and developing a brain tumor with $\geq$50 mGy of radiation. Limitations included using standardized CT machine settings as a proxy when assessing radiation exposure due to missing data regarding machine-specific settings. However, the use of a cohort from Great Britain's national database ensured a large study group with low risk of loss to follow-up. This was the first cohort study to investigate the potential association between lower doses of radiation than the estimated 100 mGy of radiation exposure experienced by many Japanese atomic bomb victims. While the overall incidence of these malignancies is small within the pediatric population, this study does indicate significant risks associated with over-imaging developing children. With this in mind, the Alliance for Radiation Safety in Pediatric Imaging within the United States has started the "Image Gently" campaign, a movement designed to increase awareness of healthcare practitioners and caregivers to the benefits of reducing unnecessary radiation exposure.

In-Depth [retrospective cohort]: A total of 355 191 patients seen at a Great Britain National Health Service hospital without a history of prior malignancy, but who underwent a first CT scan between 1985-2002 at ages younger than 22, were included in the study. The study group was divided such that 178 604 patients were investigated with respect to leukemia and 176 587 patients were studied with respect to brain tumors. Malignancies investigated included acute lymphoblastic leukemia, acute myeloid leukemia, myelodysplastic syndromes (MDS), leukemia excluding MDS, gliomas, and meningiomas plus schwannomas. Relative risks were calculated to assess the relationship between the radiation doses expressed in mGy units and malignancy. Data were collected from a national registry and ended on December 31, 2008, at time of death, or when patients were lost to follow-up. During analysis, radiation doses were adjusted to reflect the time it typically takes to develop a malignancy. This resulted in a 2 year lag for leukemia and a 5 year lag for brain tumors.

Among the patients included in the leukemia analysis, 283 919 CT scans were completed (64% head) and 74 patients had developed leukemia on follow-up. 279 824 scans were completed for patients included in brain tumor analysis with 135 patients ultimately receiving diagnoses of brain tumors on follow-up. Significant positive associations between leukemia and CT radiation dosing ($p < 0.01$) and brain tumors and radiation ($p < 0.001$) were observed. Mean radiation dose was 51.13 mGy for patients who developed leukemia and with exposure to ≥30 mGy of radiation. Among those who received ≥30 mGy, patients were more than 3 times as likely to develop leukemia when compared to those who received <5 mGy (RR 3.18; 95%CI 1.46-6.94). Mean radiation dose for patients who received ≥50 mGy and developed brain tumors was 104.16 mGy. Those who received ≥50 mGy of radiation were at greater than 3 times the risk of developing a brain tumor when compared to those who were exposed to <5 mGy (RR 3.32; 95%CI 1.84-6.42).

Pearce MS, Salotti JA, Little MP, McHugh K, Lee C, Kim KP, et al. Radiation exposure from CT scans in childhood and subsequent risk of leukaemia and brain tumours: a retrospective cohort study. Lancet. 2012 Aug 4;380(9840):499–505.

VII. Infectious Disease

Prophylactic penicillin reduces septicemia in sickle cell patients

1. This randomized, placebo-controlled, double-blinded trial demonstrated an 84% reduction in the incidence of pneumococcal septicemia among patients with sickle cell taking prophylactic penicillin when compared to those taking placebo.

2. Fifteen severe, Streptococcus pneumoniae-related infections occurred during the study with 13 occurring in patients taking placebo, 3 of which resulted in death. No patients taking prophylactic penicillin died during the study course.

Original Date of Publication: June 1986

Study Rundown: Children with sickle cell disease are at increased risk for severe, often deadly septicemia secondary to Streptococcus pneumoniae. This study investigated the use of oral penicillin prophylaxis to prevent pneumococcal sepsis. Previous research indicated the potential benefit of penicillin injections in decreasing pneumococcal septicemia in patients with compromised splenic function; however, no controlled trial of oral penicillin existed. This multicenter, randomized, double-blinded, placebo-controlled trial compared the use of twice daily penicillin to placebo vitamin C tablets using serious infection secondary to S. pneumoniae as the primary endpoint and was terminated early on account of the clear benefit of the treatment. In total, 15 cases of pneumococcal sepsis were reported, of which 13 cases occurred in patients taking placebo. Of note, 3 placebo-treated patients died from their infections. This study initiated the recommendation for all patients to undergo screening for sickle cell at birth and, for those found to be positive, to have prophylactic penicillin therapy initiated in conjunction with pneumococcal vaccination. Presently, twice daily penicillin prophylaxis from 3 months of age through 5 years old is recommended, although whether or not to stop at 5 years of age is controversial.

In-Depth [randomized controlled trial]: A total of 215 children with sickle cell disease diagnosed on hemoglobin electrophoresis and aged 3 to 36 months were recruited from 33 clinical centers and included in final analysis. Recruitment started in August 1983 and ended in February 1985. Participants needed to be asymptomatic at the time of enrollment and were randomized to receive either 125 mg of penicillin V potassium 2 times daily or a placebo of 50 mg vitamin C tablets twice daily. Patients were seen by a practitioner on study

244

enrollment and then every 3 months. At each visit, patients were examined, had a complete blood count drawn, had their pills counted, and underwent penicillin-sensitive urine testing (to ensure compliance). Patients were nasopharyngeal swabbed for pneumococcal antibodies. While the purpose of this study was not to evaluate the efficacy of the pneumococcal vaccination, patients required vaccine administration and were given the first dose at 1 year of age and then at 2 years of age. The primary endpoint of the study was a severe infection such as bacteremia, meningitis, or pneumonia resulting in hospitalization secondary to S. pneumoniae with a severe infection due to any other organism considered a secondary endpoint.

The study was concluded 8 months earlier than planned after 15 episodes of pneumococcal septicemia were reported, with 13 cases among patients taking placebo and 2 among those taking penicillin. These were the only S. pneumoniae-related infections and amounted for an 84% reduction in pneumococcal septicemia with significantly less penicillin-treated patients experiencing S. pneumoniae infections compared to those on placebo ($p < 0.005$). Three of the placebo-treated patients died as a result of their pneumococcal infection, despite all having been vaccinated according to the recommended regimen. No children receiving prophylactic penicillin died from infectious causes during the trial. No adverse effects of the treatment were noted.

Gaston MH, Verter JI, Woods G, Pegelow C, Kelleher J, Presbury G, et al. Prophylaxis with Oral Penicillin in Children with Sickle Cell Anemia. New England Journal of Medicine. 1986 Jun 19;314(25):1593–9.

Albumin in cirrhotic patients with spontaneous bacterial peritonitis

1. In cirrhotic patients with spontaneous bacterial peritonitis (SBP), albumin infusion on days 1 and 3 of treatment, in addition to antibiotics, significantly reduced the risk of developing renal impairment and mortality when compared with antibiotics alone.

Original Date of Publication: August 1999

Study Rundown: Renal impairment during SBP is a known risk factor for in-hospital mortality and is thought to be due to low effective circulating volume (ECV). This reduction in ECV is likely due to third-spacing, as well as excessive vasodilation resulting from systemic inflammatory response. Albumin is able to increase the ECV by providing higher oncotic pressures in the vasculature. This randomized, controlled study sought to determine the benefits of albumin in patients treated for SBP. A total of 126 patients with SBP were randomized to receive antibiotics with albumin infusions, or albumin alone. The study found that patients treated with both antibiotics and albumin had significantly lower rates of renal impairment and mortality when compared to those receiving antibiotics alone.

In-Depth [randomized controlled trial]: This study involved 126 patients with cirrhosis who were diagnosed with SBP and randomized them to receive 1) antibiotics with albumin infusion or 2) antibiotics alone. Patients were recruited from 7 university hospitals in Spain. Patients in the albumin group received a 1.5 mg/kg dose of albumin on day 1 within 6 hours of enrollment in the study, and this was followed by a 1 mg/kg dose on day 3 of the study. All patients were treated with intravenous cefotaxime (dose-adjusted based on serum creatinine). After the resolution of infection, all patients were started on norfloxacin 400 mg daily prophylaxis. All investigators were blinded to treatment group assignment. Patients were included in the study if they had a polymorphonuclear cell count in the ascitic fluid $>250/mm^3$, were between 18-80 years of age, had no antibiotic treatment within 1 week before the diagnosis of SBP (except for norfloxacin prophylaxis), did not have other infections/shock/gastrointestinal bleeding/ileus/grade 3 or 4 hepatic encephalopathy/organic nephropathy (i.e., proteinuria, hematuria, abnormal renal ultrasound), did not have human immunodeficiency virus infection, and had serum creatinine ≤265 µmol/L. Primary endpoints of the study were development of renal impairment (i.e., non-reversible deterioration of renal function during hospitalization) and mortality. Patients receiving both antibiotics and albumin experienced significantly lower rates of renal impairment, when compared with patients being treated with antibiotics alone (10% vs. 33%, p = 0.002). Moreover, patients in the antibiotics and albumin group experienced significantly lower mortality both in-hospital (10% vs. 29%, p = 0.01) and at 3 months (22% vs. 41%, p = 0.03), when compared with patients receiving antibiotics alone.

Sort P, Navasa M, Arroyo V, Aldeguer X, Planas R, Ruiz-del-Arbol L, et al. Effect of Intravenous Albumin on Renal Impairment and Mortality in Patients with Cirrhosis and Spontaneous Bacterial Peritonitis. New England Journal of Medicine. 1999 Aug 5;341(6):403–9.

Adjuvant dexamethasone improves outcomes in adult bacterial meningitis

1. Treatment with dexamethasone significantly reduced morbidity and mortality in adults with bacterial meningitis.

2. There was no significant difference in risk of adverse events with corticosteroid treatment.

Original Date of Publication: November 2002

Study Rundown: Bacterial meningitis is a neurological emergency with high fatality rates and results in neurologic deficits in nearly a third of survivors. Streptococcus pneumoniae and Neisseria meningitidis are the most common causes of bacterial meningitis, accounting for 80% of adult cases. Pneumococcal meningitis refers to infection caused by S. pneumoniae while meningococcal meningitis refers to infection by N. meningitidis. Bacterial meningitis is suspected in patients presenting with the classic triad of fever, neck stiffness and altered mental status. The triad has a low sensitivity but almost all patients present with at least two of four symptoms: headache, fever, neck stiffness and altered mental status. Culture and stain of a cerebrospinal fluid (CSF) obtained by lumbar puncture is the definitive method of diagnosis and identification of the etiologic agent. However, there is a significant risk of brain herniation with the lumbar puncture due to high cranial pressure. Thus neuroimaging, typically by cranial computed tomography (CT), is recommended before lumbar puncture to detect brain shift. Antibiotic therapy is initiated as soon as possible.

This study found that early adjuvant dexamethasone (10 mg every 6 hours for four days) reduced morbidity and mortality in adults with acute bacterial meningitis. The beneficial effect of dexamethasone was clear in patients with pneumococcal meningitis but a significant benefit was not shown in patients with meningococcal meningitis, possibly due to the limited number of patients in this subgroup. There was some concern regarding delay in treatment initiation due to informed-consent procedures and the time required for cranial CT and lumbar puncture when it was indicated for patients. Previous studies suggested that 2- and 4-day regimens of dexamethasone therapy are equally effective. This study used and recommended a 4-day regimen, initiated before or with the first dose of antibiotics. Although the reduction in mortality in this study was not associated with a higher rate of neurologic sequelae, corticosteroids may be associated with ischemic injury to neurons and so further research should investigate cognitive impairment in adults treated with and without dexamethasone.

In-Depth [randomized controlled trial]: A total of 301 patients with suspected meningitis were randomly assigned to receive dexamethasone 10 mg intravenously Q6H or placebo for four days along with usual antibiotic therapy. Patients were eligible for the trial if they were ≥17 years of age, had suspected meningitis in combination with a cloudy CSF, bacteria in CSF on Gram staining, or CSF leukocyte count >1000/mm³. Exclusion criteria included hypersensitivity to beta-lactam antibiotics or corticosteroids, pregnancy, cerebrospinal shunt, treatment with antibiotics in the previous 48 hours, and a history of active tuberculosis or fungal infection. The primary outcome was the score on the Glasgow Outcome Scale, where a score of 5 indicates a favorable outcome and a score from 1-4 indicates an unfavorable outcome, eight weeks after undergoing randomization.

Patients in the dexamethasone group were less likely to experience an unfavorable outcome than patients in the placebo group at eight weeks after enrollment (RR 0.59; 95%CI 0.37-0.94). The absolute risk reduction for an unfavorable outcome was 10% in patients treated with dexamethasone. Mortality was also lower in the dexamethasone group than the placebo group (RR 0.48; 95%CI 0.24-0.96). Dexamethasone did not significantly improve or worsen neurologic sequelae (e.g., hearing loss) in survivors. Patients receiving dexamethasone were less likely to develop impaired consciousness (11% vs. 25%, p = 0.002) and were less likely to have seizures (5% vs. 12%, p = 0.04) or cardiorespiratory failure (10% vs. 20%, p = 0.02).

De Gans J, van de Beek D. Dexamethasone in Adults with Bacterial Meningitis. New England Journal of Medicine. 2002 Nov 14;347(20):1549–56.

The CURB-65 score: Risk stratifying patients with community-acquired pneumonia

1. Patients with community-acquired pneumonia (CAP) were stratified into mortality risk groups using a 5-point score.

2. One point was awarded for each of the following on initial presentation: confusion, urea >7 mmol/L, respiratory rate >30/min, low systolic (<90 mm Hg) or diastolic (<60 mm Hg) blood pressure, age >65 years.

3. Patients who received a score of ≥3 were found to be at a high-risk of mortality (>19%) and require admission.

Original Date of Publication: May 2003

Study Rundown: The CURB-65 score was developed as a simple 5-point clinical tool for risk stratifying patients presenting with community-acquired pneumonia. Patients with a score of 0-1 may suitable for home management (i.e., low-risk). Patients with a score of 2 may require a short inpatient stay (i.e., intermediate-risk), while those with scores ≥3 should be managed in hospital (i.e., high-risk). Compared to the 20-variable Pneumonia Severity Index (PSI), the CURB-65 score is much easier to remember and apply clinically. In the CURB-65 score, one point is awarded for each of the following: confusion, urea >7mmol/L, respiratory rate >30/min, low systolic (<90 mmHg) or diastolic (<60 mm Hg) blood pressure, and age >65 years on initial assessment. This prospective cohort study describes how the score was derived and validated. In summary, the CURB-65 score is a simple tool to aid clinical decision-making in stratifying patients presenting with community-acquired pneumonia into low-, intermediate-, and high-risk groups in terms of mortality, thereby assisting in management decisions.

In-Depth [prospective cohort]: Data from 1068 adult patients admitted with CAP in three prospective studies (conducted in the UK, New Zealand, and the Netherlands) were amalgamated. The main outcome measure was 30-day mortality. The dataset was divided into an 80% derivation cohort and a 20% validation cohort. Based on the modified British Thoracic Society (mBTS) assessment tool, the association between the "CURB" score and 30 day-mortality was examined, and prognostic variables were elucidated, including newly identified independent factors separate from CURB. Prognostic features not readily available during an initial hospital assessment were excluded from the clinical prediction rule for practical relevance. The CURB-65 (a six-point score from 0 to 5, one point for each variable present) enabled patients to be stratified according to mortality risk. The score (Figure) involved one point for each of **C**onfusion, **U**rea >7 mmol/L, **R**espiratory rate >30/min, low systolic (<90 mm Hg) or diastolic (<60 mm Hg) **B**lood pressure, and age >**65** years on initial patient assessment. All results were tested against the aforementioned validation cohort, which confirmed the increasing mortality pattern.

CURB-65 score	Mortality risk
0	0.7%
1	3.2%
2	3%
3	17%
4	41.5%
5	57%

Lim WS, Eerden MM van der, Laing R, Boersma WG, Karalus N, Town GI, et al. Defining community acquired pneumonia severity on presentation to hospital: an international derivation and validation study. Thorax. 2003 May 1;58(5):377–82.

Quadrivalent HPV vaccine in young women

1. Prophylactic use of a quadrivalent vaccine against human papillomavirus (HPV) strains 6, 11, 16, and 18 significantly reduced the incidence of HPV infection and HPV-associated genital disease 30 months after vaccination.

2. No significant adverse effects were observed secondary to the vaccinations.

Original Date of Publication: April 2005

Study Rundown: HPV infection causes cervical cancer in women worldwide, and while routine screening with Pap smears and close follow up of pre-cancerous lesions have reduced the risk of cervical cancer, it has not eliminated it. This study examined the efficacy of a quadrivalent vaccine in reducing the incidence of HPV infection due to the four most common strains: 6, 11, 16, and 18. These 4 strains have been linked with 70% of cervical cancers and 90% of genital warts. The vaccine is comprised of 3 injections months apart from each other and the participants were followed over the course of 36 months. In summary, the incidence of HPV infection and HPV-associated diseases were significantly lower in the vaccinated group when compared with the unvaccinated group 3 years post-vaccination. These results indicated that the vaccine may prevent infection and consequently reduce the prevalence of HPV-associated diseases. However, the study only followed the women for 3 years post-vaccination and could not demonstrate the vaccine's long-term efficacy.

In-Depth [randomized controlled trial]: This phase II randomized, multicenter, double-blind placebo-controlled study that randomized 552 women to either receive the quadrivalent HPV vaccine or a placebo injection in 3 doses, with the second and third doses administered at 2 and 6 months, respectively, after the first dose. All participants were between the ages of 16-23 years of age, not pregnant, had no history of abnormal Pap smears, and had 4 or fewer male sex partners in their lifetime. Women with history of cleared HPV infection were included in the study. Patients were followed for 36 months and had gynecological exams that included a Papanicolau test and HPV cervical swab testing on day 1, and at 7, 12, 24, and 36 months from the initiation of the study. The primary endpoint was the difference in incidence of HPV infection and/or HPV-associated genital disease.

Under the modified intention-to-treat analysis, the incidence of HPV infection and associated disease was significantly lower in the vaccinated group (6 vs. 48 participants, 89% efficacy difference, 95%CI 73-94%, p < 0.0001). Notably, the incidence of HPV infections, HPV-associated disease (e.g., condylomata acuminata, vulvar intraepithelial neoplasia, vaginal intraepithelial neoplasia), and cervical intraepithelial neoplasia were all significantly lower in vaccinated patients compared to those receiving placebo. All women who completed the vaccination regimen mounted an antibody response following the last dose of the vaccine, and a majority (76-100%) maintained seropositivity at 36 months (percentages differ for each HPV type). Adverse effects of the vaccination were of mild and moderate severity, with the most common being pain at the site of injection and a headache following the injection.

Villa LL, Costa RLR, Petta CA, Andrade RP, Ault KA, Giuliano AR, et al. Prophylactic quadrivalent human papillomavirus (types 6, 11, 16, and 18) L1 virus-like particle vaccine in young women: a randomised double-blind placebo-controlled multicentre phase II efficacy trial. Lancet Oncol. 2005 May;6(5):271–8.

Tenofovir-emtricitabine more effective and safer than zidovudine-lamivudine in HIV treatment

1. A significantly higher percentage of patients receiving tenofovir, emtricitabine, and efavirenz had human immunodeficiency virus (HIV) viral load <50 copies/mL, when compared to those taking zidovudine, lamivudine, and efavirenz.

2. Significantly more patients discontinued medication in the zidovudine-lamivudine group due to adverse events than in the tenofovir-emtricitabine group.

Original Date of Publication: January 2006

Study Rundown: Highly-active antiretroviral therapy (HAART) has significantly changed the clinical management and outcomes of HIV patients across the world. Prior to this study, zidovudine or tenofovir coupled with either lamivudine or emtricitabine, and efavirenz were the recommended HAART regimens. This 2006 paper took ART-naive and otherwise healthy HIV patients and randomly assigned them to either the tenofovir-emtricitabine regimen or the zidovudine-lamivudine regimen for 48 weeks and recorded the effects on viral load as well as adverse effects. Results revealed a significantly higher proportion of patients in the tenofovir-emtricitabine group achieved a viral load <50 copes/mL than their counterparts in the zidovudine-lamivudine group. More patients in the zidovudine-lamivudine group discontinued therapy due adverse effects, the most common being marked anemia. While the study was open-label, their primary and secondary objectives were objective data, which reduces the impact of potential observer bias.

In-Depth [randomized controlled trial]: This 2006 study was a multicenter, open-label, randomized controlled trial that assigned 500 patients with HIV to either the standard ART regimen of zidovudine, lamivudine, and efavirenz or to the newer drugs tenofovir, emtricitabine, and efavirenz for 48 weeks. All patients were previously diagnosed with HIV and had never taken anti-viral therapy in the past. None of the participants had any other significant lab abnormalities. There was no cutoff CD4 count. Patients were followed for 48 weeks and viral load, CD4 count, standard labs, and adverse events were recorded. The primary outcome was reaching a viral load of equal or fewer than 400 copies/mL. The secondary outcomes included HIV RNA levels of less than

50 copies/mL, a positive trend in CD4 count, and the prevalence of adverse events.

The tenofovir-emtricitabine group surpassed the zidovudine-lamivudine group in the primary and all secondary outcomes. The group also had a significantly higher percentage of patients who achieved HIV RNA levels of less than 400 copies per milliliters (84% vs. 73%, 95%CI 4.0-19.0%, p = 0.002) as well as less than 50 copies per milliliters (80% vs. 70%, 95%CI 2.0-17.0%, p = 0.02) than those in the zidovudine-lamivudine group. Those patients also had a significant increase in their CD4 cell counts (190 vs. 158 cells; 95%CI 9-55; p = 0.002) and fewer significant adverse effects from the drugs. There was also lower incidence of resistance development in the tenofovir-emtricitabine group compared to the zidovudine-lamivudine group.

Gallant JE, DeJesus E, Arribas JR, Pozniak AL, Gazzard B, Campo RE, et al. Tenofovir DF, Emtricitabine, and Efavirenz vs. Zidovudine, Lamivudine, and Efavirenz for HIV. New England Journal of Medicine. 2006 Jan 19;354(3):251–60.

Vancomycin superior to metronidazole for severe C. difficile diarrhea

1. Metronidazole and vancomycin were similarly effective in treating mild cases of Clostridium difficile (C. difficile)-associated diarrhea (CDAD).

2. Vancomycin was superior to metronidazole in treating severe cases of CDAD.

Original Date of Publication: August 1, 2007

Study Rundown: C. difficile is a leading cause of antibiotic associated diarrhea and nosocomial infection. This study was the first randomized, controlled trial of metronidazole versus vancomycin treatment for CDAD that stratified cases according to disease severity. No significant difference in efficacy was found in treating mild disease. However, vancomycin was superior to metronidazole in treating severe cases of CDAD. The findings are significant to treatment guidelines, as vancomycin is a more expensive drug and its use comes with the risk of selecting for vancomycin-resistant enterococci. Strengths of the study included its large sample size and the study design to reduce bias. In summary, the study suggests that severe cases of CDAD may benefit from treatment with vancomycin rather than metronidazole, given the higher cure rates demonstrated with vancomycin therapy.

In-Depth [randomized controlled trial]: Published in Clinical Infectious Diseases in 2007, this was the first randomized, controlled study to compare vancomycin and metronidazole treatment of C. difficile-associated diarrhea based on disease severity. Patients were classified as having severe disease if they had endoscopic evidence of pseudomembranous colitis, were treated in the intensive care unit or had two or more of the following characteristics: 1) age >60 years, 2) temperature >38.3°C, 3) albumin level <2.5 mg/dL, or 4) peripheral WBC count >15,000 cells/mm^3 within 48 hours of study entry. The investigators assessed cure as resolution of diarrhea by day 6 of treatment and negative result of C. difficile-toxin A at days 6 and 10 of treatment. In mild cases of disease, metronidazole treatment resulted in cure in 90% of patients and vancomycin treatment resulted in cure in 98% of patients (p = 0.36). In severe cases of disease, metronidazole cured 76% of patients while vancomycin cured 97% of patients (p = 0.02).

Zar FA, Bakkanagari SR, Moorthi KMLST, Davis MB. A Comparison of Vancomycin and Metronidazole for the Treatment of Clostridium difficile–Associated Diarrhea, Stratified by Disease Severity. Clin Infect Dis. 2007 Aug 1;45(3):302–7.

Early initiation of antiretroviral therapy significantly improves HIV survival

1. The relative risk of death was significantly higher in patients who deferred antiretroviral therapy compared to those who initiated treatment early on,

2. This finding remained significant after adjustment for independent risk factors of age, history of injection drug use and HCV infection.

Original Date of Publication: April 2009

Study Rundown: Published in NEJM in 2009, this study analyzed data collected by the North American AIDS Cohort Collaboration on Research and Design (NA-ACCORD). Results revealed that all-cause mortality was significantly higher in patients who deferred antiretroviral therapy until CD4+ counts fell below 2 thresholds of 350 and 500 cells/mm³. This effect remained significant after adjustment for independent risk factors of age, history of injection drug use and HCV infection. The improvement in survival associated with early treatment initiation may have been the result of earlier control of viral replication or protection of immune function. Strengths of the study included the large sample size and measurement of survival as a primary outcome. Limitations of the study included those inherent to an observational study design. It remains unclear at what point an asymptomatic HIV-infected patient should initiate antiretroviral therapy to balance the benefit of treatment with toxicity, but this study contributes to the body of evidence supporting earlier treatment.

In-Depth [prospective cohort]: Two analyses were conducted on separate patients groups. The first analysis included 8362 patients who had a baseline CD4+ count of 351 to 500 cells/mm³. The rate of death from any cause was compared in those who initiated antiretroviral therapy within 6 months of this count (early-therapy group) with those who deferred treatment until CD4+ count fell below this range (deferred-therapy group). The second analysis included 9155 patients who had a CD4+ count higher than 500 cells/mm³ and made the same comparison between those who initiated therapy early with those who deferred treatment. The relative risk of death was markedly higher in the deferred-therapy group in both analyses.

Kitahata MM, Gange SJ, Abraham AG, Merriman B, Saag MS, Justice AC, et al. Effect of Early versus Deferred Antiretroviral Therapy for HIV on Survival. New England Journal of Medicine. 2009 Apr 30;360(18):1815–26.

Fidaxomicin vs. vancomycin in C. difficile infection

1. **Fidaxomicin was non-inferior to vancomycin in achieving clinical cure of Clostridium difficile (C. difficile) infection.**

2. **Fidaxomicin therapy significantly reduced the rate of recurrence and significantly increased the rate of global cure of C. difficile infection when compared with vancomycin therapy.**

Original Date of Publication: February 2011

Study Rundown: C. difficile infection is a common complication affecting patients treated with antibiotics. The incidence of C. difficile infection is increasing rapidly and mortality from C. difficile is steadily rising. Infections manifest with a range of symptoms, from diarrhea to inflammation of the entire colon, potentially necessitating surgical management. Recent data have been concerning, as numerous studies have shown poorer response to treatments and higher rates of recurrence compared with previous decades. Currently, the commonly used antibiotics for treating C. difficile are metronidazole and vancomycin. Fidaxomicin is a newer macrocyclic antibiotic that was designed to selectively eradicate C. difficile. It is more active than vancomycin in vitro and is minimally absorbed into the bloodstream, thereby remaining in feces in high concentrations.

This phase 3, non-inferiority trial was performed to compare the effects of fidaxomicin and vancomycin in treating C. difficile infection. Results demonstrated that fidaxomicin was non-inferior to vancomycin in achieving clinical cure of C. difficile infection. Rates of recurrence were significantly lower in the fidaxomicin group when compared with the vancomycin group. The rates of global cure (i.e., cure without recurrence) were significantly higher in the fidaxomicin group. In 2011, fidaxomicin received full U.S. Food and Drug Administration approval for treating C. difficile infection. The cost of a 10-day course of fidaxomicin is typically many times more expensive than a course of oral vancomycin. Thus, the cost of fidaxomicin has been a major barrier to wider use.

In-Depth [randomized controlled trial]: This phase 3, non-inferiority trial compared fidaxomicin with vancomycin in treating C. difficile infection. A total of 629 patients were recruited from 67 sites across Canada and the United States and randomized to receive a 10-day course of fidaxomicin 200 mg orally every 12 hours or vancomycin 125 mg orally every 6 hours. Patients were eligible if they were 16 years of age or older, had a diagnosis of C. difficile infection (i.e., change in bowel habits, ≥3 unformed bowel movements in 24 hours prior to randomization), and a stool specimen positive for C. difficile toxin A, B, or both in the 48 hours prior to randomization. Patients were excluded if they had life-threatening or fulminant C. difficile infection, toxic megacolon, a history of inflammatory bowel disease (i.e., ulcerative colitis, Crohn's), or more than one occurrence of C. difficile infection in the 3 months before the study. The primary endpoint was the rate of clinical cure (i.e., resolution of diarrhea with no need for antimicrobials on the second day after treatment finished). The secondary endpoints were recurrence of C. difficile infection in the 4-week period after finishing therapy and global cure rates (i.e., resolution of diarrhea without recurrence).

In the modified intention-to-treat, 88.2% of patients treated with fidaxomicin and 85.8% of those treated with vancomycin met criteria for clinical cure. In the per-protocol analysis, the proportions experiencing clinical cure were 92.1% and 89.8% in the fidaxomicin and vancomycin groups, respectively. In both instances, criteria for non-inferiority were met. The rates of recurrence were significantly lower in the fidaxomicin group compared to the vancomycin group in both the modified intention-to-treat (15.4% vs. 25.3%, p = 0.005) and per-protocol analyses (13.3% vs. 24.0%, p = 0.004). The rates of global cure were also significantly higher in patients treated with fidaxomicin as compared with vancomycin (74.6% vs. 64.1%, p = 0.006 for modified intention-to-treat; 77.7% vs. 67.1%, p = 0.006 for per-protocol). There were no significant differences between the groups in the rates of adverse events.

Louie TJ, Miller MA, Mullane KM, Weiss K, Lentnek A, Golan Y, et al. Fidaxomicin versus Vancomycin for Clostridium difficile Infection. New England Journal of Medicine. 2011 Feb 3;364(5):422–31.

Early antiretroviral therapy reduces HIV-1 transmission in couples

1. Human immunodeficiency virus (HIV-1) transmission rates were significantly lower in the early-therapy group compared to the delayed-therapy group.

2. Patients in the early-therapy group had lower incidence of HIV-related clinical events with a lower viral load and higher CD4 cell count than those whose therapy was delayed.

Original Date of Publication: August 2011

Study Rundown: Previous studies had demonstrated that combination therapy significantly reduced the rate of HIV-1 replication and the viral load in genital secretions. Since HIV transmission is highly linked with viral concentrations in blood and genital secretions, it was hypothesized that initiating early treatment of HIV-positive individuals would reduce the likelihood of sexual transmission. This study revealed that treatment of HIV with antiretroviral therapy (ART) reduced HIV-1 transmission between serodiscordant couples. The participants who started ART early also showed a reduction in the viral load and an increase in CD4 count while those in the delayed-therapy group on average had a modest decline in CD4 counts over the course of the study. ART also proved beneficial to reducing the incidence of HIV-related clinical events. The participants in both groups did not differ with regards to gender, location, marital status, education level, self-reported sexual activity, condom use, and baseline CD4 count and viral load. The partners of HIV-infected individuals who eventually tested positive for the HIV virus were tested to ascertain whether the patient was infected heir partner. In summary, the delayed-therapy group had a significantly higher incidence of linked transmission between couples than those in the early-therapy group.

In-Depth [randomized controlled trial]: This 2011 study randomized 1763 serodiscordant couples to either early or delayed retroviral therapy for the HIV-infected partner and looked at the rate of seroconversion in the non-infected partner over a five-year period. Participants all had CD4 cell counts between 350-550 cells per cubic millimeter and had not received antiretroviral therapy in the past. The delayed therapy group was started on antiretroviral medication once their cell counts dropped below 250 or they developed an AIDS-defining infection. Antiretroviral medications varied between the sites. All participants had sexual intercourse with one monogamous partner, as per self-reported measures. The primary outcome was the seroconversion of the non-infected partner. Secondary outcomes included incidence of HIV-1 related clinical events and adverse events from ART. The study demonstrated that the rate of seroconversion in the early-therapy group was significantly lower than in the delayed-therapy group (HR 0.11; 95%CI 0.04-0.32). Moreover, there was significantly lower incidence of linked transmission between couples in the early-therapy group, as compared to the delayed-therapy group (HR 0.04; 95%CI 0.01-0.27). The early therapy group also had a lower incidence of HIV-related clinical events (HR 0.59; 95%CI 0.4-0.88). Most of the difference in HIV-related clinical events was driven by the higher incidence of extrapulmonary tuberculosis in the delayed-therapy group.

Cohen MS, Chen YQ, McCauley M, Gamble T, Hosseinipour MC, Kumarasamy N, et al. Prevention of HIV-1 Infection with Early Antiretroviral Therapy. New England Journal of Medicine. 2011 Aug 11;365(6):493–505.

Fecal transplantation in recurrent C. difficile infection

1. Treating recurrent Clostridium difficile (C. difficile) infection with an infusion of donor feces resulted in significantly higher cure rates than treating with vancomycin-alone or vancomycin with bowel lavage.

2. Adverse events after feces infusion included diarrhea, cramping, and belching.

Original Date of Publication: January 2013

Study Rundown: Previous studies demonstrated that vancomycin was superior to metronidazole in treating severe C. difficile-associated diarrhea. Additional studies also revealed that fidaxomicin was non-inferior to vancomycin in achieving clinical cure of C. difficile infection. In many patients, however, antibiotic treatment does not lead to sustained response, and these patients often require repeated or long tapering courses of vancomycin in attempts to achieve cure. While many factors have been suggested for C. difficile recurrence, one commonly cited reason is the destruction of the normal intestinal flora from repeated bouts of antibiotic therapy. Early non-randomized trials had explored the efficacy of gastrointestinal infusions of feces from healthy donors to treat recurrent C. difficile infection, and the results were promising. The purpose of this small randomized, controlled trial was to explore the efficacy of donor feces infusion in treating recurrent C. difficile infection. In summary, the study revealed that patients receiving donor feces infusion were significantly more likely to achieve cure without relapse in the 10 weeks after starting therapy. While these results are promising, larger, multicenter trials are needed to study the generalizability of these findings. Moreover, trials with longer follow-up are necessary to assess the duration of the effect.

In-Depth [randomized controlled trial]: This open-label, randomized, controlled trial was originally published in NEJM in 2013. Participants in the trial were randomized to three treatment groups: 1) infusion of donor feces (preceded by a short course of vancomycin and bowel lavage), 2) a standard vancomycin regimen, and 3) a standard vancomycin regimen with bowel lavage. Patients were eligible for the trial if they were >18 years old, had a life expectancy >3 months, and had a relapse of C. difficile after an adequate course of antibiotics (≥10 days of vancomycin or metronidazole). Exclusion criteria included recent chemotherapy, HIV infection with CD4 <240, prolonged use of prednisolone ≥60 mg daily, pregnancy, use of antibiotics for other infections, and admission to intensive care or requiring vasopressors. Patients who experienced recurrence after the first infusion were given a second infusion from a different donor. The primary endpoint was cure without relapse in the 10 weeks after starting therapy, or 10 weeks after the second infusion. A total of 43 patients underwent randomization. In the feces infusion group, 81% of patients were cured after the first infusion, and 94% were cured overall. Cure rates were 31% and 23% for the vancomycin-alone and vancomycin with lavage groups, respectively. Patients in the feces infusion group had significantly higher rates of cure ($p < 0.01$ for both comparisons after one infusion, $p < 0.001$ for overall cure rate). Most patients (94%) had diarrhea immediately after receiving donor feces, while cramping (31%) and belching (19%) were also common. These symptoms resolved within 3 hours in all patients.

Van Nood E, Vrieze A, Nieuwdorp M, Fuentes S, Zoetendal EG, de Vos WM, et al. Duodenal Infusion of Donor Feces for Recurrent Clostridium difficile. New England Journal of Medicine. 2013 Jan 31;368(5):407–15.

VIII. Nephrology

The MDRD trial: Protein intake and blood pressure control in renal insufficiency

1. Reducing protein intake and lowering blood pressure targets did not significantly delay the rate of decline of glomerular filtration rate (GFR) in patients with renal insufficiency.

2. In patients with renal insufficiency and elevated baseline proteinuria (≥ 1 g/day in moderate insufficiency, ≥ 3 g/day in severe insufficiency), lower blood pressure targets significantly delayed the progression of renal disease.

Original Date of Publication: March 1994

Study Rundown: At the time of the Modification of Diet in Renal Disease (MDRD) trial in 1994, studies had shown that dietary protein restriction and blood pressure control delayed the progression of renal disease in animal models. The MDRD trial sought to assess whether dietary and blood pressure changes can similarly delay worsening renal insufficiency in humans. The study involved both patients with moderate (GFR between 25-55 mL/min/1.73m^2) and severe renal insufficiency (GFR 13-24 mL/min/1.73m^2), and randomized patients to different levels of protein intake and blood pressure control. At the 3-year mark, the rate of decline in GFR did not significantly differ between different degrees of protein consumption or blood pressure control. In subsets of patient with elevated baseline proteinuria (≥ 1 g/day in moderate insufficiency, ≥ 3 g/day in severe insufficiency), lower blood pressure control significantly slowed the progression of renal disease. A major limitation of the study was its low recruitment of minority patients, as 85% of study participants were white. The authors remarked that the study's 53 black patients had a significantly more rapid rate of GFR decline than the rest of the participants, suggesting that renal disease progression may differ for different patient populations. In summary, the MDRD trial demonstrated that reducing protein intake and stricter blood pressure control did not significantly alter the rate of decline in GFR in patients with moderate or severe renal insufficiency.

In-Depth [randomized controlled trial]: Originally published in 1994 in NEJM, this randomized trial was comprised of 2 studies involving 840 patients. The first study examined individuals with moderate renal insufficiency (GFR 25-55 mL/min/1.73m^2), while the second involved those with severe insufficiency (GFR 13-24 mL/min/1.73m²). Eligible patients were between 18-70 years old, had creatinine concentrations within defined limits (1.2-7.0 mg/dL or 106-619 μmol/L for women, 1.4-7.0 mg/dL or 124-619 μmol/L for men) or a creatinine clearance rate <70 mL/min/1.73m² of body surface area, and a mean arterial pressure ≤125 mmHg. The exclusion criteria included pregnancy, being excessively under- or overweight (i.e., <80% or >160% of standard body weight), having diabetes mellitus and requiring insulin therapy, urinary protein excretion rate >10 g/day, and a history of renal transplantation or other chronic medical conditions.

Patients with moderate renal insufficiency (GFR of 25-55 ml/min/1.73m²) were randomized to a usual- (1.3 g/kg/day) or low-protein diet (0.58 g/kg/day), and usual- (<140/90 mmHg) or low-blood pressure control (<130/80 mmHg). Patients with severe renal insufficiency (GFR of 13-24 ml/min/1.73m²) were randomized to receive low- (0.58 g/kg/day) or very low-protein diet (0.28 g/kg/day), and usual- (<140/90) or low-blood pressure control (<130/80). GFR was measured at 2 and 4 months, and every 4 months thereafter as an indicator of renal disease progression. The primary endpoint was the rate of change in GFR. In patients with moderate renal insufficiency, there was no significant difference in the rate of decline in GFR between the diet or blood pressure groups at the 3-year mark. In patients with severe renal insufficiency, the rate of GFR decline also did not differ significantly between the diet and blood pressure groups at 3 years. Subgroup analyses were performed based on baseline proteinuria. Patients with moderate insufficiency and ≥1 g/day of proteinuria were found to have significantly slower rates of decline in GFR when they were managed to lower blood pressure targets. The rate of decline in GFR was also significantly slower in patients with severe insufficiency and baseline proteinuria ≥3 g/day when they lower blood pressure was targeted.

Klahr S, Levey AS, Beck GJ, Caggiula AW, Hunsicker L, Kusek JW, et al. The Effects of Dietary Protein Restriction and Blood-Pressure Control on the Progression of Chronic Renal Disease. New England Journal of Medicine. 1994 Mar 31;330(13):877–84.

The IDNT: Irbesartan protects from renal deterioration in diabetic nephropathy

1. Irbesartan significantly reduced the risk of doubling of serum creatinine concentration, developing end-stage renal disease, or death from all causes.

2. Serum creatinine concentration increased at a slower rate in patients receiving irbesartan compared to amlodipine and placebo groups.

Original Date of Publication: September 2001

Study Rundown: The Irbesartan Diabetic Nephropathy Trial (IDNT) assessed the ability of an angiotensin-II-receptor blocker (ARB), irbesartan and a calcium channel blocker (CCB), amlodipine to protect against renal deterioration in patients with nephropathy due to type 2 diabetes mellitus (T2DM). At the time of this publication, inhibitors of the renin-angiotensin-aldosterone system were known to be effective in patients with nephropathy due to type 1 diabetes but no major trial had investigated these agents in patients with nephropathy due to T2DM. While no significant differences were observed between the amlodipine and placebo treatment groups, irbesartan was associated with a significantly lower relative risk of a composite end point that included doubling of serum creatinine concentration, onset of end-stage renal disease, and death from any cause. Irbesartan was also associated with a slower rate of increase in serum creatinine concentration. These protective effects were found to be independent of the drug's benefit in lowering blood pressure. In summary, the ARB irbesartan carries renoprotective effects in addition to lowering blood pressure in patients with nephropathy due to T2DM.

In-Depth [randomized controlled trial]: This trial randomly assigned 1715 patients with a documented diagnosis of T2DM and hypertension to 1 of 3 treatment arms: 1) the ARB, irbesartan, 2) the CCB, amlodipine, or 3) placebo. The target blood pressure for all patients was the same (135/85 mmHg or less) and blood pressure was managed as needed with antihypertensive agents other than ACE inhibitors, ARBs, and CCBs. The primary endpoint was a composite of doubling of baseline serum creatinine concentration, development of end-stage renal disease, or death from any cause. A composite cardiovascular end point was measured as a secondary outcome. The relative risk of the primary end point was not significantly different between the placebo and amlodipine groups. Patients receiving irbcsartan had a 20% lower relative risk of the primary end point than patients in the placebo group (p = 0.02) and a 23% lower risk that those in the amlodipine group (p = 0.006). There was no significant difference in the occurrence of the composite cardiovascular outcome among the three groups. Serum creatinine concentration increased at significantly slower rates in the irbesartan group than in the placebo and amlodipine groups. Hyperkalemia requiring discontinuation of trial medication occurred more frequently in the irbesartan group than in the placebo and amlodipine groups.

Lewis EJ, Hunsicker LG, Clarke WR, Berl T, Pohl MA, Lewis JB, et al. Renoprotective Effect of the Angiotensin-Receptor Antagonist Irbesartan in Patients with Nephropathy Due to Type 2 Diabetes. New England Journal of Medicine. 2001 Sep 20;345(12):851–60.

The RENAAL trial: Losartan in diabetic nephropathy

1. In patients with type II diabetes mellitus (T2DM) and nephropathy, losartan at a dose of 50-100 mg daily significantly reduced the risk of developing end-stage renal disease (ESRD) compared to placebo.

2. While losartan was linked to a significant reduction in the degree of proteinuria in these patients, it did not have a related reduction in mortality when compared with placebo.

Original Date of Publication: September 2001

Study Rundown: Diabetic nephropathy is a leading cause of ESRD. Previous studies had shown that blockade of the renin-angiotensin system slowed the progression of renal disease in patients with type I diabetes. The Reduction of Endpoints in NIDDM with the Angiotensin II Antagonist Losartan (RENAAL) study was the one of the first to assess the effect of disrupting the renin-angiotensin system in patients with T2DM. The study demonstrated that in T2DM patients already receiving conventional anti-hypertensive therapy, the use of the angiotensin-II-receptor antagonist losartan significantly decreased the risk of ESRD. Losartan therapy also was associated with a significant decrease in the degree of proteinuria. There was no significant difference between the groups in mortality rates. One limitation of this study was the high rate at which patients discontinued the study drug. About 53.5% of patients in the placebo group and 46.5% of patients in the losartan group stopped taking their study medication early. In summary, the findings of this study support the use of losartan in delaying the progression of renal disease in patients with T2DM and nephropathy.

In-Depth [randomized controlled trial]: This trial included 1513 patients from 250 centers in 28 countries. Eligible patients were between 31-70 years of age with diagnoses of type 2 diabetes and nephropathy (i.e., urinary protein $\geq$0.5 g/24 hours and serum creatinine between 115-254 µmol/L). Patients who had type 1 diabetes, non-diabetic renal disease, or a history of heart failure were excluded. Moreover, patients who had recent myocardial infarction (MI), percutaneous coronary intervention (PCI), coronary artery bypass grafting (CABG), or cerebrovascular event were excluded. Patients received conventional anti-hypertensive therapy as needed, in addition to either losartan or placebo. Permitted anti-hypertensive therapy included calcium channel blockers, diuretics, alpha-blockers, and beta-blockers, but not angiotensin converting enzyme (ACE) inhibitors or angiotensin-II-receptor antagonists other than losartan. Treatment was administered for a mean of 3.4 years. The primary outcome measure was time to the composite endpoint comprised of ESRD (i.e., need for dialysis or renal transplantation), doubling of serum creatinine level, and death. The secondary endpoints were morbidity and mortality from cardiovascular causes, progression of renal disease, and changes in the degree of proteinuria.

The daily dose of losartan ranged from 50-100 mg daily with 71% of patients receiving 100 mg. Losartan treatment significantly reduced the incidence of the primary endpoint when compared to placebo (43.5% vs. 47.1%, 16% risk reduction, p = 0.02). This difference was driven by significant reductions in the risk of doubling serum creatinine (21.6% vs. 26.0%, 25% risk reduction, p = 0.006) and the risk of end-stage renal disease (19.6% vs. 25.5%, 28% risk reduction, p = 0.002) in the losartan group. There was no significant difference between the two groups in mortality (21.0% vs. 20.3%, p= 0.88). Moreover, there was no difference between the groups in the secondary endpoint of morbidity and mortality from cardiovascular causes. Patients in the losartan group, however, did experience significant reductions in the amount of proteinuria when compared with those receiving placebo (p < 0.001).

Brenner BM, Cooper ME, de Zeeuw D, Keane WF, Mitch WE, Parving H-H, et al. Effects of Losartan on Renal and Cardiovascular Outcomes in Patients with Type 2 Diabetes and Nephropathy. New England Journal of Medicine. 2001 Sep 20;345(12):861–9.

The CHOIR trial: Targeting lower hemoglobin levels in patients with anemia and chronic kidney disease

1. In patients with anemia and chronic kidney disease, treatment with epoetin α to a lower hemoglobin target significantly reduced the incidence of death, myocardial infarction (MI), hospitalization for congestive heart failure (CHF), and stroke.

2. Achieving the lower hemoglobin target required significantly lower doses of epoetin α.

Original Date of Publication: November 2006

Study Rundown: This study found that in patients with anemia and chronic kidney disease, treating with epoetin α to a higher hemoglobin target was linked with a significantly higher risk of negative events, including death, MI, hospitalization for CHF, and stroke when compared to a lower target. Moreover, achieving the higher target required about double the dose of epoetin α, a costly medication. While this study was a multicenter, randomized trial, it was criticized for its relatively small size, high rates of withdrawal from the study, and the fact that it was not double-blinded. In summary, treating anemia in patients with chronic kidney disease using epoetin α to a lower hemoglobin target (i.e., ≥11.3 g/dL) significantly reduced the risk of composite events compared to a high target (i.e., ≥13.5 g/dL). Significantly lower doses of epoetin α were required to achieve the lower hemoglobin target.

In-Depth [randomized controlled trial]: The Correction of Hemoglobin and Outcomes in Renal Insufficiency (CHOIR) trial was an open-label, randomized study exploring the use of epoetin α in treating anemia associated with chronic kidney disease. The trial sought to determine if treating with epoetin α to target a higher hemoglobin level (i.e., ≥13.5 g/dL) would improve outcomes when compared to a lower target (i.e., ≥11.3 g/dL). The targets were adjusted partway through the trial, as the initial targets were 13.0-13.5 g/dL for the high-hemoglobin group and 10.5-11.0 g/dL for the low-hemoglobin group. Patients were included if they were at least 18 years of age, had a hemoglobin <11.0 g/dL, and had chronic kidney disease (i.e., GFR 15-50 ml/min/1.73m^2 using MDRD). The primary endpoint was the time to a composite of death, MI, hospitalization for CHF, or stroke.

The study was terminated early in May 2005 at the second interim analysis on the recommendation of the data and safety monitoring board. At that time, 1432 participants had been enrolled from 130 states from across the United States, with 715 in the high-hemoglobin group and 717 in the low-hemoglobin group. Analyses were based on intention-to-treat, though 549 (38.3%) patients withdrew from the study prematurely. There was a significantly increased risk of composite event in the high-group compared to the low-group (HR 1.34; 95%CI 1.03-1.74). Of note, death (29.3%) and hospitalization for CHF (45.5%) accounted for 74.8% of the composite events. It was also noted that patients in the high-group required almost double the dose of epoetin α to achieve the target when compared to the dose required to achieve the low-target.

Singh AK, Szczech L, Tang KL, Barnhart H, Sapp S, Wolfson M, et al. Correction of Anemia with Epoetin Alfa in Chronic Kidney Disease. New England Journal of Medicine. 2006 Nov 16;355(20):2085–98.

The ADVANCE trial: Intensive glycemic control reduces the risk of nephropathy in diabetes

1. In diabetic patients, intensive glycemic control significantly reduced the risk of new or worsened nephropathy when compared to conventional glycemic control.

2. There was no significant reduction in major macrovascular events associated with intensive blood sugar control.

Original Date of Publication: June 2008

Study Rundown: Glycated hemoglobin (HbA1c) levels are used as a marker of glycemic control in diabetic patients. Previous studies, such as the ACCORD and UKPDS trials, demonstrated that tighter glycemic control reduced the risk of microvascular complications (i.e., nephropathy, retinopathy, and neuropathy). The ACCORD trial, however, also noted that there was significantly higher risk of mortality in patients who underwent tight glycemic control (i.e., target HbA1c <6.0%). Moreover, there was no strong evidence demonstrating that better glycemic control significantly improved rates of macrovascular complications (i.e., myocardial infarction, stroke). The Action in Diabetes and Vascular Disease: Preterax and Diamicron Modified Release Controlled Evaluation (ADVANCE) trial sought to assess the effects of intensive glycemic control (i.e., target HbA1c ≤6.5%) on vascular outcomes. The findings demonstrated that patients in the intensive group had significantly lower risk of new/worsening nephropathy and new-onset microalbuminuria when compared with standard therapy. There were no significant differences between the groups in the rates of macrovascular complications or all-cause mortality. Importantly, the risk of severe hypoglycemia was significantly higher in patients undergoing intensive therapy.

In-Depth [randomized controlled trial]: The study included 11 140 participants from 215 centers in 20 countries. Patients were eligible if they were ≥55 years of age, were diagnosed with type 2 diabetes mellitus at ≥30 years of age, and had a history of micro- or macrovascular disease. Exclusion criteria included a definite indication for or contraindication to any of the study drugs, or a definite indication for long-term insulin therapy at study entry. Included patients were randomized to either intensive glucose control (i.e., target HbA1c ≤6.5%) or standard glucose control (i.e., based on local guidelines). The intensive control group received gliclazide and other adjuvants to achieve target HbA1c, while the control group received treatment as per local guidelines. The primary outcome was a composite of macrovascular (i.e., myocardial infarction, stroke, or death from cardiovascular event) and microvascular events (nephropathy or retinopathy). Median follow-up time was 5 years. At the end of the follow-up period, the mean HbA1c levels were 6.5% and 7.3% in the intensive and standard groups, respectively. There were no significant differences between the 2 groups with regards to the incidence of major macrovascular events (HR 0.94; 95%CI 0.84-1.06) and death from any cause (HR 0.93; 95%CI 0.83-1.06). The intensive group had a significantly lower rate of major microvascular events (HR 0.86; 95%CI 0.77-0.97), which was driven by a significantly lower risk of new or worsening nephropathy (HR 0.79; 95%CI 0.66-0.93) and new-onset microalbuminuria (HR 0.91; 95%CI 0.85-0.98). There was no significant difference between the 2 groups in terms of the risk of new or worsening retinopathy. The risk of severe hypoglycaemia, however, was significantly higher in the intensive group (HR 1.86; 95%CI 1.42-2.40).

ADVANCE Collaborative Group, Patel A, MacMahon S, Chalmers J, Neal B, Billot L, et al. Intensive blood glucose control and vascular outcomes in patients with type 2 diabetes. New England Journal of Medicine. 2008 Jun 12;358(24):2560–72.

The Symplicity HTN-2 trial: Renal denervation effective for treatment-resistant hypertension

1. Renal denervation significantly reduced blood pressure in patients suffering from treatment-resistant hypertension.

2. Renal denervation was not associated with a significantly higher rate of adverse events in comparison to control.

Original Date of Publication: December 2010

Study Rundown: Approximately half of hypertensive patients do not experience a reduction in blood pressure despite treatment with pharmaceutical agents and/or lifestyle changes. Efferent sympathetic outflow from kidneys can stimulate renin release and increased tubular sodium reabsorption, thereby increasing blood pressure. Afferent sympathetic outflow from kidneys can influence central sympathetic signals and contribute to neurogenic hypertension. Previous non-randomized trials suggest that renal denervation can successfully ameliorate treatment-refractory hypertension.

The Symplicity HTN-2 trial was the first study to randomize patients with treatment-resistant hypertension (i.e., persistent hypertension despite compliance with three or more antihypertensive drugs) to receive renal denervation or not. Results revealed that renal denervation significantly reduced blood pressure in treatment-refractory patients. Treatment with renal denervation was not linked with significantly higher rates of adverse events. There was no major injury to the renal arteries or evidence of worsening renal function associated with the denervation procedure. Limitations of the study include the low percentage of patients (17%) in both experimental groups that reported having used an aldosterone antagonist prior to the study. This raises the concern that the participants' hypertension may not have been resistant to all available effective drug therapies. Additionally, study participants were only monitored for 6 months, thus the long-term effects of renal denervation were not assessed. It should be noted that more recent studies have shown similar results extended to 24 months. In summary, the results of the Symplicity HTN-2 trial suggest that catheter-based renal denervation can be safely and effectively used to reduce blood pressure in treatment-refractory hypertensive patients.

In-Depth [randomized controlled trial]: The Symplicity HTN-2 trial was a randomized, controlled trial involving 106 participants from Europe, Australia, and New Zealand. Eligible patients were between the ages of 18 and 85 with a systolic blood pressure (BP) of at least 160 mmHg, despite compliance with at least three hypertensive drugs. Exclusion criteria included a glomerular filtration rate (GFR) of less than 45 mL/min/1.73 m², type 1 diabetes mellitus, valvular heart disease, and pregnancy. Renal denervation was performed using the Symplicity catheter to apply radiofrequency treatments along both renal arteries. Changes in the baseline doses of anti-hypertensive drugs were not permitted during the trial. Patients' BP was measured at 1, 3, and 6 months using office-based and home-based blood pressure machines. Adverse effects were assessed by measuring serum creatinine concentration, cystatin C concentration, and urine albumin-to-creatinine ratio. Kidneys in the denervation group were also imaged by ultrasound. Results based on office-based BP measurements showed that renal denervation resulted in a significant BP decrease of 32/12 mmHg (p < 0.0001), while the control group experienced no significant change. At 6 months, office-based BP of patients in the denervation group was significantly lower than the control group (between-group difference of 33/11 mmHg, p < 0.0001). Home-based BP was also significantly lower in the denervation group (between-group difference of 22/12 mmHg, p < 0.001). There was no difference in estimated GFR, serum creatinine, and cystatin C levels between the two groups.

Symplicity HTN-2 Investigators, Esler MD, Krum H, Sobotka PA, Schlaich MP, Schmieder RE, et al. Renal sympathetic denervation in patients with treatment-resistant hypertension (The Symplicity HTN-2 Trial): a randomised controlled trial. Lancet. 2010 Dec 4;376(9756):1903–9.

IX. Neurology

The NASCET: Carotid endarterectomy in symptomatic stenosis

1. Carotid endarterectomy, in addition to medical therapy, significantly reduced the risk of major and fatal stroke in patients with symptomatic, high-grade (70-99%) carotid stenosis.

Original Date of Publication: August 1991

Study Rundown: The North American Symptomatic Carotid Endarterectomy Trial (NASCET) was one of the first trials to provide strong evidence in favor of carotid endarterectomy, in addition to medical therapy, in treating symptomatic carotid artery stenosis. The trial was originally conceived in response to the rising rates of carotid endarterectomy without strong evidence to support its use in prophylaxis against cerebrovascular events. Results demonstrated significant benefits for patients suffering from high-grade carotid stenosis (70-99%), who had recently experienced transient ischemic attack, monocular blindness, or non-disabling stroke. These findings were consistent with findings from the European Carotid Stenosis Trial. At the time, questions remained regarding the benefits of carotid endarterectomy in patients with asymptomatic carotid stenosis, and this has been explored in subsequent trials. In summary, carotid endarterectomy in addition to medical therapy significantly reduced the absolute risk of ipsilateral stroke and major or fatal ipsilateral stroke in patients with high-grade, symptomatic, carotid artery stenosis.

In-Depth [randomized controlled trial]: Patients were recruited from 50 centers across Canada and the United States and randomized to either medical therapy alone (i.e., antiplatelet, antihypertensive, antilipid, antidiabetic therapy, as needed), or medical therapy with carotid endarterectomy. Patients were eligible for the trial if they provided informed consent, were <80 years old, and had a cerebrovascular event (i.e., transient ischemic attack, monocular blindness, non-disabling stroke) in the previous 120 days with ipsilateral carotid stenosis of 30-99% (as per carotid ultrasonography). Patients were assessed at 30 days, every three months for the first year, and every four months subsequently for death or stroke. The trial was stopped prematurely by the monitoring and executive committees according to a pre-planned rule because of evidence demonstrating treatment efficacy in patients with high-grade stenosis (70-99%) undergoing endarterectomy. The trial involving medium-grade stenosis (30-69%) continued. A total of 659 patients with high-grade stenosis were part of the final analyses. At two years, there was a significant reduction in the absolute risk of ipsilateral stroke by 17% ($\pm3.5\%$, p < 0.001) and major or fatal ipsilateral stroke by 10.6% ($\pm2.6\%$, p < 0.001).

North American Symptomatic Carotid Endarterectomy Trial Collaborators. Beneficial effect of carotid endarterectomy in symptomatic patients with high-grade carotid stenosis. New England Journal of Medicine. 1991 Aug 15;325(7):445–53.

Interferon beta-1b reduces exacerbations in relapsing-remitting multiple sclerosis

1. **In patients with relapsing-remitting multiple sclerosis (MS), treatment with interferon beta-1b (IFNB) significantly reduced the rate of MS exacerbations in a dose-dependent fashion.**

2. **Serial magnetic resonance imaging (MRI) revealed less MS activity in patients with increasing doses of IFNB.**

3. **There was no difference in disability caused by IFNB treatment.**

Original Date of Publication: April 1993

Study Rundown: This landmark trial, conducted by the IFNB Multiple Sclerosis Study Group, randomized patients with relapsing-remitting MS to low-dose IFNB, high-dose IFNB, or placebo. Patients on IFNB experienced lower rates of disease exacerbation and were found to have less activity on serial MRI compared to placebo. Moreover, patients taking the higher dose of IFNB experienced significantly lower rates of relapse and MRI activity as compared to those on the lower dose, thereby demonstrating dose-dependent effect. Over a 3 year period, however, there was no significant difference in overall disability between the 3 groups. In summary, this study was vital in establishing the efficacy of IFNB as a treatment for relapsing-remitting MS and it remains a commonly used medication for this disease.

In-Depth [randomized controlled trial]: This trial enrolled patients with relapsing-remitting MS from 11 medical centers across the U.S. and Canada. In order to be enrolled, patients must have been suffering from the illness for at least 1 year and must not have received any treatment for 30 days prior to enrollment. Patients were randomized to receive placebo, 1.6 million international units (MIU) IFNB, or 8 MIU IFNB. The primary endpoint was the annual exacerbation rate and proportion of patients free of exacerbations. Exacerbations were defined as the appearance of a new symptom or the worsening of an old symptom that could be clinically attributed to MS. In addition, each patient had a brain MRI at baseline and on a yearly basis afterwards. At 3 years of follow-up, the exacerbation rates were 1.21 for the placebo group, 1.05 for the 1.6 MIU group, and 0.84 for the 8 MIU group (p = 0.0004). Furthermore, MRIs at the 3-year mark demonstrated a 17.1% increase in mean lesion area for patients in the placebo group and a 1.1% increase for the 1.6 MIU group, while the 8 MIU group experienced a 6.2% decrease compared to baseline MRIs. Over the 3-year period, there was no statistically significant difference between the groups with regards to total disability, as measured by the Kurtzke EDSS score.

Paty DW, Li DKB et al. Interferon beta-1b is effective in relapsing-remitting multiple sclerosis II. MRI analysis results of a multicenter, randomized, double-blind, placebo-controlled trial. Neurology. 1993 Apr 1;43(4):662–662.

The WARSS: Warfarin vs. aspirin in preventing recurrent ischemic stroke

1. **Warfarin was not superior to aspirin in preventing recurrent ischemic stroke in patients with a prior noncardioembolic ischemic stroke.**

2. **There was no significant difference in the rate of major hemorrhage when comparing warfarin to aspirin.**

Original Date of Publication: November 2001

Study Rundown: Previous studies demonstrated that warfarin was associated with lower rates of embolic stroke in patients with atrial fibrillation when compared to aspirin. Additionally, while aspirin was the treatment of choice for the prevention of recurrent events in noncardioembolic ischemic strokes, a substantial rate of recurrence was observed clinically. The Warfarin-Aspirin Recurrent Stroke Study (WARSS) therefore sought to investigate whether warfarin may be superior to aspirin in the prevention of recurrent ischemic stroke in patients with prior noncardioembolic strokes. The study showed no significant difference between warfarin and aspirin in the prevention of recurrent ischemic strokes. In other words, warfarin did not decrease the rate of recurrent stroke in patients with a prior noncardioembolic stroke, as it did for patients with atrial fibrillation. Because the WARSS study was only powered to detect a 30% relative reduction in primary outcome, it is possible that the study was underpowered to detect more modest treatment effects. Additionally, while there was no difference in rates of major hemorrhage (e.g., intracranial, intraspinal, dural/epidural bleeding) between aspirin and warfarin use, patients on warfarin had significantly more minor hemorrhages (e.g., gastrointestinal bleeding, ecchymoses). In summary, the results of the WARSS suggest that aspirin is a reasonable choice for prophylaxis against recurrent noncardioembolic ischemic stroke, given that warfarin requires closer monitoring, without being more effective.

In-Depth [randomized controlled trial]: This randomized, double-blinded clinical trial was conducted in 48 academic centers in the U.S. A total of 2206 patients aged 30-85 with a noncardioembolic ischemic stroke within the previous 30 days and scores of 3 or more on the Glasgow Outcome Scale were randomized to receive warfarin (dosed to a target INR of 1.4-2.8) or aspirin 325 mg daily. The primary endpoint was death from any cause or recurrent ischemic stroke. Rates of major hemorrhage (e.g., intracranial, intraspinal) and minor hemorrhage (e.g., gastrointestinal, ecchymoses) were also recorded. There was no significant difference between the warfarin and aspirin groups in the time to the primary endpoint (HR 1.13; 95%CI 0.92-1.38). There was also no difference in the rates of major hemorrhage (p = 0.10), though rates of minor hemorrhage were significantly higher in the warfarin group (p < 0.001). Finally, there was no significant difference in time to the primary endpoint due to patient differences in gender, ethnicity, or subtype of prior stroke.

Mohr JP, Thompson JLP, Lazar RM, Levin B, Sacco RL, Furie KL, et al. A Comparison of Warfarin and Aspirin for the Prevention of Recurrent Ischemic Stroke. New England Journal of Medicine. 2001 Nov 15;345(20):1444–51.

Aspirin vs. warfarin in atherosclerotic intracranial stenosis

1. There was no significant difference between warfarin and aspirin in preventing recurrent stroke in patients with significant atherosclerotic intracranial stenosis.

2. Warfarin therapy significantly increased the risk of major hemorrhage compared to aspirin.

Original Date of Publication: March 2005

Study Rundown: This trial randomized patients who were recently diagnosed with a stroke due to intracranial atherosclerotic stenosis to prophylactic treatment with either high-dose aspirin or warfarin. The trial was stopped early because the warfarin treatment group had a much higher incidence of major hemorrhages compared to the aspirin treatment group. There was no significant difference in the rate of stroke recurrence between the two groups. In summary, this study demonstrated that aspirin should be used for secondary prophylaxis in patients who suffered an ischemic stroke due to significant atherosclerotic intracranial stenosis. Warfarin was associated with increased risk of major hemorrhage and did not provide added benefit over aspirin in preventing a second stroke.

In-Depth [randomized controlled trial]: This trial involved enrollment of 569 patients with intracranial stenosis from 59 sites in North America. In order to participate, patients had to have experienced a transient ischemic attack (TIA) or non-disabling stroke within 90 days prior to enrollment that was attributed to 50-90% stenosis of a major intracranial artery. Patients were excluded if they had any evidence of 50-90% stenosis of the extracranial carotid artery, evidence or history of atrial fibrillation, or other non-atherosclerotic causes of intracranial artery stenosis. Patients were randomized to receive 5 mg of warfarin daily or 650 mg of aspirin twice daily. A non-blinded investigator made dosage changes based on side effects and INR value. The rest of the investigating team and the patients were blinded to the treatment arms. The primary endpoint was occurrence of ischemic or hemorrhagic stroke or death from any vascular cause. Study follow-up was expected to be 36 months, however the trial was stopped early due to a significant increase of adverse events in the warfarin group. The warfarin group experienced significantly more major hemorrhages than the aspirin group (HR 0.39 95%CI 0.18-0.84) after a mean of 1.8 years of follow up. There was no significant difference in primary endpoint outcomes between the two groups (HR 1.04, 95%CI 0.73-1.48).

Chimowitz MI, Lynn MJ, Howlett-Smith H, Stern BJ, Hertzberg VS, Frankel MR, et al. Comparison of Warfarin and Aspirin for Symptomatic Intracranial Arterial Stenosis. New England Journal of Medicine. 2005 Mar 31;352(13):1305–16.

The CARESS trial: Dual antiplatelet therapy superior to monotherapy in symptomatic carotid stenosis

1. Dual antiplatelet therapy with clopidogrel and aspirin significantly reduced the risk of microembolic events in patients with symptomatic carotid stenosis compared to aspirin alone.

2. There was no significant difference between the two groups in the risk of bleeding.

Original Date of Publication: May 2005

Study Rundown: The Clopidogrel and Aspirin for Reduction of Emboli in Symptomatic Carotid Stenosis (CARESS) trial evaluated combination antiplatelet therapy (i.e., clopidogrel and aspirin) compared to aspirin alone to prevent embolic events in patients with symptomatic carotid stenosis. The study used microembolic signals (MES) detected by transcranial Doppler (TCD) ultrasound as a surrogate marker for antiplatelet efficacy and risk of TIA or stroke. In summary, dual antiplatelet therapy was associated with a significant 39.8% relative risk reduction in the proportion of patients who were positive for MES after one week of treatment. Further, the frequency of MES was significantly reduced in the dual therapy group compared to the monotherapy group. There was no increased risk of bleeding associated with combination therapy. Although the trial did not assess a clinical end point, it demonstrated that MES detected by TCD is a feasible outcome measure.

In-Depth [randomized controlled trial]: This randomized, double-blind, multicenter study involved 11 centers located in France, Germany, Switzerland, and the United Kingdom. Eligible patients were >18 years old, had ≥50% stenosis, and had TIA or stroke in the past 3 months. These patients were evaluated for MES using TCD ultrasound. Exclusion criteria included having clinical/imaging evidence of hemorrhagic transformation, carotid endarterectomy scheduled within the next 2 weeks, acoustic window that did not allow TCD recording, atrial fibrillation or other major cardiac source of embolism, thrombolysis within the last 2 weeks, and anticoagulation within the past 3 days, amongst other factors. Patients in whom MES were detected were randomized to receive clopidogrel plus aspirin or aspirin monotherapy. Those in the dual therapy group received a loading dose of 300 mg of clopidogrel on day 1, followed by 75 mg once daily up to day 7. Both groups received 75 mg of aspirin once daily for the duration of the study. The primary endpoint was the proportion of patients who were MES positive on day 7. Secondary endpoints included the proportion of patients who were MES positive on day 2 and the rate of embolization (in number of MES per hour) on days 2 and 7. After screening for MES with TCD, 107 patients were randomized to receive either dual therapy or monotherapy.

On intention-to-treat analysis, dual therapy was associated with a significant reduction in the proportion of patients who were MES positive on day 7 (RRR 39.8%; 95%CI 13.8% to 58.0%; $p = 0.0046$). MES frequency per hour was reduced in the dual therapy group compared to the monotherapy group at both day 7 (embolization rate reduction 61.4%; 95%CI 31.6% to 78.2%; $p = 0.001$) and day 2 (embolization rate reduction 61.6%; 95%CI 34.9% to 77.4%; $p < 0.001$). There was no significant difference in bleeding between the two treatment groups

Markus HS, Droste DW, Kaps M, Larrue V, Lees KR, Siebler M, et al. Dual Antiplatelet Therapy With Clopidogrel and Aspirin in Symptomatic Carotid Stenosis Evaluated Using Doppler Embolic Signal Detection The Clopidogrel and Aspirin for Reduction of Emboli in Symptomatic Carotid Stenosis (CARESS) Trial. Circulation. 2005 May 3;111(17):2233–40.

Donepezil and vitamin E in Alzheimer's disease

1. High-dose vitamin E supplementation did not significantly slow progression in Alzheimer's disease (AD).

2. Donepezil, a cholinesterase inhibitor, significantly reduced the risk of progression to AD early in treatment.

Original Date of Publication: June 2005

Study Rundown: Around 80% of people who meet criteria for amnestic mild cognitive impairment develop AD within the next 6 years. There has been significant research focused on ways of slowing down the process of cognitive impairment, including medications such as donepezil and supplements such as vitamin E. This study compared donepezil (a cholinesterase inhibitor), high-dose vitamin E supplementation, and placebo concerning their effect at slowing down the progression to AD. The study found that while donepezil had a modest, but significant, effect early on in treatment, vitamin E was not superior to placebo. In summary, this study showed the modest effects of donepezil at reducing the progression to AD and that vitamin E was not effective in slowing down the progression of mild cognitive impairment. As shown in previous studies, this study also demonstrated that being a carrier of the APO-E e4 allele is the most significant risk factor in developing AD. Given the allele's propensity for AD, it was included as a covariate when running statistical analysis of data. However, the paper did not show any data concerning the covariate.

In-Depth [randomized controlled trial]: This multicenter, randomized, double-blind, placebo-controlled trial took 769 subjects with mild cognitive impairment from across the United States and Canada and randomized them to receive either 2000 IU of vitamin E with a placebo, 10 mg of donepezil with a placebo, or placebos for both. All patients also took a daily multivitamin. Subjects were screened for mild cognitive impairment by several independent measures and were all between 55-90 years of age. The primary end point was time to the development of possible or probable Alzheimer's disease, which was defined according to clinical criteria by multiple independent national neurological and Alzheimer's disease organizations. Secondary outcomes included scores on a variety of assessment scales testing different aspects of cognition. Patients were followed for 3 years. Results showed that there was no significant difference in progression to AD between the vitamin E group and the placebo group at any time during the 3 year trial (numerical data not provided in paper). Donepezil, on the other hand, did show modest reduction in risk of progression to AD compared to placebo, for the first 12 months of the trial (p = 0.004 at 6 months and p = 0.04 at 12 months). During years 2 and 3, the hazard ratios were lower, but still significant (p = 0.03 for both years). However, by 36 months, the three groups did not differ significantly in the number of subjects who had progressed to AD (63 in donepezil group vs. 73 in placebo group, p = 0.21). Secondary outcomes showed minor improvements in some of the assessments in the donepezil group compared to the placebo group but the differences were confined to the first 18 months of the study. The one marker that stood out was the APO-E e4 allele, with 76% of AD cases in the study occurring among carriers of the allele (p < 0.001).

Petersen RC, Thomas RG, Grundman M, Bennett D, Doody R, Ferris S, et al. Vitamin E and Donepezil for the Treatment of Mild Cognitive Impairment. New England Journal of Medicine. 2005 Jun 9;352(23):2379–88.

The ESPRIT trial: Aspirin with dipyridamole after cerebral ischemia

1. The combination of aspirin and dipyridamole was superior to aspirin alone in the secondary prevention of major vascular events.

2. Patients on combination therapy were more likely to discontinue the trial medication due to adverse effects.

Original Date of Publication: May 2006

Study Rundown: Daily aspirin as a secondary preventive measure was previously shown to reduce the risk of vascular events in patients with a history of transient ischemic attack. There was, however, uncertainty as to whether dipyridamole in combination with aspirin added any additional benefits. The European/Australasian Stroke Prevention in Reversible Ischemia (ESPRIT) trial was a large, multicenter randomized controlled trial of aspirin with dipyridamole versus aspirin alone following cerebral ischemia of arterial origin. When the results of this trial were included in a meta-analysis of combination therapy versus aspirin alone, a clear benefit was demonstrated in the prevention of vascular death, stroke, or myocardial infarction (MI). A potential limitation of the study is its non-blinded design; however, outcomes were verified by an auditing committee that was unaware of treatment assignment. In summary, the findings of the ESPRIT trial suggest that patients should be prescribed both aspirin and dipyridamole following cerebral ischemia of arterial origin.

In-Depth [randomized controlled trial]: Published in the Lancet in 2006, this randomized controlled trial assigned 2739 patients with a history of a transient ischemic attack within the past 6 months to receive a combination of aspirin and dipyridamole or aspirin alone. The primary outcome was a composite of death from all vascular causes, non-fatal stroke, non-fatal MI or major bleeding complication. Of the patients assigned to the combination treatment, 470 (34%) discontinued the trial medication largely due to adverse effects, while 184 (13%) of the patients assigned to aspirin alone discontinued their medication. The primary outcome occurred in 173 (13%) patients assigned to combination therapy versus 216 (16%) of those assigned to aspirin alone (HR 0.80; 95%CI 0.66-0.98). The investigators updated a previously conducted meta-analysis with the addition of these results and found an overall risk ratio of 0.82 (95%CI 0.74-0.91) for the composite outcome of vascular death, non-fatal stroke or non-fatal MI.

ESPRIT Study Group, Halkes PHA, van Gijn J, Kappelle LJ, Koudstaal PJ, Algra A. *Aspirin plus dipyridamole versus aspirin alone after cerebral ischaemia of arterial origin (ESPRIT): randomised controlled trial.* Lancet. 2006 May 20;367(9523):1665–73.

The SPARCL trial: Atorvastatin reduces the risk of stroke in patients with recent stroke or transient ischemic attack

1. In patients with recent stroke or transient ischemic attack (TIA), high-dose atorvastatin significantly reduced the risk of fatal stroke compared to placebo.

2. Atorvastatin also significantly reduced the risk of cardiovascular events.

Original Date of Publication: August 2006

Study Rundown: While this trial demonstrated that atorvastatin after stroke or TIA significantly reduced the risk of fatal stroke, there were several criticisms of this trial. One of the main criticisms of the study was the use of industry funding. Moreover, many of the contributors received consulting fees and grant support from various pharmaceutical companies. Lastly, the study was not powered to examine the effect on mortality. Nevertheless, the Stroke Prevention by Aggressive Reduction in Cholesterol Levels (SPARCL) trial has been influential, and has informed the AHA/ASA recommendation for statin therapy in patients with prior stroke and TIA. In summary, statins should be considered in patients soon after a stroke or transient ischemic attack to reduce the risk of subsequent stroke and cardiovascular events.

In-Depth [randomized controlled trial]: Published in NEJM in 2006, the SPARCL trial sought to determine whether atorvastatin would reduce the incidence of stroke or cardiovascular events in patients with recent stroke or TIA. A total of 4731 patients were randomized to either the treatment group receiving 80 mg of atorvastatin per day or to the placebo group. The primary endpoint was the incidence of fatal or nonfatal stroke. A number of cardiovascular events were also measured as secondary outcomes. Patients were eligible for inclusion if they were 18 years of age and had an ischemic or hemorrhagic stroke or TIA in the 1-6 month period prior to randomization. Patients were recruited from 205 different centers, and patients were followed for a mean of 4.9 years. Low-density lipoprotein (LDL) cholesterol levels were similar between the two groups at baseline and decreased by 53% in the atorvastatin group while remaining unchanged in the placebo group at one month after randomization. Atorvastatin was associated with a relative risk reduction of 16% for the primary end point of fatal or nonfatal stroke, which was significant according to the prespecified adjusted model (adjusted HR 0.84; 95%CI 0.71-0.99; p = 0.03). The statin was also associated with a significant reduction in risk of cardiovascular events, including nonfatal myocardial infarctions, acute coronary events, and revascularization (HR 0.80; 95%CI 0.69-0.92; p = 0.002). Overall mortality rates were the same in the two groups (p = 0.98).

Amarenco P, Bogousslavsky J, Callahan A, Goldstein LB, Hennerici M, Rudolph AE, et al. High-dose atorvastatin after stroke or transient ischemic attack. New England Journal of Medicine. 2006 Aug 10;355(6):549–59.

The ABCD2 score: Risk of stroke after transient ischemic attack

1. **The ABCD2 score is a validated, seven-point, risk-stratification tool to identify patients at high risk of stroke following a transient ischemic attack (TIA).**

2. **Patients with scores ≥4 were found to be at considerably higher risk of stroke in the 2-day period following a TIA. These patients may require urgent intervention as inpatients.**

Original Date of Publication: January 2007

Study Rundown: The ABCD2 score is a 7-point score for identifying patients who have suffered a TIA at the highest risk of stroke in the following 2-day period. The score was created by merging 2 previously validated clinical decision rules - the ABCD and the California scores. The ABCD score was created to estimate the 7-day risk of stroke following a TIA, while the California score predicted the 90-day risk. The 2 scores shared many features, and were combined in hopes of developing a more widely validated model to identify patients at the highest risk of stroke 2 days after a TIA, thereby allowing clinicians to determine if patients required urgent management.

Since its publication, the ABCD2 score has become widely used by front-line healthcare providers to risk stratify patients with TIA and determine how urgently these patients should be seen for subsequent assessment and treatment. While its c statistic was similar to those of the ABCD and California scores, the ABCD2 score has been more widely validated and has been shown to accurately predict the risk of stroke at 2, 7, and 90 days following a TIA. Some have criticized the ABCD2 score for only taking into account clinical features and not giving consideration to investigations. Moreover, the score has been shown to be predictive of carotid embolic sources, but less useful for cardiac sources of emboli.

In-Depth [randomized controlled trial]: Study cohorts were drawn from the Kaiser-Permanente Medical Care Plan in Northern California, United States and from Oxfordshire, United Kingdom. The c statistic was calculated to measure predictive ability. All combinations of factors from the ABCD and California scores were tested for their c statistic, and the combination with the highest statistic for 2-day risk of stroke was selected and validated. In total, the two derivation groups and four validation groups included 4809 individuals with

TIA. The new composite score was named the ABCD2 score (Figure), because it took into account age, blood pressure, clinical features, duration, and diabetes mellitus diagnoses.

Risk factor	Points
Age ≥60 years	1
Blood pressure elevation (systolic >140 mmHg and/or diastolic ≥90 mmHg)	1
Clinical features	
Unilateral weakness	2
Speech disturbance without weakness	1
Duration of symptoms	
≥60 minutes	2
10-59 minutes	1
Diabetes mellitus	1

ABCD2 scores were grouped into low-, moderate-, and high-risk categories. The rate of strokes are considerably higher with ABCD2 scores ≥4, and patients who are classified as moderate- and high-risk may require more urgent specialist assessment, investigation, and treatment to prevent stroke (Figure).

ABCD2score	Patients	2-day risk (%)	7-day risk (%)	90-day risk (%)
Low (0-3)	1,628	1.0	1.2	3.1
Moderate (4-5)	2,169	4.1	5.9	9.8
High (6-7)	1,012	8.1	11.7	17.8

Johnston SC, Rothwell PM, Nguyen-Huynh MN, Giles MF, Elkins JS, Bernstein AL, et al. Validation and refinement of scores to predict very early stroke risk after transient ischaemic attack. Lancet. 2007 Jan 27;369(9558):283–92.

X. Pediatrics

Childhood febrile seizure characteristics associated with epilepsy diagnosis

1. Children with febrile seizures, complex febrile seizures, and febrile seizures of early onset (before 6 months of age) had a variably increased risk of developing epilepsy when compared to individuals without febrile seizures.

2. Abnormal performance on neurologic testing was linked to increased epilepsy risk.

Original Date of Publication: November 1976

Study Rundown: Previous research indicated an increase in unprovoked seizures following childhood febrile seizures. The researchers in this study were the first to try to define the risk factors associated with progression from childhood febrile seizure to epilepsy. As a part of the Collaborative Perinatal Project of the National Institute of Neurological and Communicative Disorders and Stroke, researchers developed this multi-center, large prospective cohort study. Children were followed from birth to age 7, during which time febrile and afebrile seizure activity as well as overall development were examined. Results demonstrated that individuals who experienced febrile seizures with and without complex features, those who tested abnormally on developmental screening prior to their first febrile seizure, and children with early febrile seizures were significantly more likely to be diagnosed with epilepsy by the age of 7.

This study was limited by its lack of consideration of potential covariates, including whether or not a child was started on anticonvulsant therapy. Other studies have found that early first febrile seizures (before 5 years of age), repeated febrile seizures, prolonged febrile seizure length, and a family history of cerebral palsy were potential contributors to childhood epilepsy.

In-Depth [prospective cohort]: Conducted in 12 teaching hospitals, 54 000 children born to mothers enrolled in the Collaborative Perinatal Project were recruited for study inclusion. Children were followed from birth to 7 years of age. Parents were interviewed regarding the occurrence of seizures, convulsions, and changes in consciousness at 4, 8, 12, 18, and 24 months with annual follow-up continuing from 2 to 7 years of age. Interviews were completed by trained individuals. Medical records were obtained for each medically managed seizure episode. Neurologic and developmental assessments were completed throughout the study with standard physical examination at 4 months of age, psychological assessment at 8 months of age, and pediatric and neurologic assessment at 1 year of age. "Febrile seizures" were defined as any seizure occurring with fever in a child 1 month to 7 years of age. "Afebrile seizures" were defined as recurrent seizure without fever before 4 years of age or 1, isolated afebrile seizure episode after 2 years of age. "Epilepsy" was defined as recurrent afebrile seizures with at least 1 occurring after 2 years of age. No associated known acute neurologic illness could be present in order for these diagnoses to be made. Complex features of seizures were defined as seizure duration longer than 15 minutes, more than 1 seizure in 24 hours, and focal seizure activity.

Of the children included, 1706 experienced at least one febrile seizure and were followed to study completion at 7 years of age. Among these children, 550 (32%) had at least 1 more febrile seizure, but no afebrile seizure, while 52 children (3%) had at least 1 afebrile seizure during the study, and 34 (2%) met criteria for a diagnosis of epilepsy. Of the 39 179 children who did not have a febrile seizure and were followed for 7 years, 199 were diagnosed with epilepsy. Significantly more individuals were diagnosed with epilepsy following a first febrile seizure with complex features when compared to those with only afebrile seizures (41 vs. 5 per 1000, $X^2 = 70$, p < 0.001). Children with complex febrile seizures had significantly greater rates of epilepsy than those who had febrile seizures without complex features (41 vs. 15 per 1000, $X^2 = 7.8$, p < 0.01). Children with febrile seizures without complex features were diagnosed at higher rates than those who had afebrile seizures (15 vs. 5 per 1000, p < 0.001). Children with any abnormal findings on assessments prior to first seizure were significantly more likely to meet criteria for epilepsy when compared to those with normal screenings (39 v. 12 per 1000, $X^2 = 11$, p < 0.001). An 18-fold increase in risk of epilepsy was noted among children who had both complex first febrile seizure and abnormal screening performance compared to those with no febrile seizure (92 vs. 5 per 1000, $X^2 = 79$, p < 0.001). Previously normal children without complex seizures had significantly higher rates of epilepsy than those with afebrile seizures (11 vs. 5 per 1000, $X^2 = 4.0$, p < 0.05). There was a significant increase in epilepsy by 7 years of age among children who had febrile seizures during their first 6 months of life when compared to those who had them beyond the first year (57 vs. 15 per 1000, $X^2 = 7.6$, p < 0.01).

Nelson KB, Ellenberg JH. Predictors of Epilepsy in Children Who Have Experienced Febrile Seizures. New England Journal of Medicine. 1976 Nov 4;295(19):1029–33.

Initial guidelines for prolonged fever in children

1. Among 100 children presenting to one children's hospital for prolonged febrile illnesses, the majority of cases were of an infectious etiology (52 cases).

2. Febrile illness due to infectious causes were significantly more likely to occur in younger children, while those due to inflammatory conditions were significantly more likely to occur in older children.

Original Date of Publication: April 1975

Study Rundown: The issue of prolonged febrile illness in children presents a diagnostic challenge to pediatric practitioners. At the time of this study's publication, there were no guidelines for diagnosis and management of children with fevers of unknown origin (FUO), a term still without a clear definition today. It is often defined as temperature > 38.3°C for at least 8 days without any obvious cause following initial outpatient or hospital evaluation. This study investigated prolonged fever in 100 children in order to better define guidelines for the care of those with FUO, defined in this study as a temperature >38.5°C, ≥5 times during a 2-week period.

Of the 100 records included, the most common fever etiology was infection (52 cases). Findings indicated that significantly more young children had fevers of infectious etiologies, while significantly more older children had collagen-inflammatory fever etiologies. Based on the findings that 62% of children had stories and presentations consistent with etiology, researchers recognized the importance of a thorough history and physical in diagnosis. With 80% of children receiving antibiotics prior to official diagnosis and no resolution in their symptoms, the use of antibiotic therapy prior to hospitalization was discouraged and use of diagnostic cultures encouraged. In addition, erythrocyte sedimentation rate (ESR) testing and protein analysis were deemed more useful than complete blood count (CBC) and urinalysis (UA). Other procedures and imaging techniques were helpful when indicated by the history and physical.

This study was limited by its small sample size, lack of patient racial/ethnic diversity, and use of a single institution as a source of patient reports. Decades and multiple studies and reports on FUO later, many of the conclusions drawn from this landmark study still stand. Infection remains the most common cause of prolonged febrile illness. The importance of history and physical in diagnosing children with FUO continues to be emphasized; however specific recommendations for initial testing now include CBC, ESR, C-reactive protein, blood cultures, UA and culture, chest radiograph, tuberculosis testing, electrolytes, and blood urea nitrogen, creatinine, liver panel, and HIV serology.

In-Depth [retrospective cohort]: A total of 100 patient records of children (65% male and 91 white) seen at a tertiary children's hospital for prolonged fever during 1966 to 1973 were included in analysis. Prolonged fever defined as a temperature of >38.5℃ on ≥5 times during a 2-week period without final diagnosis from a referring physician. Temperatures were taken either rectally or by an equivalent method. Results were analyzed using X^2 testing with final diagnoses as determined by laboratory testing when appropriate and then categorized as "infectious-presumed viral," "infectious-nonviral," "collagen-inflammatory," "malignancy," "miscellaneous," or "undiagnosed." In addition, fever patterns, use of antipyretics, symptoms, physical findings, laboratory results, and radiologic findings were recorded.

Of 100 patients, most were diagnosed with infectious causes of their fevers (52 cases), with 17 secondary to presumed viral illness, 20 due to collagen-inflammatory disorders, 6 secondary to malignancy, and 10 from miscellaneous causes. When cases were divided by age into either younger than 6 years of age (52 cases) or older than 6 years of age (48 cases), it was found that significantly more younger patients were diagnosed with infection than older patients (34 vs. 18, $p < 0.05$), while significantly more of those diagnosed with collagen-inflammatory diseases were older than 6 years (16 vs. 4, $p < 0.05$). The most common presenting symptoms of febrile patients were head, ear, eye, nose, and throat symptoms (72 cases). Only 27 patients had physical signs directly related to their final diagnoses. White blood cell count and low hematocrit from CBC did not significantly relate to fever etiology. ESR was significantly related to non-serious fever etiology in the 20 children with ESR <10 mm/hr. Thirty-four of 74 children tested had reversed albumin-globulin ratios. Of these, significantly more patients with collagen-inflammatory disease had reversal compared to those with viral diagnoses (75% vs. 20%, $p < 0.05$). In addition, electrophoresis patterns differed significantly among patients with viral disorders showing a uniform decrease in albumin and increase in globulin.

Pizzo PA, Lovejoy FH, Smith DH. Prolonged Fever in Children: Review of 100 Cases. Pediatrics. 1975 Apr 1;55(4):468–73.

Artificial surfactant improves respiratory distress syndrome in infants

1. In 10 infants treated for respiratory distress syndrome (RDS) with artificial surfactant, significant improvements in blood pressure, acid-base status, arterial oxygenation, and radiologic findings were observed.

2. Infants also required significantly less oxygen therapy and ventilator pressure following surfactant administration.

Original Date of Publication: January 1980

Study Rundown: Hyaline membrane disease (HMD), now known as infant RDS, is a pulmonary disease of young infants most often linked to fetal immaturity. After the landmark 1959 discovery by Avery et al. connecting insufficient surfactant with RDS, methods of treating the disease were investigated. As surfactant was known to reduce lung surface tension, making it easier to maintain patent alveoli, this study built upon work in animals as the first trial of artificial surfactant treatment for RDS in human infants.

Using a mixture of natural and synthetic lipids including dipalmitoyl lecithin (the primary component of surfactant) and phosphatidyl glycerol, researchers administered artificial surfactant to 10 infants diagnosed with RDS and examined their laboratory, clinical examination, and radiologic changes. Significant reductions in systolic blood pressure (SBP), along with improvements in arterial oxygenation, arterial-alveolar oxygen concentration differences, acid-base balance, and radiologic findings were observed. Infants also required significantly less inspired oxygen and ventilator pressure after surfactant administration. This study was limited by a lack of randomization, comparison to control infants, and its small sample size. Despite these factors, this study led to future, large, randomized, clinical trials that further solidified the benefits of artificial surfactant use among infants with RDS. Antenatal corticosteroids coupled with post-delivery surfactant and ventilation are now commonplace treatments for infants in neonatal intensive care as they significantly improve clinical outcomes among infants suffering from poor lung development.

In-Depth [prospective cohort]: Ten infants with diagnosed RDS (mean gestational age = 30.2 weeks, mean birthweight = 1552 g) were included in the study. Prior to surfactant administration, ventilator settings were noted and not changed. Arterial oxygen tension (P_aO_2), carbon dioxide tension (P_aCO_2), and pH were recorded 30-90 minutes before and again 10-20 minutes before surfactant administration to provide a snapshot of each infant's physiologic state. No significant differences were noted between these 2 time periods. About 10 mL of artificial surfactant (150 μmol lipid phosphorus/kg) was suspended in normal saline and put into the infants' endotracheal tubes. Infants were then moved into different positions to ensure the solution was distributed to each lung segment and the infant was ventilated with a respirator. Up to 3 hours post-administration P_aO_2, $PaCO_2$, acid-base balance, and radiographic findings were assessed without alteration in ventilator settings. Following this assessment, ability to reduce inspired oxygen concentration (F_iO_2) and respiratory pressure were noted.

On clinical examination, significant increases in SBP post-administration was observed in the 6 infants who had continuous blood pressure monitoring (37 ± 5 mmHg pre vs. 59 ± 4 mmHg post, $p < 0.02$). PO_2 increased significantly (45 ± 7 mmHg pre vs. 212 ± 46 mmHg post, $p < 0.005$), PCO_2 decreased significantly (50 ± 4 mmHg pre vs. 33 ± 2 mm Hg post, $p < 0.005$), and pH increased significantly (7.13 ± 0.05 pre vs. 7.31 ± 0.04, $p < 0.05$). Three hours post-administration, F_iO_2 were able to decrease significantly from $81\pm7\%$ to $38\pm5\%$ ($p < 0.01$) and, within 6 hours of administration, inspiratory pressure could be reduced from 30 ± 2 cm H_2O to 22 ± 2 cm H_2O ($p < 0.02$). The difference in alveolar and arterial O_2 concentration decreased significantly as well 474 ± 49 mmHg to 189 ± 29 ($p < 0.005$) 3 hours post-administration and to 120 ± 18 mmHg ($p < 0.001$) 30 hours post-administration. At an average of 6 hours post-administration complete radiologic resolution of RDS was observed. Two of the 10 infants studied died due to causes unrelated to RDS or surfactant administration. No serious adverse events were linked to surfactant use.

Fujiwara T, Maeta H, Chida S, Morita T, Watabe Y, Abe T. Artificial surfactant therapy in hyaline-membrane disease. Lancet. 1980 Jan 12;1(8159):55–9.

Avery M, Mead J. Surface properties in relation to atelectasis and hyaline membrane disease. AMA Am J Dis Child. 1959 May 1;97(51):517–23.

IVIg with aspirin reduces coronary aneurysms in Kawasaki disease

1. Children with Kawasaki disease treated with a combined regimen of aspirin and intravenous gamma globulin (IVIg) experienced significantly lower rates of coronary artery aneurysms when compared to those receiving aspirin only.

2. Children treated with the combined regimen had significantly shorter fevers and a greater decrease in inflammatory markers when compared to those treated with aspirin alone.

Original Date of Publication: August 1986

Study Rundown: Kawasaki disease, also known as Kawasaki syndrome, is an inflammatory vascular condition characterized by persistent fever, oral erythema, conjunctivitis, lymphadenopathy, and rash with risk of lasting coronary artery aneurysm or ectasia. At the time of the current study, standard care for Kawasaki disease included aspirin, which was thought to aid in reducing inflammation without reducing the disease's cardiovascular complications. This study was the first to expand upon the proposed efficacy of high-dose IVIg in preventing Kawasaki-related cardiac problems when compared to aspirin. Prior studies used low-dose (100mg) IVIg and had poor study design.

In this study, researchers found that children receiving combined therapy had a significantly lower incidence of aneurysms, fever duration, and inflammatory markers by day 5 of treatment when compared to those receiving aspirin only. This study was limited in its lack of blinding among practitioners administering the treatment regimen and differences in hospitalization status (all patients undergoing IVIg required hospitalization, whereas those receiving aspirin only were not). This was the first study to provide evidence of the efficacy of high-dose IVIg in managing the cardiac and inflammatory outcomes of Kawasaki disease.

In-Depth [randomized controlled trial]: From February 1984 to September 1985, 168 children with diagnosed Kawasaki disease were recruited from 6 care centers throughout the United States. Kawasaki disease was diagnosed in individuals with 5 of 6 clinical features (fever, nonexudative conjunctivitis, oral changes, extremity changes, rash, and cervical lymphadenopathy). Participants were randomized into 1 of 2 treatment groups: 1) 100mg/kg of aspirin every 16 hours for 14 days (n = 84) or 2) 400mg (high-dose) IVIg for the first 4 days of treatment along with the aspirin regimen described previously (n = 84). Demographics, baseline laboratory testing, and follow-up salicylate levels of the groups did not differ significantly. Coronary artery pathology was assessed using echocardiography at enrollment as well as 2 and 7 weeks after enrollment. Secondary outcomes included fever duration and reduction in inflammatory markers (white-cell count, absolute granulocyte count, α_1-antitrypsin level, absolute neutrophil count, and platelet count). Imaging was read by 2 pediatric echocardiographers blinded to the study. T-tests to compare means and Mantel-Haenszel methods along with logistic regression were completed to assess the effect of IVIg on the treatment regimen.

A total of 311 follow-up echocardiograms were completed. At 2-week follow-up, significantly fewer children in the combined treatment group had coronary artery abnormalities when compared to those treated only with aspirin (8% vs. 23.1%, $p < 0.01$). This difference was also observed at 7-week follow-up (3.8% vs. 17.7%, $p = 0.005$). Using Mantel-Haeszel methods and logistic regression, it was determined that at 2 weeks, children who had the combined treatment regimen were one third as likely to have coronary aneurysms and, at 7 weeks, one fifth as likely when compared to children treated with only aspirin (95%CI). Children treated with a combined regimen experienced a significantly greater drop in body temperature during the first 2 days of treatment than with aspirin (1.30 ± 0.16C drop vs. 0.42 ± 0.11C, $p = 0.001$). By day 5 of treatment, those with treated with combined therapy had a significant greater decrease in white cell count ($p < 0.0001$), absolute granulocytes ($p = 0.0001$), and alpha$_1$ anti-trypsin levels ($p = 0.05$). Absolute neutrophil count and platelet count did not differ by treatment group. No serious adverse effects of IVIg were experienced.

Newburger JW, Takahashi M, Burns JC, Beiser AS, Chung KJ, Duffy CE, et al. The Treatment of Kawasaki Syndrome with Intravenous Gamma Globulin. New England Journal of Medicine. 1986 Aug 7;315(6):341–7.

Prone sleeping position and heavy bedding associated with sudden infant death syndrome

1. A significant increase in sudden infant death syndrome (SIDS) was observed among infants who slept prone as opposed to sleeping on their side or supine.

2. A significant increase in SIDS risk was observed among infants who were wrapped in more blankets, wore heavier clothing to bed, or were in a home that was heated overnight when compared to control infants.

Original Date of Publication: July 1990

Study Rundown: This study aimed to further elucidate the role of sleeping position, bedding, and environmental temperature in SIDS. Researchers found that prone position during sleep, heavy bedding/bed clothing, and overnight heating in homes significantly increased the risk of infants dying from SIDS. The study was limited in its generalizability through use of a study population from a single geographic location. Despite this, the study further supported the theories that SIDS deaths commonly resulted from prone infant position and increased infant heat exposure. Following this study and multiple other publications supporting findings regarding sleep positioning, the United States and many other countries initiated "Back to Sleep" campaigns now known as "Safe to Sleep," encouraging caretakers to place infants in the supine position to reduce SIDS incidence. Significant reductions in SIDS were seen following these campaigns. While side sleeping has not been identified as a SIDS risk factor, it is discouraged by pediatricians as infants can roll over from their sides onto their abdomens. In addition, further work has identified other SIDS-associated risk factors including loose bedding, soft sleeping surfaces, and bed-sharing.

In-Depth [case-control study]: All sudden infantile deaths in 2 counties of England were reported and, for each infant, 2 control infants living in the same neighborhood were identified. Researchers visited bereaved families soon after death and on several other occasions during the following months in order to gather a full social and medical history at the time of death. This included discussing sleeping position, sleep timing, clothing and blankets in the crib, and heating conditions in the room. To assess the heaviness of infant bedding and blankets, the thermal resistance of these materials was calculated and expressed in units of tog, where higher tog indicates heavier materials. Comparable histories were taken for control infants with attention paid to the 24 hours before the research visit. X^2 testing along with Mantel-Haenszel tests, and multiple logistic regression models were used to assess the difference between groups and risks associated with sudden death.

A total of 72 infants died suddenly during the study period (mean age = 94.4 days) and 144 control infants (mean age = 97.0 days) were included for comparison. Among the 72 infants who died, 5 were found to have pathologic causes contributing to their deaths, while the remaining 67 had no known cause and their deaths were therefore deemed secondary to SIDS. Among the 67 SIDS cases, 62 infants had been put to sleep in the prone position, while 76 of the 134 control infants slept prone. Prone positioning was associated with an 8.8 times increased risk of SIDS when compared to control infants (relative risk [RR] 8.8, 95%CI 7.0-11.0, p < 0.001). Infants who died of SIDS were wrapped in significantly heavier bedding than control infants (9.1 tog vs. 8.0 tog, p < 0.05). After controlling for sleep position, a significant increased risk with heavier bedding/heavier bed clothing was observed (RR 1.14 for each 1 tog increase above 8 tog, 95%CI 1.03-1.28, p < 0.05). Overnight home heating was seen in significantly more homes of infants who died than controls and was associated with a significantly increased risk of SIDS death (28 of 67 vs. 34 of 134, RR 2.7, 95%CI 1.4-5.2, p < 0.01).

Fleming PJ, Gilbert R, Azaz Y, Berry PJ, Rudd PT, Stewart A, et al. Interaction between bedding and sleeping position in the sudden infant death syndrome: a population based case-control study. BMJ. 1990 Jul 14;301(6743):85–9.

Lead exposure in childhood associated with worse cognitive performance

1. Among children exposed to lead early in life, serum lead levels at 24 months of age were significantly associated with decreased cognitive performance on measures of intelligence and educational achievement at 10 years old.

2. Each 0.48 µmol/L (10 µg/dL) increase in serum lead at 24 months of age was associated with a 5.8 point decline in a measure of intelligence quotient (IQ) and an 8.9 point decline in educational achievement score during cognitive testing at 10 years of age.

Original Date of Publication: December 1992

Study Rundown: At the time of this publication, prior studies investigating early, low-level lead exposure and cognition later in life had mixed findings. Previous reports assessed the potential connection between lead levels and cognitive performance into preschool years. This was the first study to investigate the effects of early low-level lead exposure on cognitive performance into school age. One hundred forty-eight children were assessed from birth to 10 years of age for serum lead levels and cognitive development through IQ testing via the Wechsler Intelligence Scale for Children-Revised (WISC-R) and the Kaufman Test of Educational Achievement Brief Form (K-TEA). Findings indicated that high serum lead levels at 24 months of age were significantly associated with lower IQ and neuropsychiatric performance at 10 years old, a finding which was upheld after controlling for covariates.

This study was limited by the potential role of bias towards children available for follow-up as multiple participants were lost from 5 years of age to 10 years old. In addition, this cohort was of higher socioeconomic status (SES) and intelligence than the average citizen, which may have allowed for an enhanced view of the cognitive effects of lead, but makes the findings less generalizable compared to previous study cohorts of lower SES. This study demonstrated that even at low levels, early lead exposure can lead to poor cognitive development through school age. Combined with previous work, these findings encouraged the Centers for Disease Control to lower the benchmark for toxic lead levels to the current level of 0.24 µmol/L (5 µg/dL).

In-Depth [prospective cohort]: Two hundred forty-nine infants born between August 1979 and August 1981 were recruited from Brigham and Women's Hospital in Boston, Massachusetts with umbilical blood lead levels in the ranges required for eligibility. Infants were considered for study inclusion if their umbilical cord blood lead levels were below the 10%ile at the time of the study (<0.15 µmol/L or 3µg/dL), around the 50%ile (0.31 µmol/L or 6.5 µg/dL), or above the 90%ile (≥0.48 µmol/L or 10 µg/dL) indicating, respectively, "low," "medium," or "high" prenatal lead exposure. Infants' lead levels and development were evaluated at 6, 12, 18, 24, and 57 months of age and then again at 10 years old. Primary cognitive outcomes were assessed through the use of the WISC-R and K-TEA.

Of the initial cohort, 148 children were included in the final analysis as they completed the entire study course. Of those, 116 had serum lead measurements at all 7 time points, including birth (mean 0.14 µmol/L or 2.9 µg/dL). Multiple regression analysis was completed with appropriate adjustment for confounders. Overall, participants had cognitive scores about 1 SD above the national average. After controlling for covariates, only the lead levels of children at 24 months of age (mean lead level <0.34 µmol/L or < 7 µg/dL) were significantly associated with cognitive performance including the full-scale WISC-R IQ and K-TEA battery composite. Each 0.48 µmol/L (10 µg/dL) increase in serum lead was associated with a 5.8 point decline in the IQ measure and 8.9 point decline in the K-TEA composite ($p < 0.01$, $p < 0.001$, respectively). No significant association between lead levels and cognitive scores was seen at any other age.

Bellinger DC, Stiles KM, Needleman HL. Low-Level Lead Exposure, Intelligence and Academic Achievement: A Long-term Follow-up Study. Pediatrics. 1992 Dec 1;90(6):855–61.

PROS network study examines pubertal onset by race/ethnic groups

1. In a study population of girls 3-12 years of age, African American females developed secondary sexual characteristics significantly earlier than white females.

2. African American females had earlier menarche at 12.16 years of age, compared to 12.88 years of age among white females.

Original Date of Publication: April 1997

Study Rundown: The onset of female pubertal changes varies greatly by race/ethnicity. As the start of secondary characteristics marks a significant physiologic and psychological change in an individual's life, being able to anticipate onset is essential to providing proper medical care. Prior to the initiation of this work, no nationally representative, racially diverse data was available to assess female pubertal status in the United States. This cross-sectional study stood as the first to investigate secondary sexual characteristics and menses onset among girls 3-12 years of age that could provide evidence representative of national norms.

This study included children form the American Academy of Pediatrics Practice-based Research in the Office Settings (PROS) Network. Researchers found that African American girls developed secondary sexual characteristics, including breast development, axillary hair, and pubic hair significantly earlier than white females. All girls started puberty 6 months to a year earlier than reported in prior studies. The average age of menarche in African American females was 12.16 years of age compared to 12.88 years in white females. This study was limited by potential selection bias with non-random sample selection, the lack of hormone testing to provide a potential endocrinologic etiology for these developmental differences, and participants being heavier and taller, on average, than girls in the nationally-representative height and weight values provided by the Health and Nutrition Examination Surveys. Findings from this study indicated that the initiation of sex education and physician counseling should be tailored accordingly to earlier pubertal changes among girls. Follow-up work to this initial paper was completed and published as documented below to dispel confusion regarding studies investigating this subject matter after 1997. Another, more recent publication supported these findings, indicating that thelarche onset differed by race/ethnicity and started earlier in those with higher BMI.

In-Depth [cross-sectional study]: A total of 17 077 female patients (90.4% white, 9.6% African American) aged 3-12 years from the PROS Network were included in the study. Sexual maturity was staged by physicians trained and assessed in their ability to use Tanner staging criteria. In addition, a survey with questions regarding demographics, medical history, presence or absence of menses, and development of breast, pubic, and axillary hair was completed. Axillary hair was designated according to an original scale with stage 1 as no hair, stage 2 as sparse hair, and stage 3 as adult, mature hair. With and without controlling for height and weight, African American girls were found to develop secondary sexual characters significantly earlier than white girls (8.87 years vs. 9.96 years for breast development, 8.78 years vs. 10.51 years for pubic hair, and 10.01 vs. 11.80 stage 2 axillary hair development; $p < 0.001$ for all findings). The average age of menses onset was 12.16 years for African American girls and 12.88 years for white girls. Significantly more African American females had menses at the age of 12 when compared to white girls (62.1% vs. 35.2%, $p < 0.001$).

Herman-Giddens ME, Slora EJ, Wasserman RC, Bourdony CJ, Bhapkar MV, Koch GG, et al. Secondary Sexual Characteristics and Menses in Young Girls Seen in Office Practice: A Study from the Pediatric Research in Office Settings Network. Pediatrics. 1997 Apr 1;99(4):505–12.

Biro FM, Greenspan LC, Galvez MP, Pinney SM, Teitelbaum S, Windham GC, et al. Onset of Breast Development in a Longitudinal Cohort. Pediatrics. 2013 Nov 4;132(6):1019-27.

Transcutaneous bilirubinometry linked to decreased serum testing and cost in infants

1. In a 2-year study period, researchers observed a significant decrease in the number of infants undergoing bilirubin serum testing after introduction of a transcutaneous bilirubinometer (TcB) in a single hospital's newborn nursery.

2. The use of the transcutaneous instrument decreased hospital costs by $1625 each year when compared to serum bilirubin measurements.

Original Date of Publication: April 1997

Study Rundown: At the time of this study, one of the most commonly completed laboratory tests in the newborn nursery was the serum bilirubin level, second only to other routine genetic and metabolic screening tests. Researchers proposed that the use of a transcutaneous instrument for bilirubin measurements would be an effective way to decrease unnecessary serum bilirubin testing as well as reduce costs in the nursery setting.

As the use of a TcB was integrated into the nursery work environment, researchers observed a significant decrease in the number of serum bilirubin measurements completed. In addition, significantly fewer low serum bilirubin (< 10 mg/dL) measurements were obtained over the course of the study, indicating a potential decrease in unnecessary serum tests secondary to TcB use. TcB monitor use was also associated with an estimated decrease in annual hospital expenses secondary to bilirubin monitoring of about $1625. This study was limited in its lack of a control group, lack of generalizability due to the study population coming from a single nursery, and complications with the practicality of the TcB device. However, the results suggested that TcB use could reduce the need for unnecessary invasive testing in addition to lowering overall costs. Today, this device is commonly used as its validity and reliability has been reaffirmed in numerous studies.

In-Depth [prospective cohort]: On November 1, 1990, the TcB meter was introduced for regular use in the William Beaumont Hospital Department of Pediatrics newborn nursery. The number of serum bilirubin measurements along with the estimated total costs for performing the tests was calculated for newborns in the nursery from July 1990 to December 1992. Costs included salary for laboratory staff, supply costs, and time required for the procedure. Information from 12 625 infant admissions were included in the analysis. Data from July 1990 to December 1990 admissions were considered "pre-jaundice meter" as hospital staff adjusted to TcB use. A 40% decrease in infants requiring at least 1 serum bilirubin test and a 56% decrease in those requiring at least 2 were seen by study completion (p < 0.0001). Over the course of the study, bilirubin levels less than 10 mg/dL decreased significantly, starting at 46% of readings progressing to 27% of readings at the study conclusion (p < 0.0001). When the costs related to serum and transcutaneous bilirubin measurements were calculated, it was found that nearly $1625 per year for a cohort of 12 625 infants would be saved through regular TcB use.

Maisels MJ, Kring E. Transcutaneous Bilirubinometry Decreases the Need for Serum Bilirubin Measurements and Saves Money. Pediatrics. 1997 Apr 1;99(4):599–600.

The ACE trial: Adverse childhood exposures associated with poor health in adulthood

1. A significant dose-response relationship was observed between childhood exposures, adult health risk behaviors and adult disease states.

Original Date of Publication: May 1998

Study Rundown: At the time of this study, researchers had just begun investigating the role of childhood trauma on the development of adult medical conditions. Through a retrospective approach, the Adverse Childhood Experiences (ACE) trial investigated the influence of childhood abuse on adult disease risk factors, disease incidence, quality of life, use of healthcare resources, and death. Overall, 8056 adults completed a standardized questionnaire addressing their exposure to various forms of adverse events including abuse and household dysfunction. Researchers found individuals who experienced adverse childhood exposures to be at increased risk of having both health-related risk factors such as smoking and obesity as well as illnesses such as ischemic heart disease and malignancy in adulthood. These risk increases were largely present in a dose-response fashion. While this study was limited by its retrospective design and reliance on self-reporting for both adverse exposures and health status, the prevalence of adverse exposures was consistent with national averages. These findings emphasized the importance of preventative measures in childhood and extending into adulthood to reduce childhood adverse exposure, the development of health risk factors, and ultimately disease development and mortality.

In-Depth [retrospective cohort]: A total of 8056 adults (mean age = 56.1 years, 52.1% female, 79.4% white) who underwent standardized medical evaluation at a large United States adult healthcare clinic from August-November of 1995 and January-March of 1996 were included. Following examination, patients received a mailed copy of the study questionnaire, which inquired about childhood psychological, physical, and sexual abuse along with household dysfunction metrics. Responses were then related to self-reported present health risk factors, adult disease conditions with high mortality rates, and overall health status. Risk factors investigated included physical inactivity (defined as no physical activity participation in the past month), severe obesity (defined as body mass index >35 kg/m²), current smoking, attempted suicide, depressed mood (defined as 2 or more weeks of depressed mood over the past year), alcohol abuse, illicit drug use, intravenous drug use, history of sexually transmitted infections, and high numbers of total sexual partners (defined as >50 partners). Logistic regression analysis was completed with adjustment for potential confounders to investigate the relationship between the number of childhood exposures to risk factors and adult medical conditions.

Overall, 52% of respondents experienced >1 adverse childhood exposure and 6.2% reported exposure to >4 adverse events. Substance abuse was the most common adverse exposure (25.6%) with a housemate being imprisoned as the least common (3.4%). Individuals who experienced 1 adverse exposure had a median probability of exposure to at least 1 more adverse exposure of 80%. Increases in number of exposures were associated with increased odds of developing health risk factors and adult disease conditions. Linear regression accounting for age, gender, race, and educational level as covariates, revealed a significant dose-response relationship between the number of adverse childhood exposures and each of the risk factors ($p < 0.001$) as well as the development of ischemic heart disease, cancer, emphysema, hepatitis or jaundice, fractures, and poor health on self-report ($p < 0.05$).

Felitti VJ, Anda RF, Nordenberg D, Williamson DF, Spitz AM, Edwards V, et al. Relationship of Childhood Abuse and Household Dysfunction to Many of the Leading Causes of Death in Adults. American Journal of Preventive Medicine. 1998 May 1;14(4):245–58.

Sleep-disordered breathing associated with poor academics and surgical improvement

1. Sleep-associated gas exchange abnormalities were highly prevalent among a first-grade study cohort with poor academic performance. About 18% of participants had oxygenation abnormalities assessed during overnight observation.

2. School performance improved significantly among children who received surgical intervention for abnormal breathing patterns during sleep.

3. Symptoms of disordered sleep were significantly worse among children who did not undergo surgical tonsillectomy and adenoidectomy.

Original Date of Publication: September 1998

Study Rundown: Previous studies indicated that a substantial portion of children suffered from obstructive sleep apnea (OSA) and primary snoring (PS), disorders linked to pulmonary hypertension, failure to thrive, systematic hypertension, and behavioral disturbances. To prevent these negative outcomes, children with sleep disorders often underwent tonsillectomy and adenoidectomy. Despite prior research, no prospective, controlled trial had investigated the potential cognitive outcomes of individuals with OSA. Researchers in this study aimed to determine whether or not sleep-associated gas exchange abnormalities (SAGEA) among children performing poorly in school was related to academic difficulties and whether or not surgical intervention aided in resolution of cognitive and disordered sleep symptoms.

Results demonstrated that a large number of cohort participants had PS (22.2%) and SAGEA (18.1%) and that both school performance and symptoms could improve through surgical intervention. This study was limited in the use of SpO_2 as a measure of oxygenation, which does not indicate whether obstruction or a lower respiratory process is responsible for desaturation and in the use of academic performance as the sole measure of cognition. Despite these limitations, this study added evidence obtained in a prospective, controlled manner to mostly case study-based findings. Current recommendations encourage adenotonsillectomy to prevent the physical, behavioral, and cognitive complications discussed here, with particular attention paid to assessing for potential residual disease requiring further intervention.

In-Depth [prospective cohort]: Two hundred ninety-seven first-grade students in the lowest 10%ile of their class were recruited for study participation in an overnight study. To assess sleep-disordered breathing symptoms, parents completed an OSA Syndrome (OSAS) questionnaire regarding childhood sleep behavior and respiratory compromise. Subsequently, the children underwent overnight respiratory analysis including pulse oximetry (SpO_2) and transcutaneous carbon dioxide tension (T_{CCO2}). SAGEA was diagnosed based upon a high score on the questionnaire along with 2 desaturations (periods of > 5% reductions in baseline SpO_2 or $SpO_2 < 90\%$) per hour and/or an elevated $T_{CCO2} > 8$ mmHg compared with normal, waking values during an overnight study. Children without changes in SpO_2 or T_{CCO2}, but an elevated questionnaire score were diagnosed with PS. Children testing positive for SAGEA were followed 3 months and then 1 year after diagnosis date to assess if patients underwent surgical intervention. Cognitive outcomes were assessed through school records both 1 year before and 1 year after completion of the overnight study. For analysis, children were grouped into those who had no abnormalities on overnight study (CO), those with PS, those with SAGEA who went untreated (NT), and those who were treated surgically (TR). Two-way analyses of variance, Newman-Keuls tests, and paired *t* tests were completed.

Of the 297 children tested, 66 met criteria for PS (22.2%) and 54 for SAGEA (18.1%). Twenty-four had surgical treatment for their disorder (TR), while 30 went untreated (NT). In comparing academic scores between groups, mean grades among the TR group increased significantly from first to second grade (2.43 ± 0.17 in first grade vs. 2.87 ± 0.19, $p < 0.001$). Only 2 of the 24 children in the TR group remained in the lowest 10%ile following intervention. Those in the NT group had no significant improvement in grades. Upon follow-up questionnaire administration to parents of NT and TR children, untreated children scored significantly higher, indicating worse symptoms, compared to surgically treated children (10.4 ± 2.6 in NT vs. 1.7 ± 2.4 in TR, $p < 0.001$).

Gozal D. Sleep-Disordered Breathing and School Performance in Children. Pediatrics. 1998 Sep 1;102(3):616–20.

The Bogalusa Heart Study: Childhood weight status and cardiovascular risk factors

1. In children, a higher body mass index (BMI) was associated with increased frequencies of cardiac risks factors

2. Among the cardiovascular risk factors assessed, overweight youth had the highest odds of having elevated insulin levels.

Original Date of Publication: June 1999

Study Rundown: The Bogalusa Heart Study was initiated in 1972 in Bogalusa, Louisiana, and stands as the longest running biracial study of children. Although an abnormal BMI was an established risk factor for multiple adverse health outcomes at the time of the investigation, this study added insight into the connection between early weight risk and cardiovascular health. It was also one of the first trials to factor sex, race/ethnicity, and age into analysis. Eleven percent of the 9167 children included in the study were overweight. Cardiac risk factors increased in prevalence as BMI increased beyond the 85%ile, with considerable risk elevations as BMI increased from the 95%ile to 97%ile and beyond. Among the risk factors, overweight youth were found to have the highest odds of having elevated insulin levels. Being overweight was considered an effective screening tool for cardiovascular risk with over 50% of overweight participants having at least 1 risk factor (positive predictive value [PPV] > 50%). Differences between African Americans and whites were noted when examining diastolic blood pressure (DBP) and insulin levels. Low density lipoprotein cholesterol (LDLC), DBP, and systolic blood pressure (SBP) differed significantly between age groups. While BMI is a useful surrogate for assessing weight status, it has limited accuracy among certain populations including those with very high or low levels of muscle mass. Despite this limitation, this study produced results agreeing with previous findings and strengthened the evidence to support prevention and early intervention for overweight youth.

In-Depth [cross-sectional study]: Nine thousand one hundred sixty-seven children, 5-17 years of age (mean age = 11.9 years; 48% female; 36% black) were drawn from 7 cross-sectional studies completed during 1973-1994 within the larger Bogalusa Heart Study. Age, race/ethnicity, weight, height, triceps and subscapular skinfolds measurements, total cholesterol (TC), triglycerides (TG), LDLC, high-density lipoprotein cholesterol (HDLC), SBP, DBP, and fasting insulin levels were all included in analysis. Logistic regression analyses were completed to assess the association between risk factors and BMI. Eleven percent of study participants were categorized as overweight with a BMI greater than the 95%ile. As BMI increased, the number of associated risk factors increased. For example, among all children, elevated insulin levels, defined as above the 95th age-, race-, and sex-adjusted percentile, increased from 1% to 27% as BMI increased from 25 to > 97%ile with the largest increase observed between the increase from 95-97 to > 97%ile (10% vs. 27% among 5-10 year olds, 10% vs. 25% among 11-17 year olds). The sensitivity of being overweight and having a cardiovascular risk factor varied from 23% for elevated DBP to 62% for elevated insulin levels. The PPV of being overweight also varied from 9% for elevated DBP to 24% for elevated triglycerides (TG > 130mg/dL). The largest calculated odds ratios (ORs) were seen with elevated insulin levels as overweight youth were 12.6 times more likely to have elevated insulin than youth of normal weight. Being overweight was considered effective in screening for cardiovascular risk with 61% of overweight 5- to 10-year-olds having at least 1 elevated risk factor and a 58% PPV of being overweight and having cardiovascular risk factors among 11- to 17-year-olds. Significant differences between race/ethnicity were seen between DBP and insulin levels with whites having elevated ORs in both when compared to blacks. As indicated by X^2 values above 20.5, elevated LDLC, SBP, and DBP values differed significantly by age group (p < 0.001). Additional analyses indicated that triceps skinfold thickness did not add additional information when BMI was known.

Freedman DS, Dietz WH, Srinivasan SR, Berenson GS. The Relation of Overweight to Cardiovascular Risk Factors Among Children and Adolescents: The Bogalusa Heart Study. Pediatrics. 1999 Jun 1;103(6):1175–82.

Antibiotic Group B Streptococcus prophylaxis linked with reduced neonatal infection

1. **During the 1990-1998 study period, which included the 1996 initiation of national Group B Streptococcus (GBS) guidelines, a significant, 65% decrease in early-onset neonatal disease was observed.**

2. **During the study's final year, an estimated 3900 early-onset neonatal GBS cases, along with 200 early- and late-onset neonatal deaths, were estimated to have been prevented by the recommended antibiotic prophylaxis.**

Original Date of Publication: January 2000

Study Rundown: With the identification of GBS as a maternally-transmitted pathogen leading to significant neonatal morbidity and mortality, the United States instituted a national advocacy group and guideline recommendations to prevent and manage perinatal GBS infection during the 1990s. This study was the first to assess trends in GBS disease following the issuance of 1996 American Academy of Pediatrics (AAP)-, American College of Obstetricians and Gynecologists-, and Centers for Disease Control (CDC)-approved guidelines instructing practitioners on intrapartum antibiotic prophylaxis. Based on a high transmission risk or positive 35-37 week screening, women received intrapartum antibiotics. Researchers found a significant, 65% reduction in GBS early-onset neonatal disease, defined as disease manifesting before 7 days of life, but no difference in neonatal disease diagnosed at 7-89 days of life. When these findings were projected upon 1998 national data, it was estimated that about 3900 early-onset cases and 200 deaths due to neonatal GBS infection had been prevented. A significant, 21% reduction in GBS disease among pregnant women and girls was also seen.

This study was limited in its generalizability due to lack of racial diversity, particularly in its low numbers of Hispanic participants and in the likely higher alertness of practitioners in the study to GBS positivity. However, this large, multi-state study did allow for assessment of the guidelines among many laboratory-confirmed GBS cases. With this research indicating the effectiveness of preventative strategies in decreasing early-onset neonatal GBS infection, continued efforts to promote prevention, appropriate antibiotic intervention, and to determine why these strategies fail was and still are necessary. Antibiotic resistance, lack of education, and decreased compliance continue to be problematic today. The 1996 guidelines were later updated by the CDC in 2010 and an AAP policy statement followed in 2011.

In-Depth [cross-sectional study]: During 1993 to 1998, GBS cases in Maryland, California, Georgia, Tennessee, Connecticut, Minnesota, Oregon, and New York were reported through a laboratory-based surveillance protocol. Additional data from California, Georgia, and Tennessee for 1990-1993 were included to provide a greater temporal context for GBS rates prior to guideline initiation. GBS cases were reported if individuals tested positive for GBS in normally sterile body fluid. GBS isolated from either placenta, amniotic fluid, or urine was not included. GBS disease was classified by time of onset as follows: early-onset neonatal disease (< 7 days old), late-onset (7-89 days old), childhood disease (90 days to 14 years of age), or adult disease (> 15 years old). Disease in pregnancy was considered separately. National estimates of GBS incidence were calculated based on known population sizes.

During the 5-year study period, 7867 GBS cases were reported (84% from blood, 4% from cerebrospinal fluid, 4% from joint fluid, and the remainder from other sites). Early-onset disease remained constant throughout 1990-1993 and then declined by a significant 65% during 1993-1998 (1.7 per 1000 births in 1993 vs. 0.6 per 1000 in 1998, $X^2 = 121.0$, p < 0.001). African Americans had higher early-onset disease rates, but also underwent a steeper reduction during the study period than whites, with a 75% reduction in the difference between the 2 groups by 1998. No significant change in late-onset disease incidence took place in 1990-1998. Among pregnant women and girls, a significant, 21% reduction in GBS incidence was seen over the study course (0.29 per 1000 births in 1993 vs. 0.23 per 1000 births in 1998, $X^2 = 4.86$, p < 0.03). After projecting 1998 incidence from the selected states onto national data, it was estimated 3900 neonatal early-onset GBS cases and 200 early- and late-onset neonatal deaths were prevented through antibiotic usage.

Schrag SJ, Zywicki S, Farley MM, Reingold AL, Harrison LH, Lefkowitz LB, et al. Group B Streptococcal Disease in the Era of Intrapartum Antibiotic Prophylaxis. New England Journal of Medicine. 2000 Jan 6;342(1):15–20.

Parental input in oncology-related palliation and pain relief for children

1. When interviews with parents whose children died from cancer were compared to patient hospital records, researchers found that many children experienced substantial suffering toward the end of life with poorly managed symptoms.

2. There was significant discordance between parent and physician reports of patient discomfort, with parents being significantly more likely to report patient symptoms than physicians.

Original Date of Publication: February 2000

Study Rundown: While researchers previously investigated the quality of end-of-life care among adult oncology patients, no study explored palliative care for children. This study was the first to delve into the state of pediatric end-of-life care through interviews with parents whose children died from cancer and retrospective chart analysis of patient care. Results demonstrated that many children received aggressive care at the end of their lives, with nearly half dying in the hospital and many dying in the intensive care unit. In addition, 89% of children experienced substantial suffering in their last month of life, most of which went unresolved despite treatment attempts.

Through this retrospective analysis, it was found that parents were significantly more likely to report their child's fatigue, poor appetite, constipation, and diarrhea when compared to physicians. Parents were also significantly more likely to report their child to be in pain if they believed the child's oncologist to be less involved in direct end-of-life care. These findings suggested that care providers may not be optimally treating these patients due a lack of recognized patient discomfort. Also, results showed that earlier discussions of hospice care were significantly associated with parental descriptions of children as calm in the last month of life.

This study was limited by use of parental report and chart review. However, its findings had many implications for patient care. By encouraging early, direct discussions between physicians and patient families regarding symptoms, discomfort, and goals of care, researchers recognized that patient quality of life might improve as a patient progressed toward the end of life. Today, palliative care is better defined as care of the whole patient, involving an interdisciplinary team that is introduced to patients and their families at the time of a serious diagnosis

In-Depth [retrospective analysis]: A total of 103 parents (91% white, 86% female) of children who had died of cancer during 1990-1997 were interviewed by researchers based out of a large, tertiary children's hospital. The interview information was then combined with data obtained from chart reviews. In interviews, parents were asked to assess many aspects of his or her child's end-of-life care including, but not limited to, physical symptoms and suffering during the last month of life, treatment of these symptoms, and the perception of physician involvement at the end of life. Chart review was then completed to collect demographic data along with treatments administered, cancer care course, symptoms in the last month of life, cause and place of death, medical interventions close to the time of death, and discussions regarding end-of-life planning such as hospice and do not resuscitate orders (DNR).

Interviewed parents had children who died of leukemia or lymphoma (n = 50, 49%), brain tumors (n = 23, 22%), or other solid tumors (n = 30, 29%). Eighty-one children died from progressive disease, 21 died from treatment-related complications, with 1 child's records unavailable for review. On chart review, physicians discussed hospice care with 66% of children with progressive disease. Sixty-six percent of children had DNR orders in their charts. Nearly half, 49%, of patients died in the hospital and, of those, 45% died in the intensive care unit. From parental interview, nearly 100% of patients had at least 1 symptom toward the end of life with fatigue, pain, dyspnea, and poor appetite being the most common. Eighty-nine percent of children had "a great deal" of suffering as a result of 1 or more symptoms. Pain and dyspnea were the most commonly treated symptoms (76% and 65%, respectively), but few patients experienced relief from treatment (27% and 16%, respectively). During the last month of life, 21% of children were described by parents as being afraid. With regard to end-of-life discussions, the length of time between hospice care discussions and death were significantly longer for children whose parents found them to be calm during most of the last month of life (p = 0.01). Based upon parental report, lack of oncologist involvement in end-of-life care was associated with significantly more pain in the last month of a child's life (OR 2.6, 95%CI 1.0-6.7). In comparing parental interview to chart review, parents reported fatigue (p < 0.001), poor appetite (p < 0.001), constipation (p < 0.001) and diarrhea (p < 0.05) in their children significantly more often than physicians.

Wolfe J, Grier HE, Klar N, Levin SB, Ellenbogen JM, Salem-Schatz S, et al. Symptoms and Suffering at the End of Life in Children with Cancer. New England Journal of Medicine. 2000 Feb 3;342(5):326–33.

Laboratory values and treatment associated with DKA-related cerebral edema in children

1. Among children admitted diabetic ketoacidosis (DKA) management, elevated serum urea nitrogen concentrations and low partial pressures of carbon dioxide were associated with a significantly increased risk of developing cerebral edema.

2. Lack of pronounced serum sodium rise and the use of bicarbonate for treatment were also associated with significantly increased cerebral edema risk.

Original Date of Publication: January 2001

Study Rundown: Among children presenting in DKA, about 1% will experience cerebral edema. At the time of this study, mortality occurred in 40-90% of these individuals, accounting for 50-60% of type 1 diabetes mellitus (T1DM)-related childhood deaths. However, before this study's publication, there was limited information regarding cerebral edema risk factors among children with T1DM. Researchers found that elevated serum urea nitrogen concentrations and low partial pressures of carbon dioxide were associated with significantly increased risk of children hospitalized for DKA developing cerebral edema. In addition, lack of pronounced increases in serum sodium with treatment and use of bicarbonate were also associated with significantly increased risk of cerebral edema development.

This study was limited by an inability to detect the possible influence of other confounders as well as to detect the potential role of variables that did not produce noticeable changes in clinical data. This was the first large, controlled study to investigate the role of cerebral edema-associated risk factors among children treated for DKA. It was proposed that each of these factors likely resulted in the development of cerebral edema due to potential contributions to cerebral ischemia. While this study helped lay the foundation for our understanding of cerebral edema risk, no exact pathophysiologic mechanism has been confirmed. Other risk factors found not to be statistically significant in this study have proven influential in subsequent studies. These include young age and DKA as the first presenting symptom of DM.

In-Depth [case-control study]: Through a review of records at 10 pediatric hospitals, all children with DM-related cerebral edema treated between1982-1997 were included in analyses. The record of any child who had died during admission in this time period was also included in analysis. Records of included patients had evidence of confirmed DKA (serum glucose >300 mg/dL, venous pH <7.25 or serum bicarbonate <15 mmol/L, and urine ketones), altered mental status, and a radiologic or pathologic diagnosis of cerebral edema or clinical improvement following cerebral edema treatment. For each child with cerebral edema, 6 control patients were included for comparison: 3 patients selected randomly among the other patients with DKA and 3 patients matched by age among the other patients with DKA. Demographics, treatments, laboratory values, and calculated laboratory results were included for analysis. One-way analysis of variance was completed to analyze continuous variables and X^2 tests were used to analyze categorical variables.

Of the 6977 DKA-related admissions to the 10 centers, 61 (0.9%) had cerebral edema. After controlling for covariates, comparison of children with cerebral edema to the random control group revealed a 1.7 times increased cerebral edema risk per increase in urea nitrogen of 9 mg/dL from presentation. A 3.4 times increased risk of cerebral edema per 7.8 mmHg decrease in carbon dioxide partial pressure from presentation was also appreciated (RR 1.7, p < 0.003; RR 3.4, p < 0.001, respectively). Multivariate analysis, showed a significantly increased risk of cerebral edema with high urea nitrogen (RR 1.8 per 9 mg/dL increase, p < 0.01), low arterial carbon dioxide (RR 2.7 per decrease of 7.8 mmHg, p < 0.01), slow increases in serum sodium concentration during therapy (RR 0.6 per increase of 5.8 mmol/L/hr, p < 0.0.5), and bicarbonate treatment (RR 4.2, p < 0.01).

Glaser N, Barnett P, McCaslin I, Nelson D, Trainor J, Louie J, et al. Risk Factors for Cerebral Edema in Children with Diabetic Ketoacidosis. New England Journal of Medicine. 2001 Jan 25;344(4):264–9.

Earlier diagnosis and improved cystic fibrosis nutritional status with newborn screening

1. Among infants randomized to undergo either newborn screen with cystic fibrosis (CF) testing or undergo normal pediatric surveillance, those who underwent the screen were diagnosed with CF significantly earlier.

2. Infants diagnosed based on surveillance were significantly more likely to be severely malnourished compared to those diagnosed by newborn screen.

Original Date of Publication: January 2001

Study Rundown: CF is an autosomal recessive disease responsible for multi-system organ involvement most commonly secondary to impaired chloride channel transport. At the time of this study's publication, many patients were diagnosed through sweat testing following recognition of signs/symptoms linked to the disease. In 1996, the average age of diagnosis was 5 years and this delay in diagnosis was associated with worse nutritional status and lung disease. This clinical trial investigated the potential benefits of neonatal screening on nutritional outcomes. Infants were diagnosed using testing for elevated immunoreactive trypsinogen (IRT), which was later modified to include both IRT and DNA testing. A total incidence rate of 1:3938 was seen in the cohort, and those who underwent newborn screening were diagnosed significantly earlier than those diagnosed by surveillance. In addition, those who were diagnosed on newborn screening were at significantly lower risk of being severely malnourished when compared to those diagnosed by surveillance.

While strengthened by a randomized design, the study was limited secondary to the change of diagnostic technique partway through the study. Regardless, the study aided in establishing the value of early diagnosis and early intervention in the care of children with CF. Since the introduction of newborn screening, every state in the United States has adopted use of either IRT or combined IRT-DNA testing. Today, nearly 60% of cases of CF are diagnosed by newborn screen, increased from under 10% in 2001, with the average age of diagnosis under 2 years.

In-Depth [randomized controlled trial]: From April 1985 to 1998, 2 CF centers along with a newborn screening program in Wisconsin began a randomized clinical trial examining the effects of early screening for CF on nutritional and pulmonary outcomes. Children were randomized to either undergo newborn screening or traditional pediatric follow-up (i.e., monitoring for signs or symptoms of CF during acute and health maintenance visits). Initial newborn screening included the use of IRT analysis, with testing later modified in June 1991 to add DNA testing for ΔF508, the most common CF-related genetic mutation. All children were screened and then randomized such that the control group's lab results were blinded. These results were eventually unblinded. Positive testing on either the IRT or DNA testing in the screening group resulted in pediatrician-parental contact with the recommendation for a follow-up sweat test when the child was 4 to 6 weeks of age. Children with sweat chloride tests of ≥60 mEq/L were diagnosed with CF, those with 40-60 mEq/L were considered to have an indeterminate diagnosis, and those with sweat tests ≤40 mEq/L were not diagnosed with CF. Patients presenting with meconium ileus were also assigned to the "other CF group." Children diagnosed with CF (both through newborn screening and at a later age) were given the option to enroll for study inclusion. They then underwent standardized nutritional and pulmonary assessments along with therapeutic disease management starting at the time of diagnosis. Surveillance of patient outcomes was performed through healthcare provider-completed surveys and review of birth and death certificates.

A total of 650 341 babies born during the study period were randomized to either undergo newborn CF screening or be in the control group. Overall, 325 121 infants were included in the screening group and 325 120 were included in the control group. Among those in the screening group, 220 862 underwent IRT and 104 308 underwent both IRT and DNA testing. A total of 157 patients were identified as having CF. Additional diagnoses on autopsy and from sweat chloride testing in the 40-60 mEq/L range, resulted in a total incidence of CF in this cohort was 1:3938. Children who underwent initial newborn screen (n = 56) were diagnosed significantly earlier than those in the control group (n = 107; 13±37 weeks in screening group vs. 107±117 in control group, p < 0.001). At the time of diagnosis, those screened had significantly higher length (p < 0.001), weight (p < 0.05), and head circumference (p < 0.01) than those in the control group. Throughout the study, significantly greater odds of being severely malnourished, as determined by having a weight and height below the 10th percentile, was observed in the control group when compared to the screening group (odds ratio for weight = 4.12, 95%CI 1.64-10.38; odds ratio for height = 4.62, 95%CI 1.70-12.61). Odds of being below the 10th percentile for height disappeared by 9 years of age for those who were screened early.

Farrell PM, Kosorok MR, Rock MJ, Laxova A, Zeng L, Lai H-C, et al. Early Diagnosis of Cystic Fibrosis Through Neonatal Screening Prevents Severe Malnutrition and Improves Long-Term Growth. Pediatrics. 2001 Jan 1;107(1):1–13.

MMR vaccine not associated with autism

1. **Among children born in Denmark during a 7-year study period, no increase in risk of developing autism was seen in those who were vaccinated against measles, mumps, and rubella (MMR) relative to unvaccinated children.**

Original Date of Publication: November 2002

Study Rundown: There is considerable controversy surrounding the possible connection between the MMR vaccine and the development of autism in children. While previous studies did not find any associations, this was the first study on this topic to have adequate statistical power and appropriate design. In this retrospective cohort study, 537 303 files from children born in Denmark were analyzed to determine the relative risk of autism with MMR vaccination. No increased risk of autism diagnosis was seen among those receiving the vaccine nor was any association between the timing of vaccination and autism risk observed. This study provided strong evidence from a large cohort sample that an association between MMR vaccination and autism risk does not exist. Historically, the authors noted that the increase in autism incidence occurred much later than the release of the MMR vaccine - a temporal rift that makes a cause and effect relationship unlikely.

In-Depth [retrospective cohort]: Records from national registries of all children born between 1991 and 1998 in Denmark were studied and MMR vaccination status at 15 months of age, the typical age of first dose completion, was recorded. The primary outcome investigated was autism diagnosis. In total, 537 303 children, 440 655 vaccinated and 96 649 unvaccinated, were included in the study. Among those, 5811 children were diagnosed with autism or an autism-related disorder. A subgroup of diagnosed cases were validated with 93% meeting the Diagnostic and Statistic Manual of Mental Disorders-IV's criteria for autistic disorders. A log-linear Poisson regression model was used to assess the RR associated with the vaccine. When adjusted for potential confounding factors such as demographics and family socioeconomic status, no increase in relative risk of autism or related disorders was seen among those who received the vaccination (aRR 0.92, 95%CI 0.68-1.24 for autism and aRR = 0.83, 95%CI 0.65-1.07 for other autism-spectrum disorders). No associations were found between autism development and age at vaccination, time since vaccination, or year of vaccination.

Madsen KM, Hviid A, Vestergaard M, Schendel D, Wohlfahrt J, Thorsen P, et al. A Population-Based Study of Measles, Mumps, and Rubella Vaccination and Autism. New England Journal of Medicine. 2002 Nov 7;347(19):1477–82.

Clinical prediction rule stratifies pediatric bacterial meningitis risk

1. A Bacterial Meningitis Score (BMS) of 0 accurately identified all children with aseptic meningitis in the study's validation group.

2. The negative predictive value of a BMS score of 0 was 100% with a specificity of 73% in predicting bacterial meningitis. A BMS score of ≥ 2 was found to have a sensitivity and positive predictive value of 87% in predicting bacterial meningitis.

Original Date of Publication: October 2002

Study Rundown: Bacterial meningitis is associated with significant morbidity and mortality. At the time of this study, many children found to have CSF pleocytosis were admitted for intravenous antibiotic therapy and blood culture monitoring while distinguishing bacterial from aseptic meningitis. As individuals diagnosed with viral meningitis may be managed as outpatients, this study sought to create and validate a clinical prediction rule to aid in identifying patients at low risk for bacterial meningitis. This was the first study to create such a scoring system in the post-Haemophilus Influenzae Type b vaccination era. Researchers were able to create a scoring system that accurately stratified patients at low and high risk for bacterial meningitis diagnosis. This study was limited in both its design and potential referral bias as evidenced by the high percentage of patient participants with bacterial meningitis (18%). Through use of this prediction rule, clinicians may be able to better identify patients who could be cared for outside of the hospital setting. Of note, this scoring system was further validated in a follow-up analysis published in JAMA in 2007.

In-Depth [retrospective cohort]: A total of 696 patients from 29 days to 19 years old diagnosed with bacterial, viral, fungal, or tuberculous meningitis as identified by hospital diagnostic codes were recruited from 8 years of hospital records at a large, pediatric hospital. Patients were randomized into either a derivation or validation set. Patients were considered to have bacterial meningitis if their CSF sample grew bacteria or if they had CSF pleocytosis with a positive blood culture or positive CSF latex agglutination test. Patient charts were reviewed and analyzed for information regarding CSF characteristics, seizure occurrence, complete blood count data, CSF and blood culture results, and latex agglutination testing. One hundred and twenty-five (18%) of the patients identified were diagnosed with bacterial meningitis and 571 (82%) with aseptic meningitis. Positive gram stain, CSF protein ≥ 80 mg/dL, seizure upon or prior to presentation, peripheral ANC $\geq$10,000 cells/mm³, and CSF ANC $\geq$10,000 cells/mm³ were identified as predictors of bacterial meningitis, with positive gram stain as the most significant predictor. A BMS ranging from 0 to 6 was created with presence of each predictor receiving 1 point except for a positive gram stain, which received 2 points. When applied to the validation set participants, a score of 0 accurately identified all children with aseptic meningitis and did not misclassify any cases of bacterial meningitis. The negative predictive value of a BMS score of 0 was 100% for bacterial meningitis with a specificity of 73%. A BMS score of $\geq$2 was found to have a sensitivity and positive predictive value of 87% in predicting bacterial meningitis.

Nigrovic LE, Kuppermann N, Malley R. Development and Validation of a Multivariable Predictive Model to Distinguish Bacterial From Aseptic Meningitis in Children in the Post-Haemophilus influenzae Era. Pediatrics. 2002 Oct 1;110(4):712–9.

Nigrovic LE, Kuppermann N, Macias CG, et al. Clinical prediction rule for identifying children with cerebrospinal fluid pleocytosis at very low risk of bacterial meningitis. JAMA. 2007 Jan 3;297(1):52–60.

RSV positivity associated with less serious bacterial infection risk in infants

1. Respiratory syncytial virus (RSV)-positive infants were significantly less likely to have a serious bacterial infection (SBI) relative to those who tested negative.

2. Infants ≤28 days old were significantly more likely to have an SBI than older infants.

Original Date of Publication: June 2004

Study Rundown: SBIs, such as meningitis and bacteremia, are sources of significant morbidity and mortality in febrile infants under 2 months of age. While many studies had investigated the risk factors for SBIs, at the time of this study no groups had investigated the potential interaction of viral infection in febrile infants with a simultaneous SBI. This study investigated the risk of SBI in febrile infants diagnosed with RSV infections. RSV was associated with a lower risk of concurrent SBI; however, many RSV-positive infants had simultaneous urinary tract infections (UTIs) and younger infants (≤28 days old) were found to have statistically similar SBI rates regardless of RSV positivity. Potential clinical implications of this study include limiting testing for infants >1 month of age with RSV to urinalysis only, while continuing a full workup for younger infants regardless of their viral status.

In-Depth [cross-sectional study]: Data from 1248 patients, ≤60 days of age and with rectal temperatures ≥38°C, were gathered from 8 pediatric emergency departments over a period of 3 years. Patients underwent a history and physical examination, rapid RSV testing by nasopharyngeal aspirate, and further workup, treatment, and imaging at the discretion of their physician. Data was analyzed taking patients' RSV status into account while also considering the presence of SBI defined as bacterial meningitis, bacteremia, UTI, or bacterial enteritis. Over 11% of all study participants were found to have SBI with 0.7% having bacterial meningitis, 2% having bacteremia, 9.1% having UTI, and 1.9% having bacterial enteritis. Infants who tested positive for RSV were significantly less likely to have an SBI than those who tested negative (7% vs. 12.5%, RR 0.6, p < .05). Further analysis indicated that RSV-positive patients were at significantly lower risk for SBI. The highest concurrent bacterial infection was UTI, with 5.4% of RSV-positive infants having UTIs. In subanalyses, 82 RSV-positive infants ≤28 days old had SBIs; 6.1% of these infants had UTIs and 3.7% had bacteremia. There was no RSV-dependent significant difference between SBI rates in infants ≤28 days old. A total of 187 RSV-positive infants 29-60 days old were found to have an SBI rate of 5.5%, all of which were UTIs. Infants ≤28 days old were significantly more likely to have an SBI than older infants (10.1% vs. 5.5%).

Levine DA, Platt SL, Dayan PS, Macias CG, Zorc JJ, Krief W, et al. Risk of Serious Bacterial Infection in Young Febrile Infants With Respiratory Syncytial Virus Infections. Pediatrics. 2004 Jun 1;113(6):1728–34.

Computerized order system linked with increased pediatric mortality

1. The use of a computerized physician order entry (CPOE) program in a large, tertiary pediatric hospital was associated with over 3 times the risk of mortality when compared to patients admitted to the same center prior to CPOE implementation.

2. CPOE implementation resulted in increased physician time placing medication orders as opposed to providing patient care. It also increased delays in medication administration.

Original Date of Publication: December 2005

Study Rundown: CPOE systems were initially implemented to aid in reducing the tens of thousands of medical errors contributing to patient deaths across the United States. In 2002, the implementation of a CPOE in a large, tertiary pediatric hospital resulted in a significant reduction of adverse drug events (ADEs). This study was one of the first to evaluate long-term outcomes following CPOE implementation by examining mortality rates among children admitted to the same facility from the 2002 study. Retrospective analysis comparing patients transferred to the hospital before and after CPOE administration revealed a significant increase in mortality risk associated with care post-CPOE. Researchers attributed this result to changes in patient care following the implementation, including increased physician time spent entering orders and new challenges in acquiring medications as drugs were located in the hospital pharmacy as opposed to at the bedside.

This study was limited by its conduction in a single medical center, its short evaluation of time post-CPOE (which might have largely been an adjustment period to the new system), and potential lack of generalizability. However, these findings highlighted how promising technologic advances could pose serious underlying consequences and that decreases in ADEs are not necessarily an indication of improved clinical outcomes. This study argued that technologic advances require careful, thorough evaluation in order to ensure that unexpected consequences do not negatively influence patient care. Current CPOE implementation involves active incorporation of the findings from this study to ensure effective prevention of potential complications.

In-Depth [retrospective analysis]: From October 1, 2001 to March 31, 2003, 1942 patients (55% male, median age = 9 months) were recruited upon arrival to a tertiary care center via interfacility transport. Overall, 1394 patients were admitted before CPOE implementation and 548 after. The clinical condition for admissions, patient demographics, clinical characteristics, and mortality for each patient were recorded. Between group differences were calculated using Mann-Whitney rank sum and X^2 or Fisher's tests. Odds ratios were calculated as well. Patients were transferred for the following conditions: airway- (42.6%), infectious disease- (34.9%), and central nervous system- (19.4%) related. A total of 75 children died during the study.

Mortality increased significantly following CPOE implementation (2.80% before vs. 6.57% after, p < 0.001). Odds of mortality were increased significantly if a patient experienced shock (OR 6.24, 95%CI 2.94-13.26), was treated following CPOE introduction (OR 3.71, 95%CI 2.13-6.46), or severe coma (OR 3.43, 95%CI 1.88-6.25). Additional adjustment for covariation maintained significance between CPOE and mortality (OR 3.28, 95%CI 1.94 - 5.55). Researchers reported differences in clinical care following CPOE initiation. As the new system did not allow for orders to be entered prior to patient arrival, physicians spent longer times entering requests into the system as opposed to the shorter times required for handwritten orders. In addition, nurses were no longer at the bedside readily administering medications as CPOE implementation required all medications to be located within the pharmacy.

Han YY, Carcillo JA, Venkataraman ST, Clark RSB, Watson RS, Nguyen TC, et al. Unexpected Increased Mortality After Implementation of a Commercially Sold Computerized Physician Order Entry System. Pediatrics. 2005 Dec 1;116(6):1506–12.

Antibiotic prophylaxis and UTI prevention in children

1. Among children with low grade vesicoureteral reflex (VUR) recruited following febrile urinary tract infection (UTI) and randomized to receive either antibiotic prophylaxis or no medication, no significant difference in UTI recurrence was noted between groups.

2. Male children experienced a significant reduction in subsequent UTIs if treated with prophylactic antibiotics.

Original Date of Publication: February 2008

Study Rundown: In the years leading up to this study, physicians often prescribed antibiotic prophylaxis to children at perceived increased risk for repeat UTIs, particularly those with VUR). As multiple UTIs have been linked to renal scarring and nephropathy, preventing recurrence is highly important. However, since previous studies indicated that antibiotics might be ineffective at preventing UTIs, this study took a prospective, randomized approach to investigate the effectiveness of prophylactic antibiotics in pediatric patients with mild VUR. This randomized, multi-center prospective study found no significant difference in repeat UTI among children with mild VUR who did or did not receive prophylactic antibiotics. A significant increase in the risk for a second UTI was seen in those with grade III mild VUR and significant reduction in repeat UTI with treatment was observed in males. This study was limited in its lack of a blinded approach, lack of placebo for the control group, along with the use of potentially contaminated urine specimens from urine bags and uncircumcised males. It also lacked assessment for antibiotic compliance.

This study raised questions regarding the necessity to prescribe prophylaxis for all young children following first febrile UTI and the need to obtain voiding cystourethrograms (VCUGs) for all children in order to determine VUR presence. As unnecessary treatment is linked to potential adverse drug effects coupled with organism resistance, careful consideration should be taken in prescribing antimicrobial medication. In the time since this study's publication, many research projects have investigated UTI risk in children. The most recent American Academy of Pediatrics (AAP) practice guidelines for UTI management in young children recommend renal and bladder ultrasound prior to VCUG and VCUG only if abnormal findings are found on ultrasound. Use of prophylactic antibiotics following initial UTI is not recommended, but potential further investigation of prophylaxis value among males with higher grade VUR is proposed.

In-Depth [randomized controlled trial]: From June 2001 to December 2004, 225 patients (31% male) 1 month to 3 years of age with low grade VUR diagnosed on VCUG following febrile UTI were recruited from 17 French pediatric facilities. VUR was graded by severity into grade I, grade II, or grade III VUR and grouped by laterality (unilateral or bilateral). Participants were randomized to receive either trimethoprim (2 mg/kg)/sulfamethoxazole (10 mg/kg), also known today as Bactrim (n = 103, 46%), or no medication (n = 122, 54%). Follow-up renal ultrasound (US) was performed 9 and, 18 months after study initiation, both US and VCUG were completed. UTI was a study endpoint with children who experienced a UTI, defined as $>10^5$ bacteria per mL of urine, excluded from the study and the UTI noted.

Following study initiation, 50 children, 18 in the treatment group (17%) and 32 in the control group (26%), experienced a second UTI. There was no significant difference between the 2 groups in terms of UTI rates (p = 0.15). There was also no significant difference between groups regarding the diagnosis of febrile UTI (13 or 13% in treatment group vs. 19 or 16% of the control group, p = 0.52). The majority of UTI recurrence occurred in females (78%). Males who received prophylactic treatments had a significantly lower rate of UTIs than those who went untreated (39, 57% in untreated vs. 30, 43% in treated, p < 0.05). This effect was not seen among females. No significant differences were seen between groups when analyzed by VUR grading or by VUR laterality. Multiple regression analysis indicated that grade III VUR was a significant risk factor for repeat UTI (p < 0.01).

Roussey-Kesler G, Gadjos V, Idres N, Horen B, Ichay L, Leclair MD, et al. Antibiotic Prophylaxis for the Prevention of Recurrent Urinary Tract Infection in Children With Low Grade Vesicoureteral Reflux: Results From a Prospective Randomized Study. The Journal of Urology. 2008 Feb 1;179(2):674–9.

PECARN Prediction rules for children at a low risk of clinically-important traumatic brain injury

1. The absence of 6 established predictors was found to have a near 100% negative predictive value (NPV) for clinically-important traumatic brain injury (ciTBI) when applied to head trauma patients under 18 years of age.

2. An algorithm was proposed, applying these predictors, in order to prevent physicians from using unnecessary computed tomography (CT) in pediatric patients at low risk for ciTBI.

Original Date of Publication: September 2009

Study Rundown: TBI continues to be one of the leading causes of morbidity and mortality among the pediatric population. At the time of this study, CT was the standard imaging technique for identifying TBI patients requiring intervention after head trauma. However, given the increase in malignancy risk associated with CT scans, investigators of this trial sought to identify patients at a low risk for ciTBI to potentially reduce CT imaging. Through the use of a large study cohort from various emergency departments, researchers analyzed the NPVs and sensitivities associated with a proposed "prediction rule", defined as having none of the identified ciTBI predictors versus having any cTBI predictors. The NPV and sensitivity of this prediction rule was then analyzed. Researchers found a NPV of >98% and sensitivity >94% in the prediction of ciTBI and TBI-negative CT scans in participants of all ages. Despite the fact that researchers did not CT scan all participants and sensitivities were not found to be 100%, this large, adequately powered study found similar results among both derivation and validation participant groups. With their findings, researchers were able to construct algorithms guiding physicians on appropriate CT scans use in head-injured patients. Altered mental status (AMS) and signs of skull fracture were established as branching points for patients at highest risk for ciTBI.

In-Depth [prospective cohort]: Data was analyzed from 42 412 patients under 18 years of age (mean 7.1 years ±5.5) who had experienced blunt head trauma within 24 hours from presentation and had Glasgow Coma Scale scores of 14-15. Patients were divided into derivation (n = 33 785) and validation groups (n = 8627) by recruitment date. ciTBI was defined as TBI-related death, need for neurosurgical intervention, intubation for more than one day following injury, or hospital admission for 2 or more nights. Research coordinators reviewed patient records during hospital admissions and completed telephone surveys of patient guardians for follow-up of patients discharged within 90 days of their ED visit. Predictors were chosen based upon established selection criteria and analyses were run to account for baseline development-related radiation risk with children under 2 years of age analyzed separately from those above 2 years of age.

Predictors for children under 2 years of age included: AMS, scalp hematoma, loss of consciousness (LOC), significant mechanism of injury (MOI), potential skull fracture, and changes in behavior. Predictors for those older than 2 years old included: AMS, LOC, vomiting, significant MOI, signs of basilar skull fracture, and headache. The number of predictors and risk of ciTBI in the derivation and validation groups were then compared. A total of 14 696 (35.5%) of participants underwent CT scan. Of these patients, 780 (5.2%) were found to have TBI on imaging and 376 (0.9%) with ciTBI (15.9% required surgical intervention, 0.02% required intubation for more than one day, 0% died from their injury). Among children under 2 years of age in the validation group, the prediction rule had an NPV of 100% and sensitivity of 100% for ciTBI. Among children over 2 years of age, this prediction rule had an NPV of 99.95% and sensitivity of 96.8% for ciTBI. In addition, among children under 2 years of age, the prediction rule had an NPV of 100% and sensitivity of 100% for patients having CT scan without evidence of TBI. Among children older than 2 years of age, the prediction rule had an NPV of 98.4% and sensitivity of 94% for patients having CT scans without evidence of TBI.

Kuppermann N, Holmes JF, Dayan PS, Hoyle JD, Atabaki SM, Holubkov R, et al. Identification of children at very low risk of clinically-important brain injuries after head trauma: a prospective cohort study. Lancet. 2009 Oct 3;374(9696):1160–70.

XI. Surgery

The Lee index: Risk of perioperative cardiac events

1. The Lee index is a prospectively validated model that predicts the risk of a cardiac event in patients undergoing noncardiac surgery.

2. The 6 independent predictors are as follows: 1) high-risk surgery, 2) history of ischemic heart disease, 3) history of congestive heart failure, 4) history of cerebrovascular disease, 5) preoperative treatment with insulin, 6) preoperative serum creatinine >2.0 mg/dL (>177 µmol/L).

Original Date of Publication: September 1999

Study Rundown: Patients undergoing noncardiac surgery are at risk of major cardiovascular complications. With the number of patients undergoing major noncardiac surgery consistently increasing, the incidence of surgery-associated cardiovascular complications has steadily risen. Numerous efforts have been made to identify potential interventions to reduce the likelihood of these complications, with several studies exploring the potential perioperative use of beta-blockers, calcium channel blockers, statins, aspirin, and cardiac revascularization. Several different groups have also attempted to develop tools to stratify patients with regards to their risk of perioperative cardiovascular complications. These include the Kumar, Detsky, and Goldman indices, as well as the American College of Cardiology/American Heart Association algorithm. The Revised Cardiac Risk Index, commonly referred to as the Lee index, was developed by modifying and simplifying the Goldman index. Initially published in 1999, the Lee index is considered the best validated tool for estimating perioperative cardiovascular risk. It uses six equally-weighted criteria to predict the likelihood of a cardiovascular event, and is widely used because of its simplicity.

In-Depth [prospective cohort]: Of the 4315 patients that took part in the study, 2893 were used in the development of the Lee index. The other 1422 patients took part in the prospective validation cohort. The major cardiovascular complications assessed were myocardial infarction, pulmonary edema, ventricular fibrillation/primary cardiac arrest, or complete heart block. Through logistic regression analyses, six predictors of perioperative major cardiovascular complications were identified: 1) high-risk surgery, 2) ischemic heart disease, 3) history of congestive heart failure, 4) history of cerebrovascular disease, 5) insulin therapy for diabetes, and 6) perioperative serum creatinine >2.0 mg/dL (>177 µmol/L). The presence of any of these predictors contributes 1 point to the Lee index score. Higher Lee index scores were associated with higher rates of perioperative cardiac events.

The Lee index

Criteria	Points
High-risk surgery (e.g., emergency surgery, major thoracic procedures, cardiac procedures, aortic/major vascular procedures, procedures >4 hours)	1
Ischemic heart disease	1
History of congestive heart failure	1
History of cerebrovascular disease	1
Insulin therapy for diabetes	1
Perioperative serum creatinine >2.0 mg/dL (>177 µmol/L)	1

Cardiac Event Rates

Lee index score	Derivation cohort	Validation cohort
0	5/1071 (0.5%)	2/488 (0.4%)
1	14/1106 (1.3%)	5/567 (0.9%)
2	18/506 (3.6%)	17/258 (6.6%)
≥3	19/210 (9.1%)	12/109 (11.0%)

Lee TH, Marcantonio ER, Mangione CM, Thomas EJ, Polanczyk CA, Cook EF, et al. Derivation and Prospective Validation of a Simple Index for Prediction of Cardiac Risk of Major Noncardiac Surgery. Circulation. 1999 Sep 7;100(10):1043–9.

The NETT: Lung-volume-reduction surgery in emphysema

1. Lung-volume-reduction surgery significantly improved exercise capacity, but not overall survival, in patients with emphysema when compared with medical therapy.

2. Post hoc subgroup analyses showed that in patients with upper lobe emphysema and low baseline exercise capacity, lung-volume-reduction surgery significantly decreased mortality compared to medical therapy.

Original Date of Publication: May 2003

Study Rundown: While lung-volume-reduction surgery had been proposed as a treatment option for patients with severe emphysema, there was little evidence examining its effects. The National Emphysema Treatment Trial (NETT) was the first study to assess the morbidity, mortality, and therapeutic benefits of lung-volume-reduction surgery for emphysema patients. The findings of the trial showed that lung reduction significantly improved patients' exercise capacity compared to medical therapy, but did not significantly change overall survival. Post hoc subgroup analyses demonstrated that surgery significantly reduced mortality in patients with upper lobe emphysema and low exercise capacity and significantly increased mortality in patients with non-upper lobe emphysema and high exercise capacity when compared with medical treatment. A major criticism of this trial centers on the survival differences demonstrated in specific subgroups based on post hoc analyses, as opposed to predefined analyses. In summary, results of this study suggest that lung-volume-reduction surgery can significantly improve exercise capacity in patients with emphysema. While subgroup analyses did demonstrate survival benefits in patients with upper-lobe emphysema and low exercise capacity at baseline, these findings should be interpreted with caution given that they were performed post hoc.

In-Depth [randomized controlled trial]: This was a randomized, controlled trial that involved enrollment of 1218 patients from 17 clinics from across the United States. The list of inclusion and exclusion criteria is lengthy - generally, patients were eligible if they had clinical and radiological evidence of emphysema, were non-smokers for at least 4 months, completed all pre-rehabilitation assessments, and were considered fit for surgery. Each patient's distribution of emphysema (i.e., predominantly upper-lobe vs. predominantly non-upper-lobe) was determined by high-resolution CT. The primary outcome measures were overall mortality and maximal exercise capacity as measured by cycle ergometry. The secondary outcome measures included pulmonary function, distance walked within 6 minutes, and quality of life, as determined by self-administered questionnaires. Prior to randomization, patients underwent 6-10 weeks of supervised pulmonary rehabilitation. Patients were then randomly assigned to receive lung-volume-reduction surgery (i.e., bilateral stapled wedge resection via median sternotomy or video-assisted thoracic surgery) or medical therapy, and then re-evaluated after 6, 12, and 24 months of follow-up. Improved exercise capacity was defined as a 10 W increase in workload during cycle ergometry.

At 90 days, the mortality rate in the surgery group was significantly higher than the medical therapy group (7.9% vs. 1.3%, p < 0.001). There was no significant difference in mortality rates when comparing patients who underwent median sternotomy and video-assisted thoracic surgery (8.6% vs. 6.1%, respectively, p = 0.33). Total mortality rates were not significantly different between the two groups at a mean follow-up of 29.2 months (RR 1.01, p = 0.90). Patients receiving surgery had significantly improved exercise capacity as measured by cycle ergometry at 6 (28% vs. 4%, p < 0.001), 12 (22% vs. 5%, p < 0.001), and 24 months (15% vs. 3%, p < 0.001) than the medical-therapy group. Post hoc subgroup analyses revealed that surgery patients with upper-lobe disease and low-exercise capacity had a lower mortality rate (RR 0.47, p = 0.005) and experienced significantly improved exercise capacity (30% vs. 0%, p = 0.005) when compared with similar patients receiving medical therapy only. In patients with non-upper-lobe disease and high baseline exercise capacity, mortality was significantly higher in the surgical group (RR 2.06, p = 0.02).

Fishman A, Martinez F, Naunheim K, Piantadosi S, Wise R, Ries A, et al. A randomized trial comparing lung-volume-reduction surgery with medical therapy for severe emphysema. New England Journal of Medicine. 2003 May 22;348(21):2059–73.

The CARP trial: Preoperative revascularization prior to elective vascular surgery

1. In patients with stable coronary artery disease undergoing elective vascular surgery, preoperative revascularization did not significantly reduce short- or long-term mortality.

2. Patients undergoing revascularization experienced significant time delays prior to surgery.

Original Date of Publication: December 2004

Study Rundown: The Coronary Artery Revascularization Prophylaxis (CARP) trial demonstrated that in patients with stable coronary artery disease undergoing elective vascular surgery, pre-operative coronary revascularization did not provide any benefit in terms of reducing the risk of myocardial infarction or mortality (i.e., short- or long-term). Patients undergoing revascularization, however, waited significantly longer before having surgery compared to individuals who did not undergo revascularization (54 vs. 18 days). The findings of this study supported practice guidelines at the time, which recommended that coronary revascularization be reserved for patients with symptomatic coronary artery disease. Given the efficacy of perioperative beta-blockers and statins, medical management may be suitable alternatives to revascularization in patients with asymptomatic coronary artery disease.

In-Depth [randomized controlled trial]: Patients undergoing elective vascular surgery have a high prevalence of coronary artery disease and have high-risk of perioperative cardiac complications. The CARP trial, originally published in 2004 in NEJM, sought to explore the long-term effects of pre-operative coronary revascularization in patients undergoing elective vascular surgery, as retrospective studies until that point had mixed findings. Of the 5859 patients screened, 510 patients were eligible and underwent randomization. Patients were eligible if they were scheduled for elective vascular surgery (i.e., abdominal aortic aneurysm, severe occlusive arterial disease in the legs) and had stenosis of at least 70% in one or more major coronary artery that was suitable for revascularization (i.e., percutaneous intervention - PCI, coronary artery bypass graft - CABG). The primary endpoint was long-term mortality, as determined by follow-up. Of the 258 patients who were randomized to the revascularization group, 59% underwent PCI, while 41% underwent CABG.

The median time from randomization to surgery was 54 days in the revascularization group and 18 days in the non-revascularization group (p < 0.001). There were no significant differences between the groups in terms of the incidence of myocardial infarction or death in the 30 days following surgery. There were no significant differences between the two groups in terms of long-term mortality.

McFalls EO, Ward HB, Moritz TE, Goldman S, Krupski WC, Littooy F, et al. Coronary-Artery Revascularization before Elective Major Vascular Surgery. New England Journal of Medicine. 2004 Dec 30;351(27):2795–804.

The POISE trial: Perioperative use of beta-blockers

1. The POISE trial was a randomized controlled trial exploring the effect of perioperative beta-blockade on cardiac death, nonfatal myocardial infarctions, and nonfatal cardiac arrest.

2. Perioperative oral extended-release metoprolol was found to reduce the risk of nonfatal myocardial infarction, while increasing the risk of stroke and mortality when compared to placebo.

Original Date of Publication: May 2008

Study Rundown: With recent advances in non-cardiac surgery allowing for better treatment of diseases and improvements in quality of life, there have been substantial increases in the number of patients undergoing surgeries. These surgeries, however, are associated with increased risk of cardiac events. Numerous therapies have been investigated as prophylaxis against cardiac events in the perioperative state. The PeriOperative ISchemic Evaluation (POISE) trial was a randomized controlled trial published in 2008 exploring the effect of perioperative metoprolol in patients undergoing non-cardiac surgery. Perioperatively, beta-blockers are thought to protect against myocardial ischemia, while potentially increasing the risk of hypotension and bradycardia. In summary, the POISE trial demonstrated that perioperative beta-blockade significantly reduced the risk of perioperative myocardial infarctions compared to placebo. Patients treated with beta-blockers, however, also experienced significantly higher rates of stroke and death. Thus, patients must be carefully counseled regarding the risks and benefits of initiating perioperative beta-blockers for cardiac protection.

In-Depth [randomized controlled trial]: The final analysis involved 8351 patients from 190 hospitals in 23 countries randomized to either perioperative treatment with extended-release metoprolol or placebo. Patients were eligible for the trial if they were ≥45 years of age, were undergoing non-cardiac surgery, had expected hospitalization ≥24 hours, and had elevated risk of perioperative cardiac events (e.g., history of coronary artery disease, stroke, hospitalization for congestive heart failure, undergoing major vascular surgery). Exclusion criteria included heart rate <50 beats per minute, second/third-degree heart block, asthma, treatment with a beta-blocker, and prior adverse reaction to beta-blocker. The primary outcome was a composite of cardiovascular death, non-fatal myocardial infarction, and non-fatal cardiac arrest at 30 days. Beta-blockers were found to significantly reduce the incidence of the primary endpoint compared to placebo (HR 0.84; 95%CI 0.70-0.99), due to a significant reduction in myocardial infarctions (HR 0.73; 95%CI 0.60-0.89). Compared to placebo, perioperative beta-blockade was also found to significantly increase the risk of stroke (HR 2.17; 95%CI 1.26-3.74), clinically significant hypotension (HR 1.55; 95%CI 1.38-1.74), and clinically significant bradycardia (HR 2.74; 95%CI 2.19-3.43). Furthermore, the metoprolol group had a significantly higher risk of mortality (HR 1.33; 95%CI 1.03-1.74).

POISE Study Group, Devereaux PJ, Yang H, Yusuf S, Guyatt G, Leslie K, et al. Effects of extended-release metoprolol succinate in patients undergoing non-cardiac surgery (POISE trial): a randomised controlled trial. Lancet. 2008 May 31;371(9627):1839–47.

The PANTER trial: Open necrosectomy vs. step-up approach for necrotizing pancreatitis

1. A minimally invasive step-up approach was associated with significantly reduced rates of major complications as compared to open necrosectomy in patients with necrotizing pancreatitis.

Original Date of Publication: April 2010

Study Rundown: Necrotizing pancreatitis with infected necrotic tissue is associated with high rates of both complication and death. Though first-line treatment is open necrosectomy, this study compared this with a minimally invasive step-up approach, consisting of percutaneous drainage, endoscopic drainage, and/or minimally invasive retroperotineal necrosectomy. The incidence of multiple organ failure was significantly lower in patients who underwent the step-up approach compared with those who had open necrosectomy. Though the rate of death did not differ significantly between the two groups, patients who were assigned to the step-up approach faced significantly lower rates of both incisional hernias and new-onset diabetes. One limitation of the study was that it was not powered to detect significant differences in death between the 2 groups.

In-Depth [randomized controlled trial]: Originally published in NEJM in 2010, this multicenter, randomized, controlled study involved 88 patients with acute pancreatitis and pancreatic necrosis. They were randomized to receive treatment with either open necrosectomy or a step-up approach, which included percutaneous or endoscopic drainage, and minimally invasive retroperitoneal necrosectomy. The primary end point was a composite of complications (i.e., new-onset multiple-organ failure, multiple systemic complications, bleeding, perforation of a visceral organ) and death. Patients managed using the step-up approach experienced a significantly lower rate of the composite primary endpoint compared to those treated with open necrosectomy (RR 0.57; 95%CI 0.38-0.87). This was largely driven by a significant reduction in new-onset organ failure (12% vs. 40%, p = 0.002), as there was no significant difference between the two groups in mortality. After 6 months of follow-up, patients who underwent open necrosectomy had a higher rate of incisional hernias (RR 0.29; 95%CI 0.09-0.95), new-onset diabetes (RR 0.43; 95%CI 0.20-0.94) and use of pancreatic enzymes (RR 0.21; 95%CI 0.07-0.67) when compared to those treated with the step-up approach. The study suggests that when treating necrotizing pancreatitis patients, a minimally invasive step-up approach reduces the rate of major complications and long-term complications when compared to open necrosectomy.

van Santvoort HC, Besselink MG, Bakker OJ, Hofker HS, Boermeester MA, Dejong CH, et al. A Step-up Approach or Open Necrosectomy for Necrotizing Pancreatitis. New England Journal of Medicine. 2010 Apr 22;362(16):1491–502.

The EVAR I trial: Endovascular vs. open abdominal aortic aneurysm repair

1. The EVAR I trial compared the safety and efficacy of endovascular and open abdominal aortic aneurysm repair.

2. There were no significant differences in all-cause mortality between the 2 groups.

3. The endovascular group experienced significantly higher rates of graft-related complications and reinterventions.

Original Date of Publication: May 2010

The Endovascular Aneurysm Repair (EVAR) trials were randomized controlled trials conducted to explore the safety and efficacy of repairing abdominal aortic aneurysms using endovascular methods. Two trials were conducted simultaneously and published in the same issue of The New England Journal of Medicine.

Study Rundown: Endovascular aortic aneurysm repair was first introduced in the late 1980s as an alternative for people considered unfit for open surgery. Several randomized controlled trials have demonstrated benefits of endovascular repair with regards to 30-day mortality, and it has become increasingly used to manage patients with abdominal aortic aneurysm. There was, however, a paucity of data with regards to the long-term follow-up of endovascular repairs. The EVAR I trial was a landmark study that compared mortality and graft-related complication/reintervention rates in patients who had undergone endovascular and open aortic aneurysm repairs. There were no significant differences between the 2 groups in terms of all-cause mortality. While early aneurysm-related mortality (i.e., 0-6 months after repair) was significantly lower in the endovascular repair group, this trend reversed in the longer run. More than 4 years after the repair, the endovascular repair group had significantly higher aneurysm-related mortality than the open group. Moreover, there were significantly higher rates of graft-related complications and reinterventions in the endovascular repair group.

In-Depth [randomized controlled trial]: Patients were eligible for the trial if they were at least 60 years of age, had an abdominal aortic aneurysm with a diameter of at least 5.5 cm on computed tomography, and were anatomically and clinically suitable for either endovascular or open repair. Eligible participants were then randomized to receive either endovascular or open aneurysm repair. The primary outcome was all-cause mortality, while other outcomes were aneurysm-related mortality, graft-related complications, and graft-related reinterventions. A total of 1252 patients were recruited for the trial from 37 hospitals across the UK. Approximately 90.7% of the study participants were male. There were no significant differences between the two groups in all-cause mortality at any timepoint. With regards to aneurysm-related mortality, there were significantly fewer deaths in the endovascular repair group until 6 months after the repair (adjusted HR 0.47; 95%CI 0.23-0.93), though this difference was not observed 6 months to 4 years after the repair. More than 4 years after the repair, there were significantly more aneurysm-related deaths in the endovascular groups compared to the open repair group (adjusted HR 4.85; 95%CI 1.04-22.72). There were significantly higher rates of graft-related complications and reinterventions in the endovascular repair group compared to the open group.

The United Kingdom EVAR Trial Investigators. Endovascular versus open repair of abdominal aortic aneurysm. Maedica (Buchar). 2010 Apr;5(2):148.

The EVAR II trial: Endovascular approach when unfit for open aortic aneurysm repair

1. The EVAR II trial compared endovascular abdominal aortic aneurysm repair with no intervention in patients unsuitable for the open procedure.

2. There were significantly fewer aneurysm-related deaths in the endovascular group, compared to no intervention.

3. The rates of complication and reintervention were similar to the rates observed in EVAR I.

Original Date of Publication: May 2010

Study Rundown: Endovascular aortic aneurysm repair was first introduced in the late 1980s as an alternative for people considered unfit for open surgery. The purpose of the EVAR II trial was to assess the benefits and risks associated with endovascular aortic aneurysm repair in patients who were unfit for the open procedure. There were no significant differences between the two groups in terms of all-cause mortality, though aneurysm-related mortality was significantly lower in the endovascular repair group. This benefit was largely attributed to the significant reductions observed in the 6-month to 4-year period following the repair procedure. Notably, the graft-related complication and reintervention rates were comparable to those observed in the EVAR I trial.

In-Depth [randomized controlled trial]: The EVAR II trial, originally published in 2010 in NEJM, focused on patients who were physically unsuitable for open abdominal aneurysm repair. The trial was supported by the National Institute for Health Research of the United Kingdom (UK). Patients were eligible for the trial if they were at least 60 years of age and had an abdominal aortic aneurysm with a diameter of at least 5.5 cm on computed tomography. Moreover, eligible patients were unsuitable for open repair, but candidates for endovascular repair. Eligible participants were then randomized to receive either endovascular aneurysm repair or no intervention. Again, the primary outcome was all-cause mortality, while other outcomes were aneurysm-related mortality, graft-related complications, and graft-related reinterventions. A total of 404 patients were recruited from 33 different hospitals across the UK. Approximately 86% of the participants were male. With regards to all-cause mortality, there were no significant differences between the two groups at any timepoint following the repair. Notably, there were significantly fewer aneurysm-related deaths in the endovascular group compared to the no intervention group (adjusted HR 0.53; 95%CI 0.32-0.89). This difference was driven by significant reductions in mortality in the 6-month to 4-year period following repair (adjusted HR 0.34; 95%CI 0.16-0.72). In total, 158 graft-related complications and 66 graft-related interventions were observed during the trial, and these rates were comparable to the rates observed in the EVAR I trial.

United Kingdom EVAR Trial Investigators, Greenhalgh RM, Brown LC, Powell JT, Thompson SG, Epstein D. Endovascular repair of aortic aneurysm in patients physically ineligible for open repair. New England Journal of Medicine. 2010 May 20;362(20):1872–80.

The CREST: Stenting versus endarterectomy for carotid stenosis

1. The rate of stroke, myocardial infarction or death did not differ significantly between patients treated with carotid artery stenting (CAS) compared to carotid endarterectomy (CEA).

2. The periprocedural rate of stroke was higher with stenting, while the rate of myocardial infarction was higher with endarterectomy.

Original Date of Publication: July 2010

Study Rundown: Carotid artery stenosis occurs as a result of atherosclerosis and leads to increasing risk of embolus and stroke. CEA and CAS are 2 procedures used to treat carotid artery stenosis but the evidence regarding their comparative efficacies is indecisive. The Carotid Revascularization Endarterectomy versus Stenting Trial (CREST) is one of the largest randomized controlled trials comparing these 2 treatment modalities. Prior to publication of these results, several trials had found higher rates of stroke and death associated with CAS, leading to a trend towards endarterectomy. The CREST trial found no significant difference in a composite outcome of stroke, myocardial infarction, and death between the 2 treatment groups and achieved lower rates of complications in both groups than those observed in previous trials. This supported both procedures as safe and effective treatment options; however, these results have been attributed to the highly trained interventionists involved in the study, which limits the external validity of the results. An interesting finding of the trial was that the rate of periprocedural stroke was higher in the stenting group, while the rate of myocardial infarction was higher in the endarterectomy group. This has led to debate regarding the relative harmful effects of suffering a stroke compared to myocardial infarction with some agreement that stroke results in more debilitating long-term consequences. In summary, the results of the CREST trial did not identify a definitive superior treatment for carotid artery stenosis. Treatment decisions should be individualized to patients' characteristics and needs.

In-Depth [randomized controlled trial]: This trial enrolled 2522 patients from 117 centers in the United States and Canada with symptomatic or asymptomatic carotid stenosis and randomized participants to receive CAS or CEA. Patients were considered eligible if they were symptomatic with ≥50% stenosis on angiography, ≥70% stenosis on ultrasonography, or ≥70% stenosis on computed tomographic/magnetic resonance angiography (CTA/MRA) but

50-69% stenosis on ultrasonography. Partway through the study, eligibility criteria were expanded to include asymptomatic patients with ≥60% stenosis on angiography, ≥70% stenosis on ultrasonography, or ≥80% stenosis on CTA/MRA but 50-69% stenosis on ultrasonography. Exclusion criteria included severe prior stroke, chronic atrial fibrillation, or paroxysmal atrial fibrillation. The primary outcome was a composite of stroke, myocardial infarction, and death during the periprocedural period, or ipsilateral stroke within four years of randomization.

There was no significant difference in the 4-year rates of the primary endpoint between CAS and CEA for the sample as a whole (HR 1.11; 95%CI 0.81-1.51), nor among symptomatic or asymptomatic patients separately (p = 0.84). The rate of the primary endpoint during the periprocedural period did not differ between treatment groups; however, when components were analysed separately, the rate of stroke was higher with CAS (4.1% vs. 2.3%, p = 0.01) while the rate of myocardial infarction was higher with CEA (1.1% vs. 2.3%, p = 0.03). Treatment effect was not modified by symptomatic status or sex; however, an interaction was detected between age and treatment efficacy, with CAS more effective in younger patients and CEA more effective in older patients.

Brott TG, Hobson RW, Howard G, Roubin GS, Clark WM, Brooks W, et al. Stenting versus Endarterectomy for Treatment of Carotid-Artery Stenosis. New England Journal of Medicine. 2010 Jul 1;363(1):11–23.

The PIVOT: Radical prostatectomy versus observation

1. Prostatectomy did not significantly reduce all-cause mortality or prostate cancer mortality when compared to observation.

2. These findings supported conservative management for men with localized prostate cancer, especially for those with prostate-specific antigen (PSA) values less than 10 ng/mL and low-risk disease.

Original Date of Publication: July 2012

Study Rundown: The incidence of prostate cancer in men is relatively high, but high long-term survival rates have been observed with conservative management. The treatment of localized prostate cancer is controversial, as few trials have compared surgical intervention to observation in the time since PSA testing has become a common screening tool. The Prostate Cancer Intervention versus Observation Trial (PIVOT) found no significant difference in all-cause or prostate-cancer mortality following radical prostatectomy compared to observation. These findings suggest that observation is a safe strategy in managing localized prostate cancer and avoids the unnecessary risks of intervention. The results also showed that PSA levels and tumor risk may be useful in identifying patients who will benefit from radical prostatectomy. Strengths of the study include the representative sample and measurement of all-cause mortality as the primary outcome, which avoids biased assessments of cause-of-death. Of note, the study may have been underpowered as the investigators intended to enroll 2000 participants, but reduced the sample size to 731. In addition, a substantial number of patients did not adhere to the assigned treatment in both groups, which could influence the observed treatment effect.

In-Depth [randomized controlled trial]: The trial included 731 men and followed participants for a median of 10 years. Patients were recruited from 44 Department of Veteran Affairs sites and 8 National Cancer Institute sites. In order to be eligible for the trial, patients had to be fit for radical prostatectomy, have histologically confirmed, clinically localized prostate cancer of any grade diagnosed within the previous 12 months, have PSA <50 ng/mL, be ≤75 years of age, a negative bone scan, and life expectancy of at least 10 years from randomization. The primary outcome was all-cause mortality and a secondary outcome was prostate-cancer mortality, defined as death due to prostate cancer or prostate cancer treatment. The rate of all-cause mortality was not significantly different between the two groups (HR 0.88; 95%CI 0.71-1.08). There was also no significant difference between groups in prostate cancer mortality (HR 0.63; 95%CI 0.36-1.09). A significant interaction was found between study group and baseline PSA value. In men with a PSA value greater than 10 ng/mL, a significant reduction in all-cause mortality was observed with surgery (p = 0.04), though surgery did not reduce all-cause mortality in men with a PSA less than or equal to 10 ng/mL.

Wilt TJ, Brawer MK, Jones KM, Barry MJ, Aronson WJ, Fox S, et al. Radical Prostatectomy versus Observation for Localized Prostate Cancer. New England Journal of Medicine. 2012 Jul 19;367(3):203–13.

Index

Bibliography

This bibliography includes any references, such as original trials and follow-up trials, in this text.
References are in ascending order by publication date.

1. Avery M, Mead J. Surface properties in relation to atelectasis and hyaline membrane disease. AMA Am J Dis Child. 1959 May 1;97(5I):517–23.

2. Douglas GJ, Simpson JS. The conservative management of splenic trauma. Journal of Pediatric Surgery. 1971 Oct 1;6(5):565–70.

3. Pugh RNH, Murray-Lyon IM, Dawson JL, Pietroni MC, Williams R. Transection of the oesophagus for bleeding oesophageal varices. Br J Surg. 1973 Aug 1;60(8):646–9.

4. Pizzo PA, Lovejoy FH, Smith DH. Prolonged Fever in Children: Review of 100 Cases. Pediatrics. 1975 Apr 1;55(4):468–73.

5. Nelson KB, Ellenberg JH. Predictors of Epilepsy in Children Who Have Experienced Febrile Seizures. New England Journal of Medicine. 1976 Nov 4;295(19):1029–33.

6. Fujiwara T, Maeta H, Chida S, Morita T, Watabe Y, Abe T. Artificial surfactant therapy in hyaline-membrane disease. Lancet. 1980 Jan 12;1(8159):55–9.

7. Cohn JN, Archibald DG, Ziesche S, Franciosa JA, Harston WE, Tristani FE, et al. Effect of Vasodilator Therapy on Mortality in Chronic Congestive Heart Failure. New England Journal of Medicine. 1986 Jun 12;314(24):1547–52.

8. Gaston MH, Verter JI, Woods G, Pegelow C, Kelleher J, Presbury G, et al. Prophylaxis with Oral Penicillin in Children with Sickle Cell Anemia. New England Journal of Medicine. 1986 Jun 19;314(25):1593–9.

9. Newburger JW, Takahashi M, Burns JC, Beiser AS, Chung KJ, Duffy CE, et al. The Treatment of Kawasaki Syndrome with Intravenous Gamma Globulin. New England Journal of Medicine. 1986 Aug 7;315(6):341–7.

10. Puylaert JBCM, Rutgers PH, Lalisang RI, de Vries BC, van der Werf SDJ, Dörr JPJ, et al. A Prospective Study of Ultrasonography in the Diagnosis of Appendicitis. New England Journal of Medicine. 1987 Sep 10;317(11):666–9.

11. Tzivoni D, Banai S, Schuger C, Benhorin J, Keren A, Gottlieb S, et al. Treatment of torsade de pointes with magnesium sulfate. Circulation. 1988 Feb 1;77(2):392–7.

12. Balthazar EJ, Robinson DL, Megibow AJ, Ranson JH. Acute pancreatitis: value of CT in establishing prognosis. Radiology. 1990 Feb 1;174(2):331–6.

13. Fleming PJ, Gilbert R, Azaz Y, Berry PJ, Rudd PT, Stewart A, et al. Interaction between bedding and sleeping position in the sudden infant death syndrome: a population based case-control study. BMJ. 1990 Jul 14;301(6743):85–9.

14. Brennan TA, Leape LL, Laird NM, Hebert L, Localio AR, Lawthers AG, et al. Incidence of Adverse Events and Negligence in Hospitalized Patients. New England Journal of Medicine. 1991 Feb 7;324(6):370–6.

15. Echt DS, Liebson PR, Mitchell LB, Peters RW, Obias-Manno D, Barker AH, et al. Mortality and Morbidity in Patients Receiving Encainide, Flecainide, or Placebo. New England Journal of Medicine. 1991 Mar 21;324(12):781–8.

16. Leape LL, Brennan TA, Laird N, Lawthers AG, Localio AR, Barnes BA, et al. The Nature of Adverse Events in Hospitalized Patients. New England Journal of Medicine. 1991 Feb 7;324(6):377–84.

17. North American Symptomatic Carotid Endarterectomy Trial Collaborators. Beneficial effect of carotid endarterectomy in symptomatic patients with high-grade carotid stenosis. N Engl J Med. 1991 Aug 15;325(7):445–53.

18. The SOLVD Investigators. Effect of enalapril on survival in patients with reduced left ventricular ejection fractions and congestive heart failure. N Engl J Med. 1991 Aug 1;325(5):293–302.

19. Bellinger DC, Stiles KM, Needleman HL. Low-Level Lead Exposure, Intelligence and Academic Achievement: A Long-term Follow-up Study. Pediatrics. 1992 Dec 1;90(6):855–61.

20. Lai ECS, Mok FPT, Tan ESY, Lo C, Fan S, You K, et al. Endoscopic Biliary Drainage for Severe Acute Cholangitis. New England Journal of Medicine. 1992 Jun 11;326(24):1582–6.

21. Pfeffer MA, Braunwald E, Moyé LA, Basta L, Brown EJ, Cuddy TE, et al. Effect of Captopril on Mortality and Morbidity in Patients with Left Ventricular Dysfunction after Myocardial Infarction. New England Journal of Medicine. 1992 Sep 3;327(10):669–77.

22. Paty DW, Li DKB, Group the UMS, Group the IMSS. Interferon beta-1b is effective in relapsing-remitting multiple sclerosis II. MRI analysis results of a multicenter, randomized, double-blind, placebo-controlled trial. Neurology. 1993 Apr 1;43(4):662–662.

23. Klahr S, Levey AS, Beck GJ, Caggiula AW, Hunsicker L, Kusek JW, et al. The Effects of Dietary Protein Restriction and Blood-Pressure Control on the Progression of Chronic Renal Disease. New England Journal of Medicine. 1994 Mar 31;330(13):877–84.

24. Livraghi T, Giorgio A, Marin G, Salmi A, de Sio I, Bolondi L, et al. Hepatocellular carcinoma and cirrhosis in 746 patients: long-term results of percutaneous ethanol injection. Radiology. 1995 Oct 1;197(1):101–8.

25. Malmberg K, Rydén L, Efendic S, Herlitz J, Nicol P, Waldenstrom A, et al. Randomized trial of insulin-glucose infusion followed by subcutaneous insulin treatment in diabetic patients with acute myocardial infarction (DIGAMI study): Effects on mortality at 1 year. J Am Coll Cardiol. 1995 Jul 1;26(1):57–65.

26. Stavros AT, Thickman D, Rapp CL, Dennis MA, Parker SH, Sisney GA. Solid breast nodules: use of sonography to distinguish between benign and malignant lesions. Radiology. 1995 Jul 1;196(1):123–34.

27. The National Institute of Neurological Disorders and Stroke rt-PA Stroke Study Group. Tissue Plasminogen Activator for Acute Ischemic Stroke. New England Journal of Medicine. 1995 Dec 14;333(24):1581–8.

28. Rockall TA, Logan RF, Devlin HB, Northfield TC. Risk assessment after acute upper gastrointestinal haemorrhage. Gut. 1996 Mar 1;38(3):316–21.

29. Sacks FM, Pfeffer MA, Moye LA, Rouleau JL, Rutherford JD, Cole TG, et al. The Effect of Pravastatin on Coronary Events after Myocardial Infarction in Patients with Average Cholesterol Levels. New England Journal of Medicine. 1996 Oct 3;335(14):1001–9.

30. Smith RC, Verga M, McCarthy S, Rosenfield AT. Diagnosis of acute flank pain: value of unenhanced helical CT. American Journal of Roentgenology. 1996 Jan 1;166(1):97–101.

31. Appel LJ, Moore TJ, Obarzanek E, Vollmer WM, Svetkey LP, Sacks FM, et al. A Clinical Trial of the Effects of Dietary Patterns on Blood Pressure. New England Journal of Medicine. 1997 Apr 17;336(16):1117–24.

32. Herman-Giddens ME, Slora EJ, Wasserman RC, Bourdony CJ, Bhapkar MV, Koch GG, et al. Secondary Sexual Characteristics and Menses in Young Girls Seen in Office Practice: A Study from the Pediatric Research in Office Settings Network. Pediatrics. 1997 Apr 1;99(4):505–12.

33. Khuroo MS, Yattoo GN, Javid G, Khan BA, Shah AA, Gulzar GM, et al. A Comparison of Omeprazole and Placebo for Bleeding Peptic Ulcer. New England Journal of Medicine. 1997 Apr 10;336(15):1054–8.

34. Maisels MJ, Kring E. Transcutaneous Bilirubinometry Decreases the Need for Serum Bilirubin Measurements and Saves Money. Pediatrics. 1997 Apr 1;99(4):599–600.

35. The Digitalis Investigation Group. The Effect of Digoxin on Mortality and Morbidity in Patients with Heart Failure. New England Journal of Medicine. 1997 Feb 20;336(8):525–33.

36. Decousus H, Leizorovicz A, Parent F, Page Y, Tardy B, Girard P, et al. A Clinical Trial of Vena Caval Filters in the Prevention of Pulmonary Embolism in Patients with Proximal Deep-Vein Thrombosis. New England Journal of Medicine. 1998 Feb 12;338(7):409–16.

37. Felitti VJ, Anda RF, Nordenberg D, Williamson DF, Spitz AM, Edwards

V, et al. Relationship of Childhood Abuse and Household Dysfunction to Many of the Leading Causes of Death in Adults. American Journal of Preventive Medicine. 1998 May 1;14(4):245–58.

38. Gozal D. Sleep-Disordered Breathing and School Performance in Children. Pediatrics. 1998 Sep 1;102(3):616–20.

39. UK Prospective Diabetes Study (UKPDS) Group. Effect of intensive blood-glucose control with metformin on complications in overweight patients with type 2 diabetes (UKPDS 34). Lancet. 1998 Sep 12;352(9131):854–65.

40. UK Prospective Diabetes Study (UKPDS) Group. Intensive blood-glucose control with sulphonylureas or insulin compared with conventional treatment and risk of complications in patients with type 2 diabetes (UKPDS 33). The Lancet. 1998 Sep 12;352(9131):837–53.

41. UK Prospective Diabetes Study (UKPDS) Group. Tight blood pressure control and risk of macrovascular and microvascular complications in type 2 diabetes: UKPDS 38. UK Prospective Diabetes Study Group. BMJ. 1998 Sep 12;317(7160):703–13.

42. Freedman DS, Dietz WH, Srinivasan SR, Berenson GS. The Relation of Overweight to Cardiovascular Risk Factors Among Children and Adolescents: The Bogalusa Heart Study. Pediatrics. 1999 Jun 1;103(6):1175–82.

43. Hébert PC, Wells G, Blajchman MA, Marshall J, Martin C, Pagliarello G, et al. A Multicenter, Randomized, Controlled Clinical Trial of Transfusion Requirements in Critical Care. New England Journal of Medicine. 1999 Feb 11;340(6):409–17.

44. Lee TH, Marcantonio ER, Mangione CM, Thomas EJ, Polanczyk CA, Cook EF, et al. Derivation and Prospective Validation of a Simple Index for Prediction of Cardiac Risk of Major Noncardiac Surgery. Circulation. 1999 Sep 7;100(10):1043–9.

45. MERIT-HF Study Group. Effect of metoprolol CR/XL in chronic heart failure: Metoprolol CR/XL Randomised Intervention Trial in-Congestive Heart Failure (MERIT-HF). The Lancet. 1999 Jun 12;353(9169):2001–7.

46. Packer M, Poole-Wilson PA, Armstrong PW, Cleland JGF, Horowitz JD, Massie BM, et al. Comparative Effects of Low and High Doses of the Angiotensin-Converting Enzyme Inhibitor, Lisinopril, on Morbidity and Mortality in Chronic Heart Failure. Circulation. 1999 Dec 7;100(23):2312–8.

47. Pitt B, Zannad F, Remme WJ, Cody R, Castaigne A, Perez A, et al. The Effect of Spironolactone on Morbidity and Mortality in Patients with Severe Heart Failure. New England Journal of Medicine. 1999 Sep 2;341(10):709–17.

48. Sort P, Navasa M, Arroyo V, Aldeguer X, Planas R, Ruiz-del-Arbol L, et al. Effect of Intravenous Albumin on Renal Impairment and Mortality in Patients with Cirrhosis and Spontaneous Bacterial Peritonitis. New

England Journal of Medicine. 1999 Aug 5;341(6):403–9.

49. Hyams JS, Markowitz J, Wyllie R. Use of infliximab in the treatment of Crohn's disease in children and adolescents. The Journal of Pediatrics. 2000 Aug 1;137(2):192–6.

50. Lau JYW, Sung JJY, Lee KKC, Yung M, Wong SKH, Wu JCY, et al. Effect of Intravenous Omeprazole on Recurrent Bleeding after Endoscopic Treatment of Bleeding Peptic Ulcers. New England Journal of Medicine. 2000 Aug 3;343(5):310–6.

51. Schrag SJ, Zywicki S, Farley MM, Reingold AL, Harrison LH, Lefkowitz LB, et al. Group B Streptococcal Disease in the Era of Intrapartum Antibiotic Prophylaxis. New England Journal of Medicine. 2000 Jan 6;342(1):15–20.

52. The Acute Respiratory Distress Syndrome Network. Ventilation with Lower Tidal Volumes as Compared with Traditional Tidal Volumes for Acute Lung Injury and the Acute Respiratory Distress Syndrome. New England Journal of Medicine. 2000 May 4;342(18):1301–8.

53. Wolfe J, Grier HE, Klar N, Levin SB, Ellenbogen JM, Salem-Schatz S, et al. Symptoms and Suffering at the End of Life in Children with Cancer. New England Journal of Medicine. 2000 Feb 3;342(5):326–33.

54. Yusuf S, Sleight P, Pogue J, Bosch J, Davies R, Dagenais G. Effects of an angiotensin-converting-enzyme inhibitor, ramipril, on cardiovascular events in high-risk patients. The Heart Outcomes Prevention Evaluation Study Investigators. N Engl J Med. 2000 Jan 20;342(3):145–53.

55. Brenner BM, Cooper ME, de Zeeuw D, Keane WF, Mitch WE, Parving H-H, et al. Effects of Losartan on Renal and Cardiovascular Outcomes in Patients with Type 2 Diabetes and Nephropathy. New England Journal of Medicine. 2001 Sep 20;345(12):861–9.

56. Cohn JN, Tognoni G. A Randomized Trial of the Angiotensin-Receptor Blocker Valsartan in Chronic Heart Failure. New England Journal of Medicine. 2001 Dec 6;345(23):1667–75.

57. Dargie HJ. Effect of carvedilol on outcome after myocardial infarction in patients with left-ventricular dysfunction: the CAPRICORN randomised trial. Lancet. 2001 May 5;357(9266):1385–90.

58. Farrell PM, Kosorok MR, Rock MJ, Laxova A, Zeng L, Lai H-C, et al. Early Diagnosis of Cystic Fibrosis Through Neonatal Screening Prevents Severe Malnutrition and Improves Long-Term Growth. Pediatrics. 2001 Jan 1;107(1):1–13.

59. Gage BF, Waterman AD, Shannon W, Boechler M, Rich MW, Radford MJ. Validation of clinical classification schemes for predicting stroke: Results from the national registry of atrial fibrillation. JAMA. 2001 Jun 13;285(22):2864–70.

60. Glaser N, Barnett P, McCaslin I, Nelson D, Trainor J, Louie J, et al. Risk Factors for Cerebral Edema in Children with Diabetic Ketoacidosis.

New England Journal of Medicine. 2001 Jan 25;344(4):264–9.

61. Kamath PS, Wiesner RH, Malinchoc M, Kremers W, Therneau TM, Kosberg CL, et al. A model to predict survival in patients with end-stage liver disease. Hepatology. 2001 Feb 1;33(2):464–70.

62. Lewis EJ, Hunsicker LG, Clarke WR, Berl T, Pohl MA, Lewis JB, et al. Renoprotective Effect of the Angiotensin-Receptor Antagonist Irbesartan in Patients with Nephropathy Due to Type 2 Diabetes. New England Journal of Medicine. 2001 Sep 20;345(12):851–60.

63. Mohr JP, Thompson JLP, Lazar RM, Levin B, Sacco RL, Furie KL, et al. A Comparison of Warfarin and Aspirin for the Prevention of Recurrent Ischemic Stroke. New England Journal of Medicine. 2001 Nov 15;345(20):1444–51.

64. Rivers E, Nguyen B, Havstad S, Ressler J, Muzzin A, Knoblich B, et al. Early Goal-Directed Therapy in the Treatment of Severe Sepsis and Septic Shock. New England Journal of Medicine. 2001 Nov 8;345(19):1368–77.

65. Schwartz GG, Olsson AG, Ezekowitz MD, et al. Effects of atorvastatin on early recurrent ischemic events in acute coronary syndromes: The miracl study: a randomized controlled trial. JAMA. 2001 Apr 4;285(13):1711–8.

66. Stiell IG, Wells GA, Vandemheen K, Clement C, Lesiuk H, Laupacis A, et al. The Canadian CT Head Rule for patients with minor head injury. Lancet. 2001 May 5;357(9266):1391–6.

67. Yusuf S, Zhao F, Mehta SR, Chrolavicius S, Tognoni G, Fox KK, et al. Effects of clopidogrel in addition to aspirin in patients with acute coronary syndromes without ST-segment elevation. N Engl J Med. 2001 Aug 16;345(7):494–502.

68. Daeppen J, Gache P, Landry U, et al. Symptom-triggered vs fixed-schedule doses of benzodiazepine for alcohol withdrawal: A randomized treatment trial. Arch Intern Med. 2002 May 27;162(10):1117–21.

69. de Gans J, van de Beek D. Dexamethasone in Adults with Bacterial Meningitis. New England Journal of Medicine. 2002 Nov 14;347(20):1549–56.

70. Fiebach JB, Schellinger PD, Jansen O, Meyer M, Wilde P, Bender J, et al. CT and Diffusion-Weighted MR Imaging in Randomized Order Diffusion-Weighted Imaging Results in Higher Accuracy and Lower Interrater Variability in the Diagnosis of Hyperacute Ischemic. Stroke. 2002 Sep 1;33(9):2206–10.

71. Fisher B, Anderson S, Bryant J, Margolese RG, Deutsch M, Fisher ER, et al. Twenty-Year Follow-up of a Randomized Trial Comparing Total Mastectomy, Lumpectomy, and Lumpectomy plus Irradiation for the Treatment of Invasive Breast Cancer. New England Journal of Medicine. 2002 Oct 17;347(16):1233–41.

72. Hypothermia after Cardiac Arrest Study Group. Mild Therapeutic Hypothermia to Improve the

Neurologic Outcome after Cardiac Arrest. New England Journal of Medicine. 2002 Feb 21;346(8):549–56.

73. Madsen KM, Hviid A, Vestergaard M, Schendel D, Wohlfahrt J, Thorsen P, et al. A Population-Based Study of Measles, Mumps, and Rubella Vaccination and Autism. New England Journal of Medicine. 2002 Nov 7;347(19):1477–82.

74. Moss AJ, Zareba W, Hall WJ, Klein H, Wilber DJ, Cannom DS, et al. Prophylactic Implantation of a Defibrillator in Patients with Myocardial Infarction and Reduced Ejection Fraction. New England Journal of Medicine. 2002 Mar 21;346(12):877–83.

75. Nigrovic LE, Kuppermann N, Malley R. Development and Validation of a Multivariable Predictive Model to Distinguish Bacterial From Aseptic Meningitis in Children in the Post-Haemophilus influenzae Era. Pediatrics. 2002 Oct 1;110(4):712–9.

76. Packer M, Fowler MB, Roecker EB, Coats AJS, Katus HA, Krum H, et al. Effect of Carvedilol on the Morbidity of Patients With Severe Chronic Heart Failure Results of the Carvedilol Prospective Randomized Cumulative Survival (COPERNICUS) Study. Circulation. 2002 Oct 22;106(17):2194–9.

77. The ALLHAT Officers and Coordinators for the ALLHAT Collaborative Research Group. Major outcomes in high-risk hypertensive patients randomized to angiotensin-converting enzyme inhibitor or calcium channel blocker vs diuretic: The antihypertensive and lipid-lowering treatment to prevent heart attack trial (allhat). JAMA. 2002 Dec 18;288(23):2981–97.

78. Wyse DG, Waldo AL, DiMarco JP, Domanski MJ, Rosenberg Y, Schron EB, et al. A comparison of rate control and rhythm control in patients with atrial fibrillation. N Engl J Med. 2002 Dec 5;347(23):1825–33.

79. Cheng Y, Wong RSM, Soo YOY, Chui CH, Lau FY, Chan NPH, et al. Initial Treatment of Immune Thrombocytopenic Purpura with High-Dose Dexamethasone. New England Journal of Medicine. 2003 Aug 28;349(9):831–6.

80. Fishman A, Martinez F, Naunheim K, Piantadosi S, Wise R, Ries A, et al. A randomized trial comparing lung-volume-reduction surgery with medical therapy for severe emphysema. N Engl J Med. 2003 May 22;348(21):2059–73.

81. Granger CB, McMurray JJV, Yusuf S, Held P, Michelson EL, Olofsson B, et al. Effects of candesartan in patients with chronic heart failure and reduced left-ventricular systolic function intolerant to angiotensin-converting-enzyme inhibitors: the CHARM-Alternative trial. Lancet. 2003 Sep 6;362(9386):772–6.

82. Lee AYY, Levine MN, Baker RI, Bowden C, Kakkar AK, Prins M, et al. Low-Molecular-Weight Heparin versus a Coumarin for the Prevention of Recurrent Venous Thromboembolism in Patients with Cancer. New England Journal of Medicine. 2003 Jul 10;349(2):146–53.

83. Lim WS, van der Eerden MM, Laing R, Boersma WG, Karalus N,

Town GI, et al. Defining community acquired pneumonia severity on presentation to hospital: an international derivation and validation study. Thorax. 2003 May 1;58(5):377–82.

84. Pitt B, Remme W, Zannad F, Neaton J, Martinez F, Roniker B, et al. Eplerenone, a Selective Aldosterone Blocker, in Patients with Left Ventricular Dysfunction after Myocardial Infarction. New England Journal of Medicine. 2003 Apr 3;348(14):1309–21.

85. Thompson IM, Goodman PJ, Tangen CM, Lucia MS, Miller GJ, Ford LG, et al. The Influence of Finasteride on the Development of Prostate Cancer. New England Journal of Medicine. 2003 Jul 17;349(3):215–24.

86. Wells PS, Anderson DR, Rodger M, Forgie M, Kearon C, Dreyer J, et al. Evaluation of D-Dimer in the Diagnosis of Suspected Deep-Vein Thrombosis. New England Journal of Medicine. 2003 Sep 25;349(13):1227–35.

87. Yusuf S, Pfeffer MA, Swedberg K, Granger CB, Held P, McMurray JJV, et al. Effects of candesartan in patients with chronic heart failure and preserved left-ventricular ejection fraction: the CHARM-Preserved Trial. Lancet. 2003 Sep 6;362(9386):777–81.

88. Cannon CP, Braunwald E, McCabe CH, Rader DJ, Rouleau JL, Belder R, et al. Intensive versus Moderate Lipid Lowering with Statins after Acute Coronary Syndromes. New England Journal of Medicine. 2004 Apr 8;350(15):1495–504.

89. Finfer S, Bellomo R, Boyce N, French J, Myburgh J, Norton R, et al. A comparison of albumin and saline for fluid resuscitation in the intensive care unit. N Engl J Med. 2004 May 27;350(22):2247–56.

90. Levine DA, Platt SL, Dayan PS, Macias CG, Zorc JJ, Krief W, et al. Risk of Serious Bacterial Infection in Young Febrile Infants With Respiratory Syncytial Virus Infections. Pediatrics. 2004 Jun 1;113(6):1728–34.

91. McFalls EO, Ward HB, Moritz TE, Goldman S, Krupski WC, Littooy F, et al. Coronary-Artery Revascularization before Elective Major Vascular Surgery. New England Journal of Medicine. 2004 Dec 30;351(27):2795–804.

92. Zhang B-H, Yang B-H, Tang Z-Y. Randomized controlled trial of screening for hepatocellular carcinoma. J Cancer Res Clin Oncol. 2004 Mar 20;130(7):417–22.

93. Chen ZM, Jiang LX, Chen YP, Xie JX, Pan HC, Peto R, et al. Addition of clopidogrel to aspirin in 45,852 patients with acute myocardial infarction: randomised placebo-controlled trial. Lancet. 2005 Nov 5;366(9497):1607–21.

94. Chen ZM, Pan HC, Chen YP, Peto R, Collins R, Jiang LX, et al. Early intravenous then oral metoprolol in 45,852 patients with acute myocardial infarction: randomised placebo-controlled trial. Lancet. 2005 Nov 5;366(9497):1622–32.

95. Chimowitz MI, Lynn MJ, Howlett-Smith H, Stern BJ, Hertzberg VS, Frankel MR, et al. Comparison of

Warfarin and Aspirin for Symptomatic Intracranial Arterial Stenosis. New England Journal of Medicine. 2005 Mar 31;352(13):1305–16.

96. de Winter RJ, Windhausen F, Cornel JH, Dunselman PHJM, Janus CL, Bendermacher PEF, et al. Early Invasive versus Selectively Invasive Management for Acute Coronary Syndromes. New England Journal of Medicine. 2005 Sep 15;353(11):1095–104.

97. Han YY, Carcillo JA, Venkataraman ST, Clark RSB, Watson RS, Nguyen TC, et al. Unexpected Increased Mortality After Implementation of a Commercially Sold Computerized Physician Order Entry System. Pediatrics. 2005 Dec 1;116(6):1506–12.

98. Lieberman JA, Stroup TS, McEvoy JP, Swartz MS, Rosenheck RA, Perkins DO, et al. Effectiveness of Antipsychotic Drugs in Patients with Chronic Schizophrenia. New England Journal of Medicine. 2005 Sep 22;353(12):1209–23.

99. Markus HS, Droste DW, Kaps M, Larrue V, Lees KR, Siebler M, et al. Dual Antiplatelet Therapy With Clopidogrel and Aspirin in Symptomatic Carotid Stenosis Evaluated Using Doppler Embolic Signal Detection The Clopidogrel and Aspirin for Reduction of Emboli in Symptomatic Carotid Stenosis (CARESS) Trial. Circulation. 2005 May 3;111(17):2233–40.

100. Petersen RC, Thomas RG, Grundman M, Bennett D, Doody R, Ferris S, et al. Vitamin E and Donepezil for the Treatment of Mild

Cognitive Impairment. New England Journal of Medicine. 2005 Jun 9;352(23):2379–88.

101. Sabatine MS, Cannon CP, Gibson CM, López-Sendón JL, Montalescot G, Theroux P, et al. Addition of Clopidogrel to Aspirin and Fibrinolytic Therapy for Myocardial Infarction with ST-Segment Elevation. New England Journal of Medicine. 2005 Mar 24;352(12):1179–89.

102. Villa LL, Costa RLR, Petta CA, Andrade RP, Ault KA, Giuliano AR, et al. Prophylactic quadrivalent human papillomavirus (types 6, 11, 16, and 18) L1 virus-like particle vaccine in young women: a randomised double-blind placebo-controlled multicentre phase II efficacy trial. Lancet Oncol. 2005 May;6(5):271–8.

103. Amarenco P, Bogousslavsky J, Callahan A, Goldstein LB, Hennerici M, Rudolph AE, et al. High-dose atorvastatin after stroke or transient ischemic attack. N Engl J Med. 2006 Aug 10;355(6):549–59.

104. ESPRIT Study Group, Halkes PHA, van Gijn J, Kappelle LJ, Koudstaal PJ, Algra A. Aspirin plus dipyridamole versus aspirin alone after cerebral ischaemia of arterial origin (ESPRIT): randomised controlled trial. Lancet. 2006 May 20;367(9523):1665–73.

105. Gallant JE, DeJesus E, Arribas JR, Pozniak AL, Gazzard B, Campo RE, et al. Tenofovir DF, Emtricitabine, and Efavirenz vs. Zidovudine, Lamivudine, and Efavirenz for HIV. New England Journal of Medicine. 2006 Jan 19;354(3):251–60.

106. Rush AJ, Trivedi MH, Wisniewski SR, Stewart JW, Nierenberg AA, Thase ME, et al. Bupropion-SR, Sertraline, or Venlafaxine-XR after Failure of SSRIs for Depression. New England Journal of Medicine. 2006 Mar 23;354(12):1231–42.

107. Singh AK, Szczech L, Tang KL, Barnhart H, Sapp S, Wolfson M, et al. Correction of Anemia with Epoetin Alfa in Chronic Kidney Disease. New England Journal of Medicine. 2006 Nov 16;355(20):2085–98.

108. Stein PD, Fowler SE, Goodman LR, Gottschalk A, Hales CA, Hull RD, et al. Multidetector Computed Tomography for Acute Pulmonary Embolism. New England Journal of Medicine. 2006 Jun 1;354(22):2317–27.

109. Trivedi MH, Fava M, Wisniewski SR, Thase ME, Quitkin F, Warden D, et al. Medication Augmentation after the Failure of SSRIs for Depression. New England Journal of Medicine. 2006 Mar 23;354(12):1243–52.

110. Boden WE, O'Rourke RA, Teo KK, Hartigan PM, Maron DJ, Kostuk WJ, et al. Optimal Medical Therapy with or without PCI for Stable Coronary Disease. New England Journal of Medicine. 2007 Apr 12;356(15):1503–16.

111. Calverley PMA, Anderson JA, Celli B, Ferguson GT, Jenkins C, Jones PW, et al. Salmeterol and Fluticasone Propionate and Survival in Chronic Obstructive Pulmonary Disease. New England Journal of Medicine. 2007 Feb 22;356(8):775–89.

112. Johnston SC, Rothwell PM, Nguyen-Huynh MN, Giles MF, Elkins JS, Bernstein AL, et al. Validation and refinement of scores to predict very early stroke risk after transient ischaemic attack. Lancet. 2007 Jan 27;369(9558):283–92.

113. Lau JY, Leung WK, Wu JCY, Chan FKL, Wong VWS, Chiu PWY, et al. Omeprazole before Endoscopy in Patients with Gastrointestinal Bleeding. New England Journal of Medicine. 2007 Apr 19;356(16):1631–40.

114. Nigrovic LE, Kuppermann N, Macias CG, et al. Clinical prediction rule for identifying children with cerebrospinal fluid pleocytosis at very low risk of bacterial meningitis. JAMA. 2007 Jan 3;297(1):52–60.

115. Wiviott SD, Braunwald E, McCabe CH, Montalescot G, Ruzyllo W, Gottlieb S, et al. Prasugrel versus Clopidogrel in Patients with Acute Coronary Syndromes. New England Journal of Medicine. 2007 Nov 15;357(20):2001–15.

116. Zar FA, Bakkanagari SR, Moorthi KMLST, Davis MB. A Comparison of Vancomycin and Metronidazole for the Treatment of Clostridium difficile–Associated Diarrhea, Stratified by Disease Severity. Clin Infect Dis. 2007 Aug 1;45(3):302–7.

117. Action to Control Cardiovascular Risk in Diabetes Study Group, Gerstein HC, Miller ME, Byington RP, Goff DC, Bigger JT, et al. Effects of intensive glucose lowering in type 2 diabetes. N Engl J Med. 2008 Jun 12;358(24):2545–59.

118. ADVANCE Collaborative Group, Patel A, MacMahon S, Chalmers J, Neal B, Billot L, et al. Intensive blood

glucose control and vascular outcomes in patients with type 2 diabetes. N Engl J Med. 2008 Jun 12;358(24):2560–72.

119. Hacke W, Kaste M, Bluhmki E, Brozman M, Dávalos A, Guidetti D, et al. Thrombolysis with Alteplase 3 to 4.5 Hours after Acute Ischemic Stroke. New England Journal of Medicine. 2008 Sep 25;359(13):1317–29.

120. Jamerson K, Weber MA, Bakris GL, Dahlöf B, Pitt B, Shi V, et al. Benazepril plus Amlodipine or Hydrochlorothiazide for Hypertension in High-Risk Patients. New England Journal of Medicine. 2008 Dec 4;359(23):2417–28.

121. Kastelein JJP, Akdim F, Stroes ESG, Zwinderman AH, Bots ML, Stalenhoef AFH, et al. Simvastatin with or without Ezetimibe in Familial Hypercholesterolemia. New England Journal of Medicine. 2008 Apr 3;358(14):1431–43.

122. POISE Study Group, Devereaux PJ, Yang H, Yusuf S, Guyatt G, Leslie K, et al. Effects of extended-release metoprolol succinate in patients undergoing non-cardiac surgery (POISE trial): a randomised controlled trial. Lancet. 2008 May 31;371(9627):1839–47.

123. Ridker PM, Danielson E, Fonseca FAH, Genest J, Gotto AM, Kastelein JJP, et al. Rosuvastatin to Prevent Vascular Events in Men and Women with Elevated C-Reactive Protein. New England Journal of Medicine. 2008 Nov 20;359(21):2195–207.

124. Roussey-Kesler G, Gadjos V, Idres N, Horen B, Ichay L, Leclair MD, et al. Antibiotic Prophylaxis for the Prevention of Recurrent Urinary Tract Infection in Children With Low Grade Vesicoureteral Reflux: Results From a Prospective Randomized Study. The Journal of Urology. 2008 Feb 1;179(2):674–9.

125. Sprung CL, Annane D, Keh D, Moreno R, Singer M, Freivogel K, et al. Hydrocortisone Therapy for Patients with Septic Shock. New England Journal of Medicine. 2008 Jan 10;358(2):111–24.

126. Tashkin DP, Celli B, Senn S, Burkhart D, Kesten S, Menjoge S, et al. A 4-Year Trial of Tiotropium in Chronic Obstructive Pulmonary Disease. New England Journal of Medicine. 2008 Oct 9;359(15):1543–54.

127. The ONTARGET Investigators. Telmisartan, Ramipril, or Both in Patients at High Risk for Vascular Events. New England Journal of Medicine. 2008 Apr 10;358(15):1547–59.

128. ACTIVE Investigators, Connolly SJ, Pogue J, Hart RG, Hohnloser SH, Pfeffer M, et al. Effect of clopidogrel added to aspirin in patients with atrial fibrillation. N Engl J Med. 2009 May 14;360(20):2066–78.

129. Andriole GL, Crawford ED, Grubb RL, Buys SS, Chia D, Church TR, et al. Mortality Results from a Randomized Prostate-Cancer Screening Trial. New England Journal of Medicine. 2009 Mar 26;360(13):1310–9.

130. Connolly SJ, Ezekowitz MD, Yusuf S, Eikelboom J, Oldgren J, Parekh A, et al. Dabigatran versus Warfarin in Patients with Atrial

Fibrillation. New England Journal of Medicine. 2009 Sep 17;361(12):1139–51.

131. Davies DA, Pearl RH, Ein SH, Langer JC, Wales PW. Management of blunt splenic injury in children: evolution of the nonoperative approach. Journal of Pediatric Surgery. 2009 May 1;44(5):1005–8.

132. Kitahata MM, Gange SJ, Abraham AG, Merriman B, Saag MS, Justice AC, et al. Effect of Early versus Deferred Antiretroviral Therapy for HIV on Survival. New England Journal of Medicine. 2009 Apr 30;360(18):1815–26.

133. Kuppermann N, Holmes JF, Dayan PS, Hoyle JD, Atabaki SM, Holubkov R, et al. Identification of children at very low risk of clinically-important brain injuries after head trauma: a prospective cohort study. Lancet. 2009 Oct 3;374(9696):1160–70.

134. NICE-SUGAR Study Investigators, Finfer S, Chittock DR, Su SY-S, Blair D, Foster D, et al. Intensive versus conventional glucose control in critically ill patients. N Engl J Med. 2009 Mar 26;360(13):1283–97.

135. Schulman S, Kearon C, Kakkar AK, Mismetti P, Schellong S, Eriksson H, et al. Dabigatran versus Warfarin in the Treatment of Acute Venous Thromboembolism. New England Journal of Medicine. 2009 Dec 10;361(24):2342–52.

136. Serruys PW, Morice M-C, Kappetein AP, Colombo A, Holmes DR, Mack MJ, et al. Percutaneous Coronary Intervention versus Coronary-Artery Bypass Grafting for Severe Coronary Artery Disease. New England Journal of Medicine. 2009 Mar 5;360(10):961–72.

137. Wallentin L, Becker RC, Budaj A, Cannon CP, Emanuelsson H, Held C, et al. Ticagrelor versus Clopidogrel in Patients with Acute Coronary Syndromes. New England Journal of Medicine. 2009 Sep 10;361(11):1045–57.

138. Bhatt DL, Cryer BL, Contant CF, Cohen M, Lanas A, Schnitzer TJ, et al. Clopidogrel with or without Omeprazole in Coronary Artery Disease. New England Journal of Medicine. 2010 Nov 11;363(20):1909–17.

139. Brott TG, Hobson RW, Howard G, Roubin GS, Clark WM, Brooks W, et al. Stenting versus Endarterectomy for Treatment of Carotid-Artery Stenosis. New England Journal of Medicine. 2010 Jul 1;363(1):11–23.

140. CRASH-2 trial collaborators, Shakur H, Roberts I, Bautista R, Caballero J, Coats T, et al. Effects of tranexamic acid on death, vascular occlusive events, and blood transfusion in trauma patients with significant haemorrhage (CRASH-2): a randomised, placebo-controlled trial. Lancet. 2010 Jul 3;376(9734):23–32.

141. De Backer D, Biston P, Devriendt J, Madl C, Chochrad D, Aldecoa C, et al. Comparison of Dopamine and Norepinephrine in the Treatment of Shock. New England Journal of Medicine. 2010 Mar 4;362(9):779–89.

142. EINSTEIN Investigators, Bauersachs R, Berkowitz SD, Brenner B, Buller HR, Decousus H, et al. Oral rivaroxaban for symptomatic venous

thromboembolism. N Engl J Med. 2010 Dec 23;363(26):2499–510.

143. García-Pagán JC, Caca K, Bureau C, Laleman W, Appenrodt B, Luca A, et al. Early Use of TIPS in Patients with Cirrhosis and Variceal Bleeding. New England Journal of Medicine. 2010 Jun 24;362(25):2370–9.

144. Jansen TC, van Bommel J, Schoonderbeek FJ, Sleeswijk Visser SJ, van der Klooster JM, Lima AP, et al. Early Lactate-Guided Therapy in Intensive Care Unit Patients. Am J Respir Crit Care Med. 2010 Sep 15;182(6):752–61.

145. Papazian L, Forel J-M, Gacouin A, Penot-Ragon C, Perrin G, Loundou A, et al. Neuromuscular Blockers in Early Acute Respiratory Distress Syndrome. New England Journal of Medicine. 2010 Sep 16;363(12):1107–16.

146. Pisters R, Lane DA, Nieuwlaat R, de Vos CB, Crijns HJGM, Lip GYH. A novel user-friendly score (has-bled) to assess 1-year risk of major bleeding in patients with atrial fibrillation: The euro heart survey. Chest. 2010 Nov 1;138(5):1093–100.

147. Stone JH, Merkel PA, Spiera R, Seo P, Langford CA, Hoffman GS, et al. Rituximab versus Cyclophosphamide for ANCA-Associated Vasculitis. New England Journal of Medicine. 2010 Jul 15;363(3):221–32.

148. Symplicity HTN-2 Investigators, Esler MD, Krum H, Sobotka PA, Schlaich MP, Schmieder RE, et al. Renal sympathetic denervation in patients with treatment-resistant hypertension (The Symplicity HTN-2 Trial): a randomised controlled trial. Lancet. 2010 Dec 4;376(9756):1903–9.

149. The United Kingdom EVAR Trial Investigators. Endovascular versus open repair of abdominal aortic aneurysm. Maedica (Buchar). 2010 Apr;5(2):148.

150. United Kingdom EVAR Trial Investigators, Greenhalgh RM, Brown LC, Powell JT, Thompson SG, Epstein D. Endovascular repair of aortic aneurysm in patients physically ineligible for open repair. N Engl J Med. 2010 May 20;362(20):1872–80.

151. Van Gelder IC, Groenveld HF, Crijns HJGM, Tuininga YS, Tijssen JGP, Alings AM, et al. Lenient versus Strict Rate Control in Patients with Atrial Fibrillation. New England Journal of Medicine. 2010 Apr 15;362(15):1363–73.

152. van Santvoort HC, Besselink MG, Bakker OJ, Hofker HS, Boermeester MA, Dejong CH, et al. A Step-up Approach or Open Necrosectomy for Necrotizing Pancreatitis. New England Journal of Medicine. 2010 Apr 22;362(16):1491–502.

153. Cohen MS, Chen YQ, McCauley M, Gamble T, Hosseinipour MC, Kumarasamy N, et al. Prevention of HIV-1 Infection with Early Antiretroviral Therapy. New England Journal of Medicine. 2011 Aug 11;365(6):493–505.

154. Granger CB, Alexander JH, McMurray JJV, Lopes RD, Hylek EM, Hanna M, et al. Apixaban versus Warfarin in Patients with Atrial

Fibrillation. New England Journal of Medicine. 2011 Sep 15;365(11):981–92.

155. Jolly SS, Yusuf S, Cairns J, Niemelä K, Xavier D, Widimsky P, et al. Radial versus femoral access for coronary angiography and intervention in patients with acute coronary syndromes (RIVAL): a randomised, parallel group, multicentre trial. Lancet. 2011 Apr 23;377(9775):1409–20.

156. Louie TJ, Miller MA, Mullane KM, Weiss K, Lentnek A, Golan Y, et al. Fidaxomicin versus Vancomycin for Clostridium difficile Infection. New England Journal of Medicine. 2011 Feb 3;364(5):422–31.

157. National Lung Screening Trial Research Team, Aberle DR, Adams AM, Berg CD, Black WC, Clapp JD, et al. Reduced lung-cancer mortality with low-dose computed tomographic screening. N Engl J Med. 2011 Aug 4;365(5):395–409.

158. Park S-J, Kim Y-H, Park D-W, Yun S-C, Ahn J-M, Song HG, et al. Randomized Trial of Stents versus Bypass Surgery for Left Main Coronary Artery Disease. New England Journal of Medicine. 2011 May 5;364(18):1718–27.

159. Patel MR, Mahaffey KW, Garg J, Pan G, Singer DE, Hacke W, et al. Rivaroxaban versus Warfarin in Nonvalvular Atrial Fibrillation. New England Journal of Medicine. 2011 Sep 8;365(10):883–91.

160. Zannad F, McMurray JJV, Krum H, van Veldhuisen DJ, Swedberg K, Shi H, et al. Eplerenone in Patients with Systolic Heart Failure and Mild Symptoms. New England Journal of Medicine. 2011 Jan 6;364(1):11–21.

161. EINSTEIN–PE Investigators, Büller HR, Prins MH, Lensin AWA, Decousus H, Jacobson BF, et al. Oral rivaroxaban for the treatment of symptomatic pulmonary embolism. N Engl J Med. 2012 Apr 5;366(14):1287–97.

162. Pearce MS, Salotti JA, Little MP, McHugh K, Lee C, Kim KP, et al. Radiation exposure from CT scans in childhood and subsequent risk of leukaemia and brain tumours: a retrospective cohort study. Lancet. 2012 Aug 4;380(9840):499–505.

163. Schoen RE, Pinsky PF, Weissfeld JL, Yokochi LA, Church T, Laiyemo AO, et al. Colorectal-Cancer Incidence and Mortality with Screening Flexible Sigmoidoscopy. New England Journal of Medicine. 2012 Jun 21;366(25):2345–57.

164. Wilt TJ, Brawer MK, Jones KM, Barry MJ, Aronson WJ, Fox S, et al. Radical Prostatectomy versus Observation for Localized Prostate Cancer. New England Journal of Medicine. 2012 Jul 19;367(3):203–13.

165. Agnelli G, Buller HR, Cohen A, Curto M, Gallus AS, Johnson M, et al. Oral Apixaban for the Treatment of Acute Venous Thromboembolism. New England Journal of Medicine. 2013 Aug 29;369(9):799–808.

166. Biro FM, Greenspan LC, Galvez MP, Pinney SM, Teitelbaum S, Windham GC, et al. Onset of Breast Development in a Longitudinal Cohort. Pediatrics. 2013 Nov 4;peds.2012–3773.

167. Davies C, Pan H, Godwin J, Gray R, Arriagada R, Raina V, et al. Long-term effects of continuing adjuvant tamoxifen to 10 years versus stopping at 5 years after diagnosis of oestrogen receptor-positive breast cancer: ATLAS, a randomised trial. Lancet. 2013 Mar 9;381(9869):805–16.

168. Guérin C, Reignier J, Richard J-C, Beuret P, Gacouin A, Boulain T, et al. Prone Positioning in Severe Acute Respiratory Distress Syndrome. New England Journal of Medicine. 2013 Jun 6;368(23):2159–68.

169. van Nood E, Vrieze A, Nieuwdorp M, Fuentes S, Zoetendal EG, de Vos WM, et al. Duodenal Infusion of Donor Feces for Recurrent Clostridium difficile. New England Journal of Medicine. 2013 Jan 31;368(5):407–15.

Statistics Abbreviations

CI: Confidence Interval
HR: Hazard Ratio
RR: Relative Risk
RRR: Relative Risk Reduction
ARI: Absolute Risk Increase
NNH: Number Needed to Harm
X^2: Chi-square

Notes

Made in the USA
Las Vegas, NV
17 April 2021

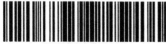